HEALTH ADMINISTRATION

ENCYCLOPAEDIA OF HOSPITAL ADMINISTRATION AND DEVELOPMENT SERIES

HEALTH ADMINISTRATION

Editor-in-Chief

Arun Kumar

INSTITUTE FOR SUSTAINABLE DEVELOPMENT
LUCKNOW

&

ANMOL PUBLICATIONS PVT. LTD.
NEW DELHI - 110 002 (INDIA)

ANMOL PUBLICATIONS PVT. LTD.
4374/4B, Ansari Road, Daryaganj
New Delhi - 110 002

Health Administration

First Edition, 2000

ISBN 81-261-0539-9

PRINTED IN INDIA

Published by J.L. Kumar for Anmol Publications Pvt. Ltd., New Delhi and Printed at Mehra Offset Press, Delhi.

Contents

Preface

'Health is wealth' as the saying goes on, Health facilities are indicator of the development stage/ status of a country.

Health, according to the constitution of India is a state subject, the main responsibility of providng health services to all people lies with the State Health Department with the assistance of local health organisations wherever these exist, e.g. Corporation, Municipalities, Panchayati Raj, and adhoc statutory bodies.

This encyclopaedia is first effort to bring together authoritative information on Hospital Management and administration.

Details of the Volumes:

- Health Administration
- Hospital Management

We are deeply beholden to all the scholars in field whose learned writings are cited or substantially made use of in this work. Our intention is to disseminate the fruits of the erudition of those scholars, which will be shared by a large readership. However we are solely responsible for any shortcomings in presentation or other way.

We are also grateful to Mr. J.L. Kumar, Managing Director, Anmol Publications Pvt. Ltd., New Delhi, for timely publication of this work despite his tight schedule of publications.

—Arun Kumar

1

Health Care Administration at the Regional State and Local Levels

A. Organisation of Health Care Administration at the Regional State Levels

Health, according to the Constitution of India, is a State subject. The main responsibility for providing health services to all people lies with the State Health Department with the assistance of local health organisations wherever these exist, e.g. Corporations, Municipalities, Panchayati Raj, ad-hoc statutory bodies like the Mines Board of Health, Employees State Insurance Corporation and so on.

The executive machinery of the government at the State level is headed by the Governor. Article 163 of the Constitution provides for a Council of Ministers with the Chief Minister as its head to aid and advice the Governor. The business of the government of the State (viz., law and order administration, the developmental functions like general administration, local government, public works, irrigation, health, education, cooperation, etc.) is allocated by the Governor amongst the Ministers in accordance with the provisions contained in Article 166(3) of the Constitution. We shall now discuss the organisation of State Health Department in one State of the Indian Union, i.e., Punjab.

Organisation of State Health Department

(a) *Political Head.* In the State of Punjab, a Minister of a Cabinet rank is the political head of the Health Department. He has to bear a heavy responsibility for formulating policies and monitoring the implementation of these policies and programmes.

The Health Minister has to perform both types of activities viz., political as well as administrative. These can be broadly discussed as follows :

(i) As a member of the State Legislature, it is his duty to support and safeguard the total policies of the Government because of the collective responsibility of the cabinet.

(ii) As a member of the Ministry, he brings all the bills pertaining to his Department for the approval of the legislature.

(iii) As political head of the Health Department, he acts as an executive and administrator. He has to see that the policies approved by the legislature are faithfully implemented.

(iv) He is the custodian of the interests of the people in general and of his constituency in particular.

(v) As a member of the Government, he performs ceremonial duties.

As far as the administrative functions of the Minister are concerned, we find that for a number of reasons these activities do not receive the time and attention they deserve. Being busy with political activities, the Minister does not find enough time for administrative works. Lack of professional knowledge and lack of aptitude are the other contributory factors.

It was also pointed out by the Administrative Reforms Commission that there was a growing feeling among the public that most of the ministers lacked interest in efficient discharge of their administrative duties and did not possess the aptitude required for the purpose. The Administrative Reforms Commission in its report on State Administration recommended that, "the head of Council of Ministers (the Chief Minister) should, in selecting his colleagues, give special attention to considerations of political stature, personal integrity, intellectual ability and capacity for taking decisions and sustained application to work. Further, in assigning a portfolio, due regard should be paid to the aptitude and capacities of an incumbent."[1] The suggestion of A.R.C. must be accepted by the Chief Ministers to bring about innovations in political leadership.

(b) ***Administrative Head***. In order to keep a record of the policies framed by the political heads and to watch over their implementation and execution, the State administration has to seek the help of an office which is known as the state secretariat. The word 'Secretariat' refers to the complex of departments which vary from State to State.

The Secretariat organisation of the State Health Department, Punjab is presently headed by an IAS officer of the rank of Commissioner who functions as Secretary to the Government in the Department of Health and Family Welfare. He is assisted by 3 Secretaries and one Under-Secretary along with other administrative staff.

The main duties and responsibilities of the health department are as under :

(i) Assisting the Minister in policy making, in modifying policies from time to time and in the discharge of his legislative responsibilities;

(ii) Framing draft legislation and rules and regulations;

(iii) Coordination and policies of programmes, supervision and control over their execution and review of results;

(iv) Budgeting and control of expenditure;

(v) Maintaining contact with the Government of India and other State Governments; and

(vi) Overseeing the smooth and efficient running of administrative machinery and initiating measures designed to develop greater personnel and organisational competence.[2]

(c) ***Technical Head***. Below the State Secretariat, there are Executive Departments.* These departments are headed mostly by the specialists and are concerned with the supervision, coordination and control of the policy framed by the State Government. Based on our personal observation and discussion, it was revealed that not-withstanding the apparently clear demarcation of functions as between the secretariat and the Executive Department a lot of duplication and overlapping still persists between the Secretariat (Health Department) and the Executive Department. This results in too much interference in the day-to-day functioning of the Executive Department. As a matter of policy the Secretariat should restrict its activities only in policy-making.

The Executive Organisation of the Health Department in Punjab is headed by the Director, Health Services, who has under him four Joint Directors—Joint Director (Family Welfare), Joint Director (Food and Drug), Joint Director (Employees Social Insurance), and Joint Director (Administration), three Deputy Directors, responsible for inspection and supervision of all the National Health Programmes and Medical Institutions in their respective zones of four districts each and five Programme Specialists, of the rank of Assistant Directors to deal with specific programmes like leprosy, eradication of malaria, planning, etc. Besides, the Director has the assistance of an Accounts Officer, who is on deputation from the State Finance Department. Similarly he has the transport officer to control the operations of the large number of transport vehicles. The Joint Directors except the Joint Director (Administration) also have Assistant Directors under them to help them in the discharge of their duties. The Director and all other officers of the Department except the Joint Director (Administration) belong to the Provincial Health Service. The Joint Director (Administration) belongs to the Punjab Civil Service cadre and is on deputation to the Health Department. Apart from allopathy, the Indian System of medicines, namely Ayurveda, Homoeopathy and Unani systems are also now beginning to receive proper attention. Their functioning is being regulated by the Director Ayurveda, Punjab. This Directorate constitutes a separate organisation and deals with all the three indigenous systems of medicines. These two Health Directorates provide technical knowledge to the Secretary and the Minister. They also coordinate, supervise and control the implementation of health programmes and projects. The success or failure of the health department depends upon the leadership of the Directors of various systems of medicine.

District Level

The district is the most/crucial level in the administration and implementation of medical/health services. At the district level there is a District Medical and Health Officer (DMHO); Chief Medical Officer who is overall responsible for the administration of medical and heath services in the entire district and for the implementation of all the national health

---

* According to the Simon Commission, the Executive Department is an administrative unit, separate from the Secretariat, which reaches its apex, usually in a single officer like the Inspector-General of Police, or the Chief Conservator of Forests outside the Secretariat altogether. Such a head of department will usually be concerned principally with a single Secretary to Government and a single... Minister, for his orders and the funds which he has to spend. It is however not necessary that every Secretariat Department must have an Executive Department. Sometimes, the Secretariat Department like Finance or Law do not have any executive departments because they are only concerned with counselling and controlling functions. [Source: *Report of the Indian Statutory Commission*, Vol. I. Survey p. 312].

and family welfare programmes. He is assisted by the Additional District Medical and Health Officers or Deputy District Medical and Health Officers along with other district officers for various national health programmes in the district. Their number varies from state to state.

Sub-Divisional Level

Each district has been divided into two or more sub-revenue divisions. In each sub-division, there is a Senior Medical Officer who is overall incharge and is responsible for supervising the activities of all health and family welfare programmes in dispensaries and Taluka Hospitals of the sub-division. He is assisted by Health Supervisors and Health Education Officer.

Primary Health Centre Level

The Primary Health Centre (PHC) is the focal point of the Health Care delivery system in the rural areas, each covering about one-lakh population. It is headed by the Medical Officer Incharge, who is responsible for carrying out all the Health and Family Welfare Programmes in the block where PHC is located.

B. Functions of State Health Department (Punjab)

(1) ***Provisions of Medical Care***

The functions of the State Department are briefly given below :

Medical care through Hospitals, dispensaries, Health Centres and Mobile Domiciliary units in both rural and urban areas, e.g., in the State of Punjab, Medical Care is provided through :

(a) MEDICAL INSTITUTIONS (Allopathic) as on 31 March 1982

		Numbers
(i)	Hospital	255
(ii)	Primary Health Centres	130
(iii)	Dispensaries	1691
	Total	2076
	Rural	1710
	Urban	366

(b)	AYURVEDIC/UNANI INSTITUTIONS	
(i)	Ayurvedic	467
(ii)	Unani	35
	Total	502
(c)	MCH CENTRES	64
(d)	FAMILY PLANNING CENTRES	161
	Rural	128
	Urban	33
	Govt. owned	152
	Other bodies	9

The patients treated in medical institutions in Punjab have increased from 2,32,921(1971) to 4,19,009 in 1981. The total number of health personnel has doubled during the last ten years i.e. the number of doctors, midwives, nurses, dais has increased from 5,239, 2,138, 2,603, 10,569 in 1971 to 9,307, 4,624, 4,712, and 17,535 in 1981. The bed population ratio has increased from 0.729 in 1971 to 1.3 in 1981. The population served by a doctor has changed from 2,585(1971) to 1,806(1981).

(2) *Arrangements for Medical Education and Research*

The following are the teaching/training institutions :

(a)	Medical Colleges	5
(b)	Nursing Training Institutions	6
(c)	A.N.M. Training Institutions	7
(d)	L.H.V. Training Institutions	1
(e)	Pharmacists Training Institutions	2
(f)	Ayurvedic College	1

In order to improve the functioning of medical education, the State health department is proposing to take the following steps :

(a) increase the out-turn of para-medical staff in view of large expansion of Rural Services;

(b) re-orientation of Medical Education with a view to progressively making the training of medical students more community-based;

(c) to make good the deficiency in the nursing/para medical/ministerial and other services staff in accordance with the norm prescribed by the Nursing Council;

(d) to improve and expand common facilities like Hospital, Pharmacy, Blood Bank, Emergency Services, Intensive Care Unit and Rehabilitation Services in the hospitals.

(e) Continuing encouragement to Research activities in Medical Colleges.[3]

(3) *Implementation of National Health Programmes*

These programmes are planned, guided and directed by the Union Health Administration. The finances for these programmes are provided by the Union Ministry of Health and Family Welfare. Only operational cost of these schemes is borne by the State. These programmes are :

(i) National Family Welfare Programme.

(ii) National Malaria Eradication Programme.

(iii) National Tuberculosis Control Programme.

(iv) National Small Pox Eradication Programme.

(v) Filariasis and its Control.

(vi) National Leprosy Control Programme.

(vii) National Trachoma Control Programme.

(viii) Applied Nutrition Programme.

(4) *Provision of Health Services*

The following personal and impersonal health services are carried out in the State namely:

(a) Immunisation Services

(b) Nutrition

(c) School Health

(d) Industrial Health

(e) Family Planning

(f) Rural and Urban Sanitation

(g Control of Fairs and Festivals

(h) Drugs and Food Control

(i) Production of Vaccines and carrying out of mass immunisation programme

(j) Emergency health services during flood, famine, earthquake, refugee influx, etc.

(5) ***Control of Food and Drug Administration***

It is the responsibility of the Health Department to control adulteration of food and drugs and enforce minimum standards of food and drugs as laid down by the State.

(6) *Collection and Dissemination of Health Information*

The Department collects and transmits information on health and vital statistics for the States.

(7) *Control Over ESI Scheme*

The Department supervises the Employees State Insurance Scheme. This scheme has been in operation since 1953. The expenditure on this scheme is shared in the ratio of 1:7 by the Government and ESI Corporation.

(8) *Enforcement of Professional Standards*

The Department determines and maintains the standards of professional education, research and practice through the statutory bodies like the University, State Medical Council and Nursing, Midwife and Pharmacy Councils, etc.

(9) *Promotion of Indigenous System of Medicine*

The Department encourages development of indigenous system of medicine, e.g. Ayurveda, Unani and Homoeopathy. As is evident from the facts give below there has been a marked increase in health services under Ayurvedic, Unani and Homoeopathic system of medicine.

(10) *Setting up of Laboratories*

The Department maintains laboratories for production and distribution of vaccines, sera and blood banks for procuring and supplying human blood for transfusion purposes.

(11) *Supervision and Control over Local Bodies*

To assist the development of health services of the local bodies (Municipalities, Corporations, Panchayati Raj, etc.) and to carry out supervision and coordination work.

(12) *Preparation for the Enactment of Health Legislation*

The Department prepares for the necessary legislation dealing with public health, medical care, environmental sanitation, nutrition, food and drug control, factory control, etc.

(13) *Provision of Family Welfare Services*

The Department provides all types of services and is ahead of many States in its performance. The present position with regard to its achievements in the field of family welfare programme could be gauged from a Punjab-India comparison of percentages of eligible couples effectively protected, as reproduced below :

	Punjab	*India*
Sterilisation	19.8	20.0
IUD	3.1	0.9
Other methods	4.5	1.6
All methods	27.4	22.5
Birth rate	3.1	34

(14) *Provision of Maternal Services*

As illustrated below, the following achievements have been made during last two years in the field of MCH.

	1976-77	*1977-78*	*1978-79*
Expectant mothers immunised against tetanus	56,666	68,778	94,838
Children given DPT	95,461	1,90,669	2,49,113
Children given DT	78,031	1,45,358	1,78,930
Women given prophylaxis against nutritional anaemia	1,17,262	1,09,405	1,94,517
Children given prophylaxis against nutritional anaemia	69,090	91,152	1,82,777
Children given Vit-A Ist dose	47,274	1,97,256	2,47,080
IInd dose	3,094	89,220	1,42,101

Local Health and Family Welfare Organisation Set-up (Punjab)
District Level

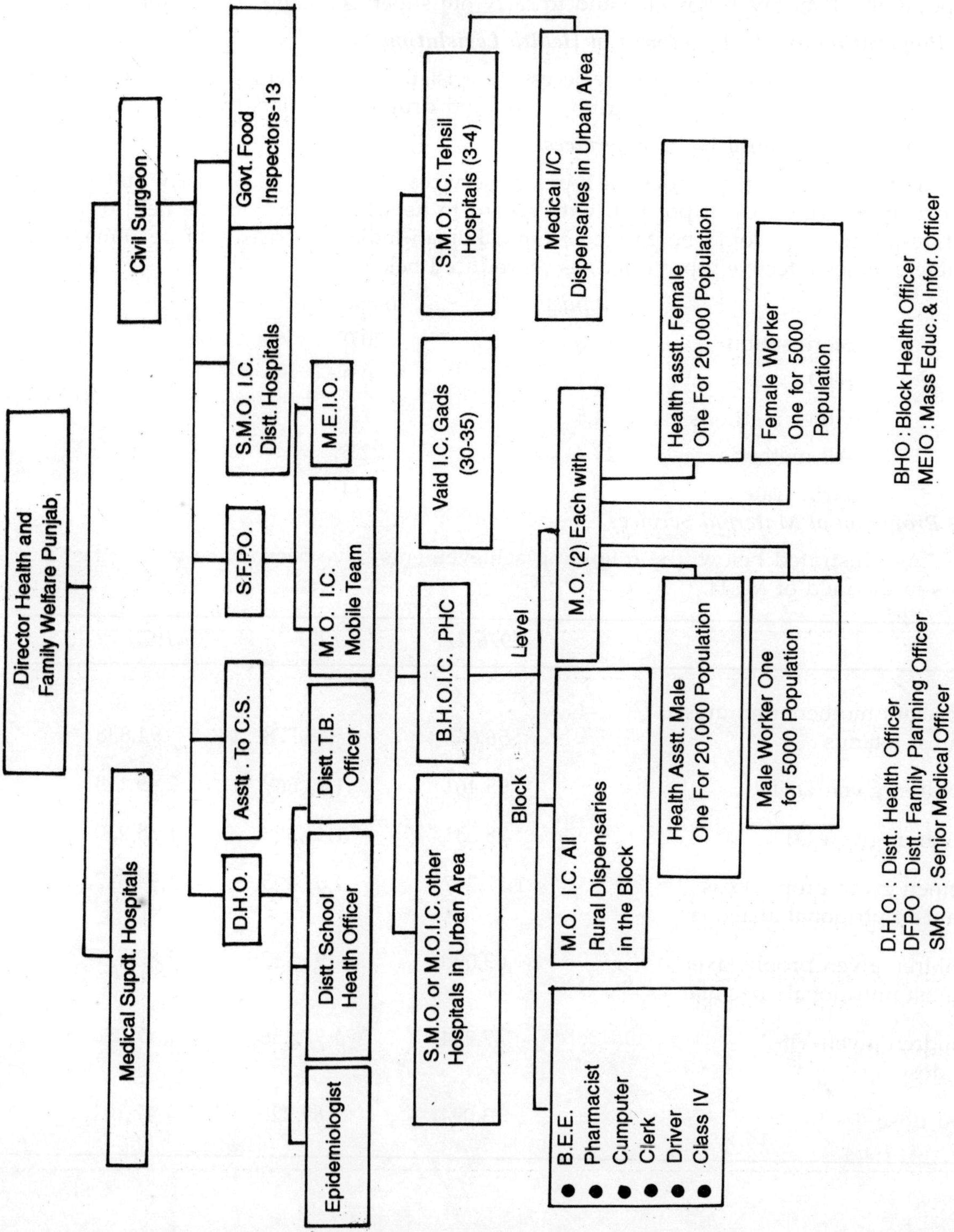

C. Local Health Administration

By Local Health Services is meant services organised in local Administrative Areas either rural or urban. We shall discuss first the Health Services in the rural areas and then in urban areas.

Health Services in Rural Areas

Eighty per cent of our population live in the rural areas consisting of villages. The Bhore Committee (1946) suggested a three-tier unit of integrated Health Services : (i) Primary Health Unit, (ii) Secondary Health Unit, (iii) Distt. Health Unit. The Central Council of Health at its first meeting in January 1953 also endorsed the Principles of the Integrated Development of Community life and a plan to establish Primary Health Centres. The Primary Health Centre (PHC) is usually located at the Block H.Qrs. or at any other convenient place well connected with other villages and a referral hospital. It covers a population of 60,000 to 1,00,000. It is the focus from where the health activities radiate to the remotest villages in the area through sub-centres. The sub-centres normally look after a population of 10,000. They provide a package of integrated health, both preventive and curative as well as family planning and nutrition services to the community. In addition to the Primary Health Centres and sub-centres there are other agencies like dispensaries under both the indigenous and modern system of medicine functioning within the Block. These have been converted into subsidiary Health Centres.

The Primary Health Centre provides accommodation for an outdoor dispensary, a consultation room, Maternal and Child Health Care and Family Planning Services, minor surgery, a small laboratory and ward of atleast 4-6 beds. Each centre today has atleast an average of 6 or more sub-centres. The existing position is as given in the table below:–

(i)	Number of PHC:	130
(ii)	Sub-centres	1034+59 opened under MPW Scheme
(iii)	Subsidiary Health Centres	846
(iv)	25/30 bedded rural hospitals	81
(v)	Mobile Eye Hospitals	39 (State) and 1 (Govt. of India)
(vi)	Dental Units at block level	68

Nature of Duties Performed by Doctors

There is a provision of three Medical Officers in each PHC, the senior most is the incharge, while the remaining two assist the Medical Officer Incharge in efficient functioning of the PHC. The Medical Officers have three areas of work—clinical, administrative and supervisory. Let us discuss them briefly :

DUTIES OF MEDICAL OFFICER (INCHARGE)

I. *Clinical*

1. Organising and conducting the outpatient clinics at PHC.
2. Organisation of indoor service.
3. Attending to medico-legal cases.
4. Attending to emergency cases.
5. Organising the laboratory service at the PHC.
6. Referring cases to hospital.

II. *Administrative*

1. Guide and check the preparation of tour programmes of staff.
2. All matters relating to management of personnel.
3. Reporting the progress of activities under all programmes to the Chief Medical Officer.
4. Liaison with other officials and agencies in the block.
5. All matters relating to indents, receipts and maintenance of supplies.

III. *Supervisory*

1. Check and guide the male workers in the field as well as in the main centres.
2. Attend to problem cases referred by field staff and arrange for appropriate services.

DUTIES OF 2ND MALE MEDICAL OFFICER

I. *Clinical*

1. Organising and conducting the out-patient clinics at PHC.
2. Organisation of the indoor service.
3. Attending to emergency cases.
4. Organising the laboratory services.
5. Attending to medico-legal cases.
6. Referring cases to hospital.

II. *Administrative*

1. Any work as and when assigned by Medical Officer Incharge.

III. *Supervisory*

1. Check and guide the male workers in the field as well as in the main centres.
2. Attend to problem cases referred by field staff and arrange for appropriate services.

DUTIES OF THE LADY MEDICAL OFFICER*

I. *Clinical*

1. Organise and conduct out-patient clinics at PHC.
2. Organisation of indoor service.
3. Attending to medico-legal cases.
4. Attending to emergencies.
5. Referring cases to hospital.
6. Conducting clinics at sub-centres and seeing referred cases and arranging for their treatment.

II. *Administrative*

1. Guide and check the preparation of tour programmes of the female staff.
2. Reporting the progress of activities under all programmes of the female staff to the Medical Officer Incharge.

III. *Supervisory*

1. Check and guide the ANMs and LHVs in the performance of their duties and maintenance of records.
2. Provide appropriate service to cases referred in the field by the peripheral staff.

Let us describe this pattern in detail.

(i) *Multipurpose Workers Scheme*. Under this scheme one male and one female multipurpose worker is provided for every 5,000 rural population. These two workers provide promotive, preventive and curative services to a localised population of 5,000 under the direct supervision of the local medical officer I/C subsidiary Health Centre, seven districts, viz., Ropar, Kapurthala, Jullundur, Sangrur, Bhatinda, Hoshiarpur and Faridkot have already been covered under the scheme and there is a proposal to extend the scheme to the remaining 5 districts by the end of the current financial year, viz., 1979-80.

(ii) *Health Guide Scheme*. Under the scheme one voluntary community level worker is to be provided for every 1,000 rural population. This is a 100 per cent centrally sponsored scheme and it was implemented in the state of Punjab in 20 Community Development Blocks on 2 October 1977. It was extended to additional 20 Community Development Blocks on 1 December 1978. So far 2506 Community Health Workers have been trained and positioned in their respective villages. The entire State is likely to be covered under the Community Worker Scheme by the end of the 6th Plan period.

(iii) *Training of Indigenous Dais*. Under another centrally sponsored scheme during 1977-78 over 2,495 indigenous dais were trained. During 1978-79 about 2,500 indigenous dais were trained. It is hoped that by the end of the 6th Plan period, over 12,000 indigenous dais,

* In case the services of the Lady Medical Officer are not available, the work of supervising female staff will be decided by the Medical Officer (Incharge).

i.e. at least one dais per village, would have been trained in the State of Punjab under this scheme.

(iv) *Subsidiary Health Centres.* The Subsidiary Health Centre is manned by an MBBS doctor, a pharmacist, an ANM, one laboratory worker and two helpers. Besides, it supplements its field services through two or four multipurpose health workers. In addition to functioning as a unit for general curative work, a subsidiary health centre is supposed to cater to the medical needs of cases referred to it by the sub-centres under its control. It also refers all the cases needing higher treatment to the nearby block hospital.

All subsidiary health centres in the State have been allotted two villages in their jurisdiction each of which is visited once a week by its doctor and para-medical staff. During these fixed day visits, the medical team arranges : (a) on the spot treatment of minor ailment cases; (b) immunisation of mothers and children; (c) prevention and cure of anaemia in mothers and children; and (d) health education of rural masses.

Thus, a Subsidiary Health Centre gives practical shape to the new concept of preventive, promotive and rehabilitative health services right in the villages. There were only 516 Subsidiary Health Centres upto 1976-77 but within a short span of the last two years, the present government has been able to open 330 more such institutions, thereby raising the total to 846.

Last but not least, the State government in order to provide integrated rural health structure, has recently upgraded the post Medical Officer Incharge Primary Health Centre from PCM S-II to PCM S-I, so that all the medical institutions falling within the jurisdiction of the Community Development Block should be placed under his administrative and technical control.

3. *Future Rural Health Services Plan*

In planning the future of rural health services we have to emphasise on the following:

(i) Correct the existing imbalance between the availability of medical facilities and manpower in urban and rural areas;

(ii) Provide total health coverage to the rural population;

(iii) Provide integrated health care services through integrated health structure; and

(iv) Provide basic specialists services to community nearer their homes.

The long-term health plan (1978-88) envisages the following health structure :

1. *Village level.* Every village will have some local voluntary health functionary (trained dai or community health worker) who will function as a contact person between the health staff and the village community in addition to providing certain basic services to the village community under the supervision of the multipurpose workers.

2. 5,000 *Population level.* There would be subsidiary health centre for every 5,000 population which will serve as the base unit; it will have one doctor, one dispenser, four class IV employees and one male and one female multipurpose workers. This base unit will provide a package of promotive, preventive and curative services in its area. It is envisage that the subsidiary health centre will develop and maintain family folders of all families in

5,000 population. Thus, on an average about 1,000 family folders will have to be maintained. This family folder will contain a complete health record of all members of the family. All vital events, viz., sickness, immunisation, birth, death and marriage, etc., will be recorded when the multipurpose worker visits the households. Once the family folder is prepared in respect of every family, it becomes a permanent record with the health authorities to be used as a reference as and when any member of the family has some health problem. In addition, the record so maintained will be very useful to measure various indices regarding the health status of the community which in turn will enable the health planners to formulate meaningful policies.

It is also proposed to provide a motor-bike to the medical officer of the subsidiary Health Centre to ensure his mobility so that he could extensively visit all the villages falling in his jurisdiction to provide services to the community as well as to give necessary support to the multipurpose workers and the local village health functionaries.

3. 25,000 *Population Level*. There would be one 25 bedded rural hospital for every 25,000 population so that this serves as the first tier in the referral system for the five Subsidiary Health Centres in its area. It will also be the headquarters of the male and female multipurpose supervisors (health assistants).

4. *Block level*. There would be a 50-bedded rural hospital in each block which will serve as the second tier in the referral system for four to five 25-bed hospitals in its area. This block level hospital would be adequately equipped and staffed so that it is able to provide basic specialist services relating to medicine, surgery, obstetrics and gynae, eye and ENT, paediatrics, anaesthesia and dental alongwith X-Ray and laboratory facilities.

It is also envisaged that the 50-bed hospital will send a team of specialists periodically according to a well chalked out programme to the peripheral units for providing specialists services to the community as near their homes as possible. This team will hold camps at suitable places within the blocks to provide specialised medical services.

Finances

During 1974-78 an expenditure of Rs 1129.08 lakhs was incurred on Public Health and Sanitation. An outlay of Rs. 5846.65 lakhs has been provided for the Sixth Five-Year Plan (1978-83). For 1979-80, a provision of Rs. 680.00 lakhs has been made. The sector-wise details of the expenditure outlay are give below:

Sector	*1974-78 (actual expenditure)*	*1978-83 (provision in lakhs)*	*1980-81 (outlay)*	*1981-92 (outlay)*
Research and Medical Education	360.51	1484.35	359.52	263.84
Public Health	738.79	4086.35	434.81	558.00
ISM and Homoeopathy	29.78	275.95	21.42	35.80
Total	1129.08	5846.65	816.15	875.65

The budget only for Health was Rs. 23.84 crores in 1976-77 and 31.6 crores during 1978-79. Per capita expenditure on health comes to Rs. 15.61(1976-77) and 19.50(1978-79), while per capita expenditure on medicine was Rs. 1.62(1976-77) and Rs. 1.92(1978-79).

D. Critical Appraisal of Working of the Health Administration at the State Level

We have already examined the organisation and functions of the Punjab State Health Department. From the quantitative analysis, it becomes quite clear that the department is doing well. On qualitative examination, it appears that the progress is superficial, unplanned and not directed to the needs of the clients. We give here some facts and suggestions which can help in the improvement of the organisation and functions of the health administration at the State Level.

(1) ***Serious Imbalance between the Rural and Urban Areas***

The mid '78 rural population of Punjab is estimated to be 1.20 crores living in 12,188 villages. There has been an imbalance in the availability of medical facilities and health manpower. Rural people have become conscious of their rights. They demand and deserve good quality health services. Even the Government itself is critical of this situation. It was stated officially that "it is an unfortunate fact that thirty years (1947-77) of health services development resulted in concentration of 80 per cent of medical manpower and facilities in urban areas where just 24 per cent of the total population resides. Paradoxically enough, Punjab's rural areas where 76 per cent of the State's total population lives were getting just 20 per cent institutional health services. Even 80 per cent of the total health budget was being spent on urban hospitals, etc. So the challenge of providing primary health care services to the ruralites was quite sizable in magnitude."[4]

What is being done to ensure health care to the rural people? The State governments are diverting more funds to develop infrastructure for providing health care to the rural people especially during the last five years. The basic question is how to ensure whether the rural people are being benefited or not. It is a common ill of Indian Administration that the people are not getting benefits because of the apathy of the personnel associated with the programmes. It is high time that we must ensure the fruitful working of our health schemes benefiting the villagers. Otherwise there is a likelihood of this imbalance increasing further. Health programmes could no more look mere political lollipops. These ought to be structured and designed in a fashion that meets the needs of the people.

(2) ***Status and Role of the Director of Health Services***

In the execution of health policy, programmes and activities, one person who has an exceedingly important role to play is the Director of Health Services. Thus a great deal depends on his competence, method of approach and managerial ability. If he has the right kind of leadership qualities, there is no reason why he should not succeed in the implementation of programmes under his control. If one has to identify factors affecting the role or performance of a Director of Health Services at the State level, one cannot possibly miss the most important factor related to his relative inferior position as compared to the prestigious position of the Secretary of Health Services. The Secretary/Deputy Secretary/ Under-Secretary of Health Services as a rule is a senior member of the Indian Administrative

Service. The Director is generally the seniormost member belonging to the State Medical Service cadre. The issues which involve them in conflicts range from decision-making regarding health programmes to their actual implementation in the field. The Director often feels that by virtue of his professional knowledge and competence his judgement is better than the judgement of his administrative counterpart. The domination of technocrats by the administrators in their day-to-day work has been debated in many national forums. The scientists feel that if they are given the freedom to decide, they can take much more interest and take rational decisions. The administrative Reforms Commission (1966-70) pointed out "An effort is needed to match jobs with the men possessing the needed qualifications, which means that the preference for the generalist, pure and simple should give place to a preference for those who have acquired competence in the concerned field."[5]

The Fulton Committee which was set up in Great Britain in 1966 and which submitted its report in 1968 similarly said, "Many scientists, engineers and members of other specialists classes get neither the full responsibilities and corresponding authority, nor the opportunities they ought to have. Too often they are organised in a separate hierarchy while the policy and financial aspects of the work are reserved for a parallel group of generalist administrators, and their access to higher management and policy-making is restricted. In the New Civil Service a wider and more important role must be opened up for specialists trained and equipped for it."[6]

Thus, the specialists should be given parity with the Indian Administrative Service in the matter of conditions of service. Besides, they must be given top positions at the policy-making levels in Government. This would raise the morale of the technocrats and would improve the efficacy of the Government.

3. ***Absence of Comprehensive Health Legislation***

In the States, legal provisions in regard to health lies scattered over a number of acts. At present there is only one State—Tamil Nadu— which has a comprehensive public health Act satisfying reasonably the requirements of the modern health administration. The present corpus of health legislation is inadequate resulting in piecemeal decisions. Regulations are lacking in many vital subjects. In several respects the legislation is ineffective and outdated. There is need for comprehensive legislation embracing all aspects of health in a State. This would result into good health policies and plans.

4. ***Medical Education not Oriented to Rural Needs***

A group on medical education and support manpower set up in 1974 noted with concern that "Medical Education in India over the years has been essentially urban-oriented, relying heavily on curative method and sophisticated diagnostic aids, with little emphasis on preventive and promotional aspects of community health. Programmes of training in the field of nutrition, family welfare planning, maternal and child health have tended to develop in isolation from medical education and thus do not subserve the total needs of the community. Although the number of doctors has speedily increased over the successive plan periods, the alienation of doctors from the rural environment has deprived the rural communities of total medical care." The same feeling was voiced in the Fifth Five Year Plan. The Sixth Plan also went on to point out that, "the basic problem is to produce a doctor who will be able to provide good health care and medical service to the community and will be able to work effectively in rural areas." Thus, it is high time for the State Governments to take policy decisions to reorient medical education with a view to progressively make the training of the medical students more community-based. It is suggested that the internship of medical college students may be arranged in villages. The students may be asked to execute a bond to serve in the villages atleast for a period of five years. The curriculum may be curtailed and may be oriented to the community needs.

5. ***Lack of Community Health and Health Administrative Researches***

Huge sums of money are poured out annually on clinical hospital-based research in most States of India. One would not underestimate the importance of this type of research because it adds to knowledge. However, one has to think in terms of defining the priorities of research. A country, where the bulk of people are living in the rural areas, should normally involve the greater number of doctors doing researches in community health. India is one country which cannot boast of even a single good epidemiological study of such communicable diseases as tuberculosis, from which a sizeable number of people suffer every year. In fact, the area of community health research does not encourage clinicians to work in the rural areas. The problems of community health, no doubt, are vast and intriguing. Yet, the country cannot afford to ignore them. India lives primarily in the villages and it is the villagers who are the recipients of probably the poorest quality of medical care. The future of India also depends on the progress made in the villages, particularly in the area of health. One has to watch and see how different States plan and administer their health programmes so that their rural beneficiaries are not outnumbered by their urban beneficiaries. Thus the present trend of our spending on curative medicine research has to change in favour of community health research particularly in the rural areas. This is a challenge which no State of India can afford to ignore.

Further, the health administration at the State level is poorly equipped. Most of the health administrators have got no training in the modern knowledge of management. There is no effort on the part of the personnel working in health departments to use modern methods to improve health care delivery. Moreover, the health departments, training institutions, medical colleges, nursing colleges do not seriously concern themselves with finding methods for optimum utilisation of resources. Health services research should be multidisciplinary, involving not only medical professionals and experts but also system analysts, operational researchers, social scientists, health economists, public administrators, anthropologists, etc. The State health department may encourage research in consonance with priority problems of its health care delivery system. The health department may encourage researches which affect programme delivery. Some areas are mentioned below :

(a) Health manpower—their training, development, utilisation, availability, needs and demands, etc., including experimentation with the development of various categories of health manpower.

(b) Equipment, materials, etc., their availability, utilisation, needs and demands.

(c) Organisational and management process in health and family welfare services, their linkages, etc., including referral systems.

(d) Performance and impact of health and family welfare services.

(e) Needs and demands of population for health and family welfare services.

(f) Perception, attitude, utilisation factors (promoters and barriers) effecting utilisation, etc., of population towards health and family welfare services.

(g) Problems and bottlenecks in the existing organisational systems and redesigning of existing systems to eliminate the same.

(h) Information systems for health and family welfare.

(i) Cost-benefit and cost-effectiveness analysis of health and family welfare services, programmes and projects.

(j) Cost-analysis of health and family welfare services, programmes and projects.

(k) Development and testing of technology suited to the Indian health scene and needs.

(l) Studies focused on the interphase between community and health services organisations.

(m) Studies on health status and social and economic development.

(n) Materials Management in a hospital.

(o) Working of Intensive-care units.

(p) Cost of running hospital services.

(q) Staffing of emergency services.

(r) Utilization of operation theatres.

(s) Enlisting of community participation.

(t) Development of planning and management techniques.

(u) Identification of goals and priorities of the health services.

6. ***Absence of Well-Designed Management Information System***

Many State governments have performed the ritual of setting up statistical bureaus dealing with health. Huge health statistics have also been collected but these have been put to a bare minimum use in terms of utilising this information for developing a realistic health care delivery system. Thus the ever-widening gap between accumulation of health statistics and their utilisation for improving health services has of late acquired new significance. While in the developed countries management information system is increasingly being given the importance it deserved, in the developing countries it has not yet become an integral part of the state health system. It would indeed be very profitable for all the States to organise data banks and critically examine the quality of their health services. Because of the many uses of health statistics in scientific analysis, planning, administration and evaluation, the health statistician must begin to think in terms of a fully coordinated health information system, in which all relevant data are collected, compiled stored, retrieved, analysed and published.[7]

However, the Health Information System has to be planned properly. A Health Information System was defined by Conference on Health Information Systems held by WHO in Copenhagen from 18-22 June, 1973, as,

> "A mechanism for the collection, processing, analysis and transmission of information required for organising and operating health services and also for research and training."[8]

We must ensure the accuracy of data, otherwise the whole of our planning would go wrong. Goddard has rightly said, "One of the greatest possible contributors to wastage of our precious resources, whether at the local, national or international levels, is the failure of those at any level of administration, and at all stages in the management of the activity, to base all decisions on verifiable facts. There should be no tolerating errors in administrative action which occur because someone failed to get all of those facts. In the evolution, execution and control of work plans, obtaining the factural evidences should always be the first step."[9]

(7) *Inadequate Financial Resources*

It is one thing to define health needs of a given population and another thing to adequately plan health services in accordance with their needs. No aspect of planning health services appears to be more important than the consideration of finance. The paucity of financial resources because of poor allocations has often proved to be a major obstacle in the execution of health programmes. With the meagre resources, one cannot expect much. At present the health department of Punjab is being allocated only 3-4 per cent of the total resources for the promotion of health. The task of providing health care to improve the quality of life of the people is challenging. The State governments must allocate at least 10 per cent of their total budget for health. Besides, there is a need to make the best use of the resources already allocated.

(8) *Non-availability of Dedicated Doctors/Workers to Serve in the Villages*

The doctors prefer to serve in the cities than in the villages. When they are forced to work in the villages, their mind is always in the cities. This results in lower efficiency of the Primary Health Centres. It is suggested that the Government while selecting the students for medical education must ensure that a large number of students should come from villages, i.e., rural areas. The missionary zeal may be cultivated among the doctors during their education so that they take up the rural assignments with dedication.

(9) *Under-utilisation of Indigenous System of Medicine*

Indian health problems are of such magnitude that if left only to the allopathic system of medicine, one cannot possibly hope to achieve much success. In the past, a policy of drift has been followed with regard to Ayurveda and other Indian systems of medicine. The supporters of Ayurveda and homoeopathy feel that this system could not get a chance to demonstrate its utility. It has been claimed by the practitioners of the indigenous system of medicine that the facilities provided to them have been too patchy and the services were inadequately supplied to prove the true worth of the system. The Punjab government has shown its keenness to promote the system but the tempo is very slow. The government should take a bold decision to encourage these systems which can provide health care to a large number of people with little cost.

(10) ***Unsatisfactory Management of Employees State Insurance Scheme***

Employees State Insurance Scheme has not been functioning well. The shortage of doctors and medicines is the common ill of these institutions. There had been complaints from the beneficiaries about the malfunctioning of these hospitals. It was mentioned in the *Tribune* by C.M. Kumbhkarni with reference to E.S.I. Hospital, Jullundur :

> "The indoor patients take their meals like beggar on paper and towel. The hospital is provided with stainless steel utensils but these are kept under lock and key."

Besides, it is widely felt that there is a lot of corruption among the doctors working in these hospitals. The State government must tighten the control over these hospitals and monitor the reactions and feeling of the patients to streamline the functioning of the ESI scheme.

(11) ***Poor Nutritional Status of the People.***

Punjab is an economically well-off State but the majority of the people suffer from diseases arising from nutritional deficiencies and malnutrition.

The following recommendations were made by the South-East Regional Committee to solve the problems of nutritional deficiencies which need the immediate attention of the State health department :

(1) Nutrition activities should be recognised as crucial components of health programmes, particularly of those directed at the mother and child.

(2) The nutrition activities of health programmes should be very clearly defined and their implementation at all levels and especially at the local level, should receive sufficient attention and allocation of resources.

(3) In the package of services, nutrition should receive the same priority as other components, so that it is not relegated to a position of secondary importance as has been many times the case.

(4) the delivery system for nutrition activities catering to the needs of the under-served population should be rationalised applying the principles of primary health care and using primary health workers within the context of national health administration.

(5) Nutrition education relevant to the local situation as a part of health education of the community and its inclusion in formal and non-formal education need to be improved.

(6) Service-oriented nutrition research to solve public health nutrition problems must receive priority.

(7) To fulfil the inter-sectoral and intra-sectoral responsibilities of health in nutrition, the role of the nutrition unit at the central level of the health services needs to be

considerably strengthened with its increased participation in health planning and programming.[10]

Finally, there are a large number of other problems in the areas concerning Health Planning, Health Manpower Planning, Health Project Management, Hospital Management, Administration of Health Education and Environmental Sanitation Programmes which would be discussed in the relevant chapters.

References

1. GOI : *Report of Administration of State Level Administrative Reforms Commission*, New Delhi 1969, p.10.
2. *Ibid*., p.19.
3. Government of Punjab, Deptt. of Planning, *Annual Plan*, 1979-80, p.112.
4. Government of Punjab, *Bold Planning and Solid Action : Health Services in Punjab*, 1979.
5. Administrative Reforms Commission, Report on Personnel Administration, New Delhi, Manager of Publication 1969, p.10.
6. *Report of the Committee on Civil Services* (The Fulton Committee) Cmnd : 3638, London H.M.S.C, 1968, p.12.
7. Forrest E.Linder, Director, International Programme of Laboratories for Population Statistics, School of Public Health, University of North California at Chapel Hill, N.C, USA "Recent Trends in Health Statistics" in *WHO Chronicle*, 30:58 63 (1976).
8. M.R.Aderson, Honorary Director, Medical Information Unit, Wessex Regional Hospital Board Winchester, U.K.:"Health Information System" in *WHO Chronicle*, 1974, 28,52-54.
9. H.A. Goddard, *Principles of Administration Applied to Nursing Service*, World Health Organisation, Geneva, 1958, p. 84.
10. SEA/RC20/pp.39-40.

2

National Health Policy

Introductory

The Constitution of India envisages the establishment of a new social order based on equality, freedom, justice and the dignity of the individual. It aims at the elimination of poverty, ignorance and ill-health and directs the State to regard the raising of the level of nutrition and the standard of living of its people and the improvement of public health as among its primary duties, securing the health and strength of workers, men and women, sepecially ensuring that children are given opportunities and facilities to develop in a healthy manner.

Since the inception of planning process in the country, the successive Five Year Plans have been providing the framework within which the States may develop their health services infrastructure, facilities for medical education, research, etc. Similar guidance has sought to be provided through the discussions and conclusion arrived at in the Joint Conferences of the Central Councils of Health and Family Welfare and the National Development Council. Besides, central legislation has been enacted to regulate standards of medical education, prevention of food adulteration, maintenance of standards in the manufacture and sale of certified drugs etc.

While the broad approaches contained in the successive Plan documents and discussions in the forums referred above may have generally served the needs of the situation in the past, it is felt that an integrated, comprehensive approach towards the future development of medical education, research and health services requires to be established to serve the actual health needs and priorities of the country. It is in this context that the need has been felt to evolve a National Health Policy.

Our Heritage

India has a rich, centuries-old heritage of medical and health sciences. The philosophy of Ayurveda and the skills enunciated by Charaka and Shushruta bear testimony to our ancient tradition in the scientific health care of our people. The approach of our ancient medical systems was of a holistic nature, which took into account all aspects of human health and disease. Over the centuries, with the intrusion of foreign influences and mingling of cultures, various systems of medicine evolved and have continued to be practised widely. However, the allopathic system of the medicine has, in a relatively short period of time, made a major impact on the entire approach to health care and pattern of development of the health services infrastructure in the country.

Progress achieved

During the last three decades and more, since the attainment of independence, considerable progress has been achieved in the promotion of the health status of our people. Smallpox has been eliminated; plague is no longer a problem; mortality from cholera and related diseases has decreased and malaria brought under control to a considerable extent. The mortality rate per thousand of population has been reduced from 27.4 to 14.8 and the life expectancy at birth has increased from 32.7 to 52. A fairly extensive network of dispensaries, hospitals and institutions providing specialised curative care has developed and a large stock of medical and health personnel, of various levels, has become available. Significant indigenous capacity has been established for the production of drugs and pharmaceuticals, vaccines, sera, hospital equipment, etc.

The existing picture

In spite of such impressive progress, the demographic and health picture of the country still constitutes a cause for serious and urgent concern. The high rate of population growth continues to have an adverse effect on the health of our people and the quality of their lives. The mortality rates for women and children are still distressingly high; almost one-third of the total deaths occur among children below the age of 5 years; infant mortality is around 129 per thousand live births. Efforts at raising the nutritional levels of our people have still to bear fruit and the extent and severity of malnutrition continues to be exceptionally high. Communicable and non-communicable diseases have still to be brought under effective control and eradicated. Blindness, Leprosy and TB continue to have a high incidence. Only 31 per cent of the rural population has access to potable water supply and 0.5 per cent enjoys basic sanitation.

High incidence of diarrhoeal diseases and other preventive and infectious diseases, specially amongst infants and children, lack of safe drinking water and poor environmental sanitation, poverty and ignorance are among the major contributory causes of the high incidence of diseases and mortality.

The existing situation has been largely engendered by the almost wholesale adoption of health manpower development policies and the establishment of curative centres based on the western models, which are inappropriate and irrelevant to real needs of our people and the socio-economic conditions obtaining in the country. The hospital-based disease, and cure-oriented approach towards the establishment of medical services has provided benefits to the upper crusts of society, specially those residing in the urban areas. The proliferation of this approach has been at the cost of providing comprehensive primary health care services to the entire population, whether residing in the urban or the rural areas. Furthermore, the continued high emphasis on the curative approach has led to the neglect of the preventive, promotive, public health and rehabilitative aspects of health care. The existing approach, instead of improving awareness and building up self-reliance, has tended to enhance dependency and weaken the community's capacity to cope with its problems. The prevailing policies in regard to the education and training of medical and health personnel, at various levels, has resulted in the development of a cultural gap between the people and the personnel providing care. The various health programmes have, by and large, failed to involve individuals and families in establishing a self-reliant community. Also, over the years, the planning process has become largely oblivious of the fact that the ultimate goal of achieving a satisfactory health status for all our people cannot be secured without involving the community in the identification of their health needs and priorities as well as in the implementation and management of the various health and related programmes.

Need for evolving a health policy—the revised 20 Point Programme

India is committed to attaining the goal of "Health For All by the Year 2000 A.D." Through the universal provision of comprehensive primary health care services. The attainment of this goad requires a thorough overhaul of the existing approaches to the education and training of medical and health personnel and the reorganisation of the health services infrastructure. Furthermore, considering the large variety of inputs into health, it is necessary to secure the overall national socio-economic development process, specially in the more closely health related sectors, e.g., drugs and pharmaceuticals, agriculture and food production, rural development, education and social welfare, housing, water supply and sanitation, prevention of food adulteration, maintenance of prescribed standards in the manufacture and sale of drugs and the conservation of the environment. In sum, the contours of the National Health Policy have to be evolved within a fully integrated planning framework which seeks to provide universal, comprehensive primary health care services, relevant to the actual needs and priorities of the community at a cost which the people can afford, ensuring that the planning and implementation of the various health programmes is through the organised involvement and participation of the community, adequately utilising the services being rendered by private voluntary organisation active in the health sector.

It is also necessary to ensure that the pattern of development of the health services infrastructure in the future fully takes into account the revised 20-point Programme. The said Programme attributes very high priority to the promotion of family planning as a people's programme, on a voluntary basis; substantial augmentation and provision of primary health care facilities on a universal basis; control of Leprosy, TB and Blindness; acceleration of welfare programmes for women and children; nutrition programmes for pregnant women, nursing mothers and children, especially in the tribal, hilly and backward areas. The Programme also places high emphasis on the supply of drinking water to all problem villages, improvements in the housing and environment of the weaker sections of society; increased production of essential food items; integrated rural development; spread of universal elementary education; expansion of the public distribution system, etc.

Population stabilisation

Irrespective of the changes, no matter how fundamental that may be, brought about in the overall approach to health care and the restructuring of the health services, not much headway is likely to be achieved in improving the health status of the people unless success is achieved in securing the small family norm, through voluntary efforts, and moving towards the goal of population stabilisation. In view of the vital importance of securing the balanced growth of the population, it is necessary to enunciate, separately, a National Population Policy.

Medical and Health Education

It is also necessary to appreciate that the effective delivery of health care services would depend very largely on the nature of education, training and appropriate orientation towards community health of all categories of medical and health personnel and their capacity to function as an integrated team, each of its members performing given tasks within a coordinated action programme. It is, therefore, of crucial importance that the entire basis and approach towards medical and health education, at all levels, is reviewed in terms of national needs and priorities and the curricular programmes restructured to produce personnel of various grades of skill and competence, who are professionally equipped and socially motivated to effectively deal with day-to-day problems, within the existing constraints. Towards this end, it is necessary to formulate, separately, a National Medical and Health Education Policy which (i) sets out the changes required to be brought about in the curricular contents and training programme of medical and health personnel, at various levels of functioning; (ii) takes into account the need for establishing the extremely essential interrelations between functionaries of various grades; (iii) provides guidelines for the production of health personnel on the basis of realistically assessed manpower requirements; (iv) seeks to resolve the existing sharp regional imbalances in their availability; and (v) ensures that personnel at all levels are socially motivated towards the rendering of community health services.

Need for providing primary health care with special emphasis on the preventive, promotive and rehabilitative aspects.

Presently, despite the constraint of resources, there is disproportionate emphasis on the establishment of curative centre—dispensaries, hospitals, institutions for specialist treatment—the large majority of which are located in the urban areas of the country. The vast majority of those seeking medical relief have to travel long distance to the nearest curative centre, seeking relief for ailments which could have been readily and effectively handled at community level. Also, for want of a well established referral system, those seeking curative care have the tendency to visit various specialist centres, thus further contributing to congestions, duplication of efforts and consequential waste of resources. To put an end to the existing all-around unsatisfactory situation, it is urgently necessary to restructure the health services within the following broad approach :

1. To provide, within a phased, time-bound programme, a well dispersed network of comprehensive primary health care services, integrally linked

within the extension and health education approach which takes into account the fact that a large majority of health functions can be effectively handled and resolved by the people themselves, with the organised support of volunteers, auxiliaries, para-medicos and adequately trained multi-purpose workers of various grades of skill and competence, of both sexes. There are a large number of private, voluntary organisations active in the health field, all over the country. Their services and support would require to be utilised and intermixed with the governmental efforts, in an integrated manner.

2. To be effective, the establishment of the primary health care approach would involve large scale transfer of knowledge, simple skills and technologies to Health Volunteers, selected by the communities and enjoying their confidence. The functioning of the front line workers, selected by the community would require to be related to definitive action plans for the translation of medical and health knowledge into practical action, involving the use of simple and inexpensive interventions which can be readily implemented by persons who have undergone short periods of training. The quality of training of these health guides/workers would be of crucial importance to the success of this approach.

3. The success of the decentralised primary health care system would depend vitally on the organised building up of individual self-reliance and effective community participation, on the provision of organised, back-up support of the secondary and tertiary levels of the health care services, providing adequate logistical and technical assistance.

4. The decentralisation of services would require the establishment of a well worked out referral system to provide adequate expertise at the various levels of the organisational setup nearest to the community, depending upon the actual needs and problems of the area, and thus ensure against the continuation of the existing rush towards the curative centres in the urban areas. The effective establishment of the referral system would also ensure the optimal utilisation of expertise at the higher levels of the hierarchical structure. This approach would not only lead to the progressive improvement of comprehensive health care services at the primary level but also provide for timely attention being available to those in need of urgent specialist care, whether they live in the rural or the urban areas.

5. To ensure that the approach to health care does not merely constitute a collection of disparate health interventions but consists of an integrated package of services seeking to tackle the entire range of poor health conditions, on a broad front, it is necessary to establish a nationwide chain of sanitary-cum-epidemiological stations. The location and functioning of these stations may be between the primary and secondary levels of the hierarchical structure, depending upon the local situations

and other relevant consideration. Each such station would require to have suitable trained staff equipped to identify, plan and provide preventive, promotive and mental health care services. It would be beneficial, depending upon the local situations, to establish such stations at the Primary Health Centres. The district health organisation should have, as an integral part of its setup, a well organised epidemiological unit to coordinate and superintend the functioning of the field stations. These stations would participate in the integrated action plans to eradicate and control diseases, besides tackling specific local environmental health problems. In the urban glomerations, the municipal and local authorities should be equipped to perform similar functions, being supported with adequate resources and expertise, to effectively deal with local preventable public health problems. The aforesaid approach should be implemented and extended through community participation and contributions, in whatever form possible, to achieve meaningful results within a time-bound programme.

6. The location of curative centres should be related to the populations they serve, keeping in view the densities of population, distances, topography, transport connections. These centres should function within the recommended referral system, the gamut of general specialities required to deal with the local disease patterns being provided as near to the community as possible, at the secondary level of the hierarchical organisation. The concept of domiciliary care and the field-camps approach should be utilised to the fullest extent, to reduce the pressures on these centres, specially in efforts relating to the control and eradication of blindness, tuberculosis, leprosy, etc. To maximise the utilisation of available resources, new and additional curative centres should be established only in exceptional cases, the basic attempt being towards the up gradation of existing facilities, at selected locations, the guiding principle being to provide specialist services as near to the beneficiaries as may be possible, within a well-planned network. Expenditure should be reduced through the fullest possible use of cheap locally available building materials, resort to appropriate architectural designs and engineering concepts and by economical investment in the purchase of machineries and equipment, ensuring against avoidable duplication of such acquisitions. It is also necessary to devise effective mechanisms for the repair, maintenance and proper upkeep of all bio-medical equipments to secure their maximum utilisation.

7. With a view to reducing governmental expenditure and fully utilising untapped resources, planned programmes may be devised, related to the local requirements and potentials, to encourage the establishment of practice by professional, increased investment by non-governmental agencies in establishing curative centres and by offering organised

logistical, financial and technical support to voluntary agencies active in the health field.

8. While the major focus of attention in restructuring the existing governmental health organisations would relate to establishing comprehensive primary health care and public health services, within an integrated referral system, planned attention would also require to be devoted to the establishment of centres equipped to provide speciality and super-speciality services, through a well dispersed network of centres, to ensure that the present and future requirements of specialist treatment are adequately available within the country. To reduce governmental expenditures involved in the establishment of such centres, planned efforts should be made to encourage private investments in such fields so that the majority of such centres, within the governmental set-up, can provide adequate care and treatment to those entitled to free care, the affluent sectors being looked after by the paying clinics. Care would also require to be taken to ensure the appropriate dispersal of such centres, to remove the existing regional imbalances and to provide services within the reach of all, whether residing in the rural or the urban areas.

9. Special, well-coordinated programmes should be launched to provide mental health care as well as medical care and the physical and social rehabilitation of those who are mentally retarded, deaf, dumb, blind, physically disabled, infirm and the aged. Also, suitable organised programmes would require to be launched to ensure against the prevention of various disabilities.

10. In the establishment of the re-organised services, the first priority should be accorded to provide services to those residing in the tribal, hilly and backward areas as well as to endemic disease affected populations and the vulnerable sections of the society.

11. In the re-organised health service scheme, efforts should be made to ensure adequate mobility of personnel, at all levels of functioning.

12. In the various approaches, set out in (1) to (11) above, organised efforts would require to be made to fully utilise and assist in the enlargement of the services being provided by private voluntary organisations active in the health field. In this context, planning encouragement and support would also require to be afforded to fresh voluntary efforts, specially those which seek to serve the needs of the rural areas and the urban slums.

Re-orientation of the existing health personnel

A dynamic process of change and innovation is required to be brought about in the entire approach to health manpower development, ensuring the emergence of fully integrated bands of workers functioning within the "Health Team" approach.

Private practice by government functionaries

It is desirable for the States to take steps to phase out the system of private practice by medical personnel in government service, providing at the same time for payment of appropriate compensatory non-practising allowance. The States would require to carefully review the existing situation, with special reference to the availability and dispersal of private practitioners, and take timely decision in regard to this vital issue.

Practitioners of indigenous and other system of medicine and their role in health care

The country has a large stock of health manpower comprising of private practitioners in various systems, for example, Ayurveda, Unani, Siddha, Homoeopathy, Yoga, Naturopathy, etc. This resource has not so far been adequately utilised. The practitioners of these various systems enjoy high local acceptance and respect and consequently exert considerable influence on health beliefs and practices. It is therefore, necessary to initiate organised measures to enable each of these various systems of medicine and health care to develop in accordance with its genius. Simultaneously, planned efforts should be made to dovetail the functioning of the practitioners of these various systems and integrate their services, at the appropriate levels, within specified areas of responsibility and functioning, in the overall health care delivery system, specially in regard to the preventive, promotive and public health objectives. Well considered steps would also require to be launched to move towards a meaningful phased integration of the indigenous and the modern systems.

Problems requiring urgent attention

Besides the recommended restructuring of the health services infrastructure, reorientation of the medical and health manpower, community involvement and exploitation of the services of private medical practitioners, specially those of the traditional and other systems, involvement and utilisation of the services of the voluntary agencies active in the health field, etc., it would be necessary to devote planned, time-bound attention to some of the more important inputs required for improved health care. Of these, priority attention would require to be devoted to :

(i) *Nutrition* : National and regional strategies should be evolved and implemented, on a time bound basis, to ensure adequate nutrition for all segments of the population through a well developed distribution system, specially in the rural areas and urban slums. Food of acceptable quality must be available to every person in accordance with his physical needs. Low cost, processed and ready-to-eat foods should be produced and made readily available. The overall strategy would necessarily involve organised efforts at improving the purchasing power of the poorer sections of the society. Schemes like employment guarantee scheme, to which the government is committed could yield optimal results if these are suitably linked to the objective of providing adequate nutrition and health cover to the rural and the urban poor. The achievement of this objective is dependent on integrated socio-economic development leading to the generation of productive employment for all those constituting the labour force. Employment guarantee scheme and similar efforts would require to be specially enforced to provide social security for identified vulnerable sections of the society. Measures aimed at improving eating habits, inculcation of desirable nutritional practices, improved and scientific utilisation of available food materials and effective popularisation of improved cooking practices would require to be implemented. Besides, a nationwide programme to promote breast-feeding of infants and eradication of various social taboos detrimental to the promotion of health would need to be initiated. Simultaneously, the problems of communities afflicted by chronic nutritional disorders should be tackled through special schemes including the organisation of supplementary feeding programmes directed to the vulnerable section of the population. The force and effect of such programmes should be ensured by delivering them within the setting of fully integrated health care activities, to ensure the inculcation of the educational aspects, in the over-all drugs.

(ii) *Prevention of food adulteration and maintenance of the quality of drugs* : Stringent measures are required to be taken to check and prevent the adulteration and contamination of foods at the various stages of their production, processing, storage, transport, distribution, etc. To ensure uniformity of approach, the existing laws would require to be reviewed and effective legislation enacted by the Centre. Similarly, the most urgent measures require to be taken to ensure against the manufacture and sale of spurious and sub-standard drugs.

(iii) *Water supply and sanitation* : The provision of safe drinking water and the sanitary disposal of waters, human and animal wastes, both in urban and rural areas, must constitute an integrated package. The enormous backlog in the provision of these services to the rural population and in the urban agglomerations must be made up on the most urgent basis. The provision of water supply and basic sanitation facilities would not automatically improve health. The availability of such facilities should be accompanied by intensive health education campaigns for the improvement of personal hygiene, the economical use of water and the sanitary disposal of waste in a manner that will improve individual and community health. All water-supply schemes must be fully integrated with efforts at proper water management, including the drainage and disposal of waste waters. To reduce expenditure and for achieving a quick headway it would be necessary to devise appropriate technologies in the planning and management of the delivery systems. Besides, the involvement of the community in the implementation and management of the systems would be of crucial importance, both for reducing costs as well as to see that the beneficiaries value and protect the services provided to them.

(iv) *Environmental protection* : While preventive, promotive, health services are established and the curative services reorganised to prevent, control and treat diseases, it would be equally necessary to ensure against the haphazard exploitation of resources which cause ecological disturbances leading to fresh health hazards. It is, therefore, necessary that economic development plans, in the various sectors, are devised in adequate consultation with the central and the state health authorities. It is also vitally essential to ensure that the present and future industrial and urban development plans are centrally reviewed to ensure against congestions, the unchecked release of noxious emissions and the pollution of air and water. In this context, it is vital to ensure that the siting and location of all manufacturing units is strictly regulated, through legal measures, if necessary. Central and State health authorities must necessarily be consulted in establishing locational development and urbanisation programmes. Environmental appraisal procedures must be developed and strictly applied in according clearance to the various developmental projects.

(v) *Immunisation programme* : It is necessary to launch an organised, nationwide immunisation programme, aimed at cent per cent coverage of targeted population groups with vaccines against preventable and communicable diseases. Such an approach would not only prevent and reduce disease and disability but also bring down the existing high infant and child morality rate.

(vi) *Maternal and child health services* : A vicious relationship exists between high birth rates and high infant mortality, contributing to the desire for more children. The highest priority would, therefore, require to be devoted to efforts at launching special programmes for the improvement of maternal and child health, with a special focus on the less privileged sections of society. Such programmes would require to be decentralised to the maximum possible extent their delivery being at the primary level, nearest to the doorsteps of the beneficiaries. While efforts should continue at providing refresher training and orientation to the traditional birth attendants, schemes and programmes should be launched to ensure that progressively all deliveries are conducted by competently trained persons so that complicated cases receive timely and expert attention within a comprehensive programme providing ante-natal, intra-natal and post-natal care.

(vii) *School health programme* : Organised school health services, integrally linked with the general, preventive and curative services would require to be established within a time-limited programme.

(viii) *Occupational health services* : There is urgent need for launching well-considered schemes to prevent and treat diseases and injuries arising from occupational hazards, not only in the various industries but also in the comparatively un-organised sectors like agriculture. For this purpose,

ORGANIZATIONAL CHART

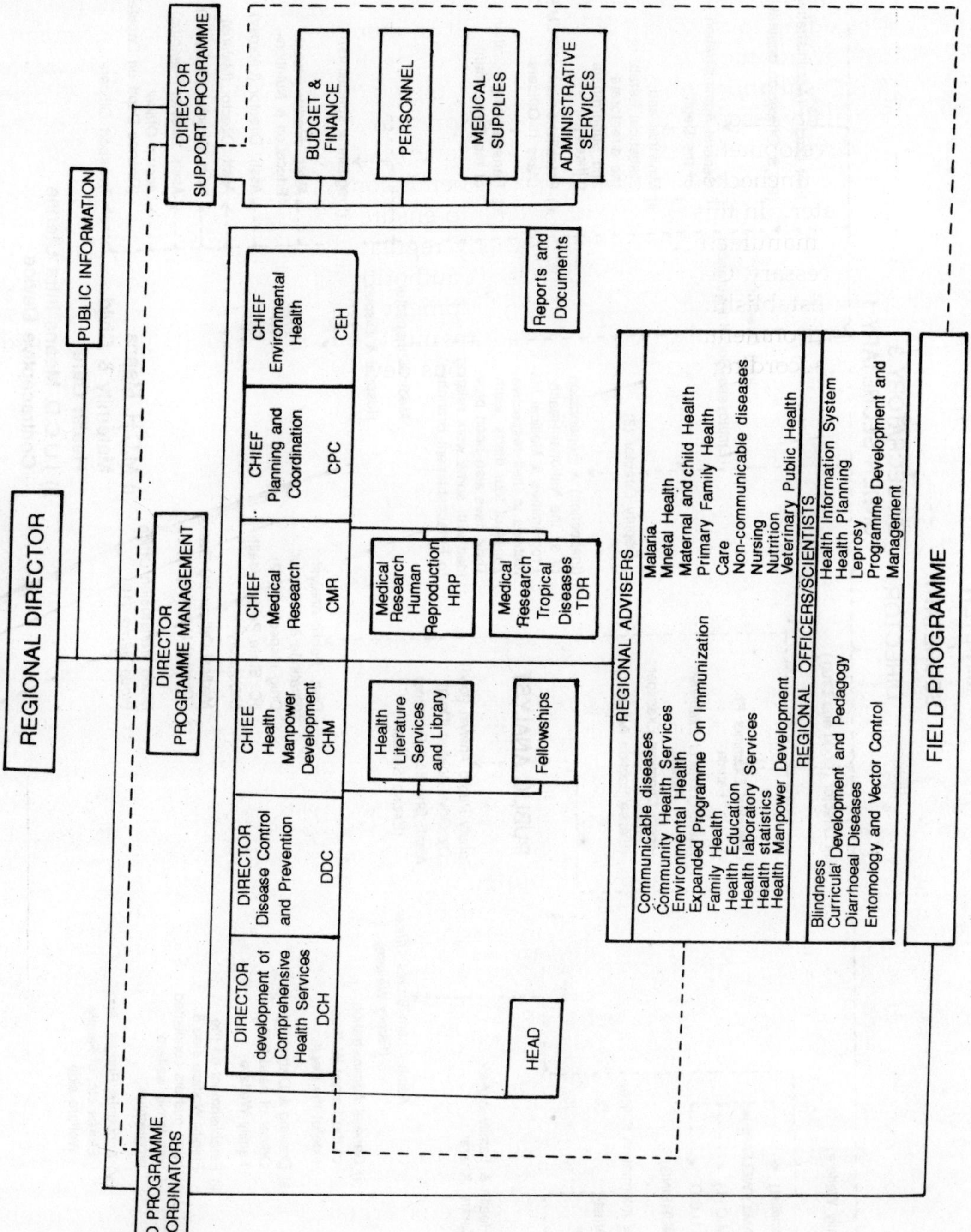

ORGANISATION OF HEALTH AND FAMILY WELFARE PUNJAB
STATE DIRECTORATE LEVEL

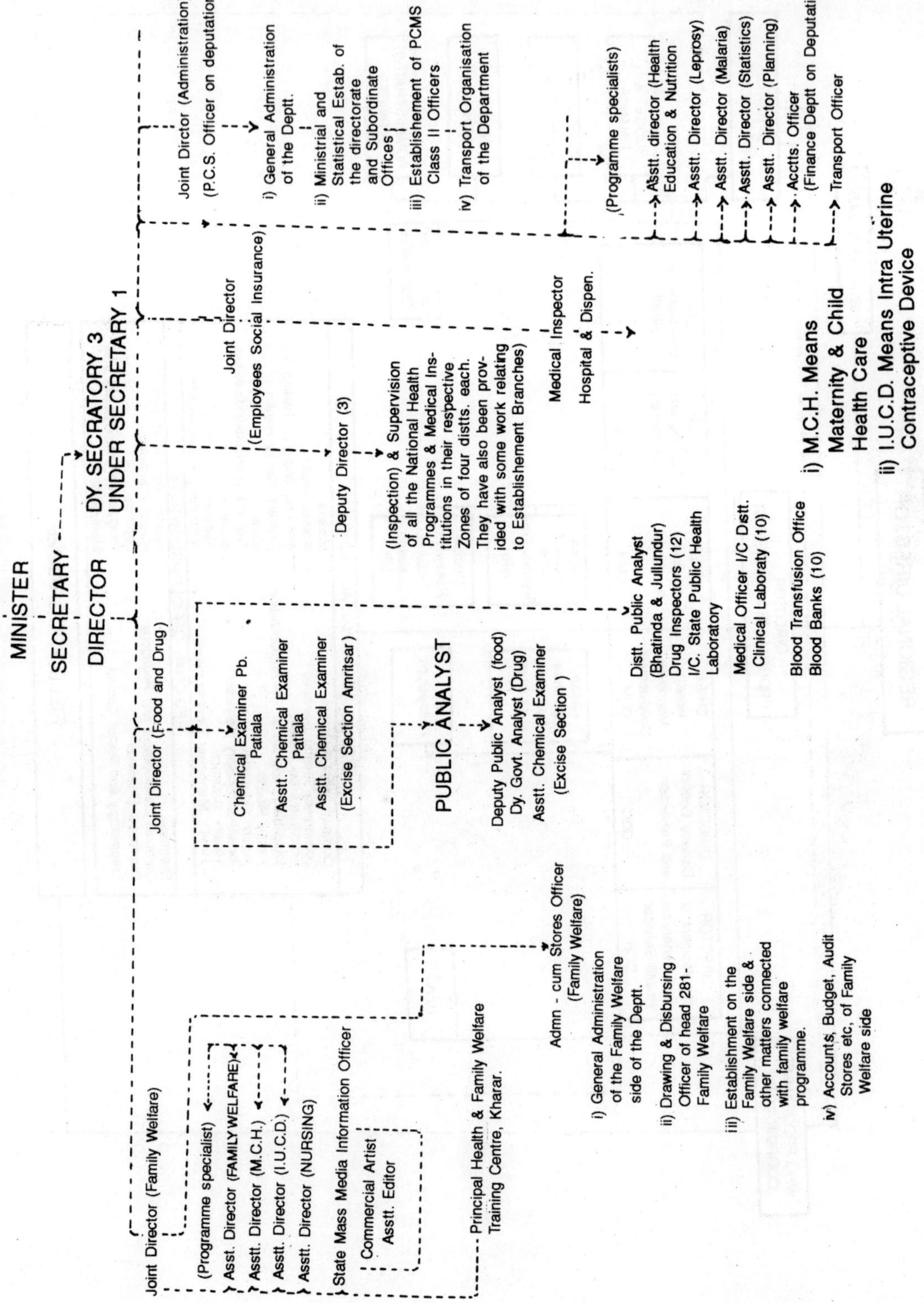

the coverage of the Employees State Insurance Act, 1948, may be suitably extended ensuring adequate coordination of efforts with the general health services. In their respective spheres of responsibility, the Centre and States must introduce organised occupational health services to reduce morbidity, disabilities and mortality and thus promote better health and increased welfare and productivity on all fronts.

Health education

The recommended efforts, on various fronts, would bear only marginal results unless nation-wide health education programmes, backed by appropriate communication strategies are launched to provide health information in easily understandable form, to motivate the development of an attitude for healthy living. The public health education, programmes should be supplemented by health, nutrition and population education programmes in all educational institutions, at various levels. Simultaneously, efforts would require to be made to promote universal education, specially adult and family education, without which the various efforts to organise preventive and promotive heath activities, family planning and improved maternal and child health cannot bear fruit.

Management information system

Appropriate decision making and programme planning in the health and related fields is not possible without establishing an effective health information system. A nationwide organisational set up should be established to procure essential health information. Such information is required not only for assisting in planning and decision making but also to provide timely warnings about emerging health problems and for reviewing, monitoring and evaluating the various ongoing health programmes. The building up of a well conceived health information system is also necessary for assessing medical and health manpower requirements and taking timely decision on a continuing basis, regarding the manpower requirements in the future.

Medical Industry

The country has built sound technological and manufacturing capability in the field of drugs, vaccines, bio-medical equipments.The available know-how requires to be adequately exploited and increase the production of essential and life saving drugs and vaccines of proven quality to fully meet the national requirements specially in regard to the national programmes to combat Malaria, TB, Leprosy, Blindness, Diarhoeal diseases, etc. The production of the essential, life-saving drugs under their generic names and the adoption of economical packaging practices would considerable reduce the unit cost of medicines bringing them within the poor section of society, besides significantly reducing the expenditure being incurred by the governmental organisation on the purchase of drugs. In view of the low cost of indigenous and herbal medicines, organised efforts may be launched to establish herbal gardens, producing drugs of certified quality and making them easily available.

The practitioners of the modern medical system rely heavily on diagnostic aids involving extensive use of costly, sophisticated bio-medical equipment. Effective mechanisms should be established to identify essential equipment required for extensive use and to promote and enlarge their indigenous manufacture, for such devices being readily available, at reasonable prices, for use at the health care centres.

Health insurance

Besides mobilising the community resources, through its active participation in the implementation and management of national health and related programmes, it would be necessary to devise well considered health insurance schemes, on a State-wise basis, for mobilising additional resources for health promotion and ensuring that the community shares the cost of the services, in keeping with its paying capacity.

Health legislation

It is necessary to urgently review all existing legislation and work towards a unified, comprehensive legislation in the health field, enforceable all over the country.

Medical research

The frontiers of the medical sciences are expanding at a phenomenal pace. To maintain the country's lead in this field as well as to ensure self-sufficiency and generation of the requisite competence in the future, it is necessary to have an organised programme for the building up and extension of fundamental and basic research in the field of bio-medical and allied sciences. Priority attention would require to be devoted to the resolution of problems relating to the containment and eradication of the existing, widely prevalent diseases as well as to deal with emerging health problems. The basic objective of medical research and the ultimate test of its utility would involve the translation of available know-how into simple, low-cost, easily applicable appropriate technologies, devices and interventions suiting local conditions, thus placing the latest technological achievements, within the reach of health personnel, and to the front line health workers, in the remotest corners of the country. Therefore, besides devotion to basic, fundamental research, high priority should be accorded to applied, operational research including action research for continuously improving the cost effective delivery of health services. Priorities would require to be identified and laid down in collaboration with social scientists, planners and decision-makers and the public. Basic research efforts should devote high priority to the discovery and development of more effective treatment and preventive procedures in regard to communicable and tropical diseases—Blindness, Leprosy, TB, etc. Very high priority would also have to be devoted to contraception research to urgently improved the effectiveness and acceptability of existing methods as well as to discover more effective and acceptable devices. Equally high attention would require to be devoted to nutrition research, to improve the health status of the community. The overall effort should aim at the balanced development of basic, clinical and problem-oriented operational research.

Inter-sectoral cooperation

All health and human development must ultimately constitute an integral component of the overall socio-economic developmental process in the country. It is thus of vital importance to ensure effective co-ordination between the health and its more intimately related sectors. It is, therefore, necessary to set up standing mechanisms, at the Centre and in the States, for securing intersectoral coordination of the various efforts in the fields of health and family planning, medical education and research, drugs and pharmaceuticals, agriculture and food, water supply and drainage, housing, education and social welfare and rural development. The coordination and review committees, to be set up, should review progress, resolve bottlenecks and bring about such shifts in the contents and priorities of programmes as may appear necessary, to achieve the overall objectives. At the community level, it would be desirable to devise arrangement for health and all other developmental activities being coordinated under an integrated programme of rural development.

Monitoring and review of progress

It would be of crucial importance to monitor and periodically review the success of the efforts made and the results achieved. For this purpose, it is necessary to urgently identify the base line situation and to evolve a phased programme for the achievement of short and long term objectives in the various sectors of activity. Towards this end, the current level of achievement as well as the broad indicators for the achievement of certain basic health and family welfare goals are set out in the annexed tabular statement. These goals, as well as other allied objectives, would require to be further worked upon and specific targets for achievement established by the Central and the State Governments in regard to the various areas of functioning.

S.No	*Indicator*		*Current level*	*1985*	*1990*	*2000*
1	2		3	4	5	6
1	Infant mortality rate	Rural	136(1978)	12		
		Urban	70(1978)	60		
		Total	125(1978)	106	87	below 60
	Perinatal mortality		67(1976)			30-35
2.	Crude death rate	Around	14	12	10.4	9.0
3.	Pre-school child (1-5 yrs.) mortality		24(1976-77)	20-24	15-20	10
4.	Maternal mortality rate		4-5 (1976)	3-4	2-3	below 2
5.	Life expectancy at birth (yrs.)	Male	52.6(1976-81)	55.1	57.6	64
		Female	51.6(1976-81)	54.3	57.1	64
6.	Babies with birth weight below 2,500 gms. (percentage)		30	25	18	10
7.	Crude birth rate	Around	35	31	27.0	21.0
8.	Effective couple protection (percentage)		23.6 (March, 82)	37.0	42.0	60.0

Contd..

1 2	3	4	5	6
9. Net Reproduction Rate (NRR)	1.48 (1981)	1.34	1.17	1.00
10.Growth rate (annual)	2.24(1971-81)	1.90	1.66	1.20
11.Family size	4.4(1975)	3.8		2.3
12.Pregnant mothers receiving ante-natal care(%)	40-50	50-60	60-75	100
13.Deliveries by trained birth attendants (%)	30-35	50	80	100
14.Immunisation status (% coverage)				
TT (for pregnant women)	20	60	100	100
TT (for school children)				
10 years		40	100	100
16 years	20	60	100	100
DPT(Children below 3 yrs)	25	70	85	85
Polio (infants)	5	50	70	85
BCG (infants)	65	70	80	85
DT (new school entrants 5-6 years)	20	80	85	85
Typhoid (new school entrants 5-6 years)	2	70	85	85
15. Leprosy — percentage of disease-arrested cases out of those detected	20	40	60	80
16. TB — percentage of disease arrested cases of those detected	50	60	75	90
17. Blindness — incidence of(%)	1.4	1	0.7	0.3

3

Health Policy and Administration

1. INTRODUCTION

General

The axiom "Health is Wealth" is relevant in all ages, for it is on the health of the people, that the wealth of a nation and the survival of its people depends. In developing countries, health care and social welfare education has to go forward to reach rural areas where, it is said, only a small percentage of health budget is spent. It is a matter of concern that in developing countries where there is 75 per cent of the world population, only 6 per cent of the world's health expenditure is spent. This fact reveals the distance these countries have to travel to provide health care to all people and to achieve the goal of excellence in health and welfare.

The theme 'Health for All by 2000 AD', a call made by the World Health Organisation as early as 1977, will be the right goal to developing countries to provide adequate health facilities to the people, particularly, the majority of the poor people, the working people, the sick people and the village people living in rural areas. There is therefore an imperative need to have a fresh look at the Health Policy and Administration of our country to doubly ensure that it is moving towards the goal of 'Health for All by 2000 AD'. The objective of health for all is, to put in the words of the Director General of WHO "Health for All does not mean that, in the year 2000 AD, doctors and nurses will provide medical repairs for everybody in the world for all their existing ailments, nor does it mean that in the year 2000 nobody will be sick or disabled. It does mean that health begins at home, in schools and in factories. It does mean that there will be an even distribution among the population of whatever health resources are available. And it does mean that essential health care will be accessible to all individuals and families, in an acceptable and affordable way, and with their full involvement."

The most important factor that is necessary to achieve the goal is full co-operation between the Government, Voluntary Agencies, International Health Organisations, and last but not the least, the people and the community. Another factor that is equally important is public awareness and public involvement. There is no gain-saying the fact that without giving due weightage to these aspects, tangible and satisfactory results cannot be obtained in the field of Health Administration. There is therefore need for injecting a sense of public awareness and dynamism in the Health Policy and Administration to make it more people oriented.

In the Health Policy of a nation, Preventive method should be considered as a very broad concept. Then, people of all categories should be involved in the implementation of the Health Policy in order to make them understand that about 80 per cent of the diseases in India are water-born. This can very well be prevented through the supply of safe and pure drinking water to every home, properly designed sanitary lines, clean surroundings and living environment, personal cleanliness and hygiene and availability of safe food items to the people. If the Health Administrators consider these elements as the basic foundation of the Nation's health, it is possible to achieve the goal aimed at by 2000 AD.

Another important factor is the policy concerning the prevention and eradication of diseases like leprosy, tuberculosis, etc. The success in this direction also would to a great extent depend upon the involvement and co-operation of the people, as removal of social prejudices are more important than treatment in case of these diseases. There is need for a special emphasis of this espect in the Health Policy and Administration of the country.

The non-availability of essential food, which is not within the reach of the majority poor people and even if it is, they cannot afford to buy it, is a matter causing serious concern to the Health Policy Makers of the country. Consequent upon this, the mental and physical structure of the children gets weakened making the susceptible to various diseases very easily. The majority of the children in the third world, they say, are victims of malnutrition. There is an urgent requirement to give top priority to the health of these children, as if we fail to make them healthy citizens of tomorrow, there will be no future for the country. It is therefore desirable to have a National Health Policy for children alone within the Master Health Policy so that we will be able to provide needed health protection to the children.

The Health Policy should also give deserving priority to welfare and rehabilitation of the handicapped whose number is tremendously going up day by day. The Administrators should help them to bring back their life to an average socio-economic status. There should be special programmes to employ the handicapped people so that apart from getting means to live in, they will also be able to contribute to the socio-economic growth of the country in a small way.

Systematic monitoring, and evaluation of the progress made has to be a primary factor in administering health programmes. There should be health policy indicators, socio-economic indicators etc. specially designed for the experts to measure the health status of the people at frequent intervals. Developments of necessary infrastructure and manpower resources should also form part of the central core of the Health Policy. So also should be the distribution of the resources to urban and rural areas.

The work ahead is really hard and arduous for the Health Administrators and people. It calls for dynamism, sacrifice and understanding. The magnitude of the problem can be judged when the Director General of WHO speaks "yet how can we speak of progress when a new born child in some African countries has only 50-50 chances of surviving through adolescence, when four-fifth of the world's population living in slums and rural areas have no access to any permanent form of health care; when only one in three persons in developing countries has reasonable access to safer water and adequate sanitation."

Thus the life situation in developing countries in general and in India in particular only points to the imperative need for a broad-based, comprehensive, and result-oriented Health Policy with pre-determined goals, sufficient infrastructure and manpower resources, supported and supplemented by Dynamic Administrators and public involvement.

In the following pages, an attempt has been made to peep into the health status of India and the challenging health problems before the nation and to suggest some ways and means towards the Health Policy and Administration. From all points of view, the Nation has to give top priority to the Health of the people. This is required precisely because, it is the healthy people who work hard to increase productivity and wealth of the Nation. So much so, the success in achieving the goal of 'Health for All by 2000 AD' would mean laying a strong foundation for the socio-economic development of India.

National Importance and Achievements

National Importance : Health of people is the natural wealth of a nation. It is an inseparable element in the development process of a nation. It is necessary that every nation should have an integrated approach to the Health and Economic Policy of the country. It should be a national objective to attain the highest possible standard of health as good health is the basic foundation for the promotion of creativeness, self-discipline, self-confidence, and dynamism in people which are necessary to increase the productive capacity of the nation.

Poor people who form the majority of the population and who are victims of ill-health become a liability to the nation in several ways. Because of their sickness, they are unable to work hard and to contribute constructively for the nation building process. Similarly, Government has got responsibility to provide adequate health protection to all people at its own cost. When people of a nation fall victims of diseases in large numbers, it brings bad name to the country. So all these factors only indicate the importance of Health in the national affairs and the top priority it deserves in National Planning.

Good health is *sine qua non* to fulfil the human aspirations and to enjoy better quality of life and to move ahead of others in professional efficiency, progress and development and also to give a balanced socio-economic status to the individual, the family and the community as a whole. There is, therefore, need to mobilise and to make effective use of all the human resources for the economic development of the nation. But this is possible only if the human resources are healthy and talented. It is also essential that each and every citizen should be concerned with the health problems and they should not resort to life styles that will damage their health but should contribute significantly in preventing the diseases and solving the health problems. The National Health Policy and Administration should have pre-determined plans to take this message to the people everywhere and to bring them close to the Health programmes.

National Achievement : India has made notable achievement in the medical and health services since independence. The fact that the average life of an Indian has increased from 27 to 58 is an indication of the progress made. This has become possible primarily because of the importance and priorities the health programmes received in our five year plans and programmes and the co-operation and support received from the UN Aided Health Agencies and other International Organisations.

The Seventh Five Year Plan emphasises on preventive and promotive aspects and organising effective and efficient health services which are comprehensive in nature, easily and widely available and accessible to people. Accordingly, broad objectives of the Health Policy have been formulated to control and eradicate communicable diseases, to provide preventive and curative and promotive health services to the people and to widen the scope for primary health care in rural and tribal areas. However, in spite of the great achievements made by India not only in the field of Medicine and General Health, Primary Health care and eradication of communicable diseases but also in Health education and Rehabilitation, there is need for a fresh look at the Health Policy and Administration strategies in the light of the new goal set to reach the Health for All by the year 2000 AD.

A peep into the Health problems of India would reveal that the following were the main factors that slowed down or made ineffective the Health and Medical services in India :–

(*a*) Growth of population and the consequent inadequacy of services and infrastructure.

(*b*) Lack of trained personnel and neglected of rural areas where the majority people live.

(*c*) Malnutrition and adulterated food.

(*d*) Non-availability of essential drugs in rural areas.

(*e*) Inadequate and ineffective health education to make the people health conscious.

(*f*) Large scale pollution of drinking water, non-availability of pure drinking water to majority people and absence of proper sanitary lines.

(*g*) Lack of dynamism in Rural Health administration, absence of public involvement and monitoring of results.

(*h*) Prejudices and dogma widely prevalent in Society about various diseases.

In view of the above, it is for the Planners and Health Administrators to clear these hurdles and take the health services to the people and involve them in implementing the various programmes for their own benefit and for the benefit of the society.

Components and Objectives

General: Political will and national resolve are the two basic factors in making an ambitious but practicable health policy. Involvement of experts and Organisations dealing with Health will make the policy broad-based result-oriented and workable. The Health Policy to be comprehensive and to keep abreast the advance in the field should consider :–

(*a*) Adoption of all the characters and resolutions passed by the UN Aided Health Organisations like World Health Organisation;

(*b*) Integration of the Activities with similar activities in other parts of the world to facilitate flow of benefits and information from research and development;

(*c*) Making an actual assessment of the health needs of the people, particularly in the rural areas;

(*d*) Proper planning for manpower resources development and utilisation in a balanced and need-based manner.

(*e*) A Drug policy to make available the needed and essential drugs to all sections of the populations.

The Health Policy should reflect the aspirations of all regions without any discrimination and the basis of policy implementation should be "equality and justice." It should commit itself to the principles and objectives enunciated in the constitution of WHO and the UN declaration on social Progress and Development.

The Health Policy should have clearly defined objectives which should include priorities such as Primary Health care, human resources planning and development for Health services, provision of safe drinking water and proper sanitation, promotion of maternity and child welfare, control and eradication of communicable diseases, supply of nutrious and safe food. Health education, rehabilitation and such other vital areas of human life.

The specific objective of a comprehensive and people oriented Health Policy may be summarised so under :–

(*a*) Highest priority for mobilisation and employment of funds with equality and justice.

(*b*) Manpower planning and development in order to produce need-based requirement of trained personnel avoiding excesses and shortages.

(*c*) Establishing full-fledged Primary Health Care Centre in all villages with facility for immunisation, Health Education and treatment.

(*d*) Stabilisation of population, family planning and welfare and people's involvement.

(*e*) Research and development and establishing specialised Institutions in rural areas. Also opening sufficient number of Hospitals to make the health services within the reach of all in an affordable way.

(*f*) National Health Policy for children and youth.

(*g*) To make available drugs and infrastructure in all areas.

(*h*) Provision of drinking water, sanitation, safe food in order to prevent diseases.

(*i*) Rehabilitation of handicapped people and plans their re-employment.

(*j*) To control and eliminate Smoking, Drinking and drug-addiction, particularly in the young, in order to prevent and control the diseases arising out of such habits.

It is necessary that under the administrative strategies, long-term and short-term plans to achieve the above objectives should be collectively chalked out by Government, International Health Organisations and Voluntary Agencies under the general guidelines issued by the Governments.

RESOURCES AND INFRASTRUCTURE PLANNING

Resources and infrastructure planning is the central core of a Health Policy and Administration. It is not possible to obtain clearcut and tangible results without proper resources and infrastructure planning. It is therefore necessary that the Health Policy of the nation should be based on concrete long-term and short-term resources and infrastructure planning.

In order to make the plan more result-oriented and to give the benefit of the Health services to all people with equality and justice, the planning should take each family as a unit so that it can be directly linked to the Health plan, as a matter of administrative strategy. For the purpose of discussion, Resources and Infrastructure planning can be brought under the following broad categories :

(*a*) Financial Plan for Health

(*b*) Human Resources Development in Health Planning

(*c*) Medical Education, Training and Research

(*d*) Hospitals and Treatment Centres

(*e*) Drug and Medicine

(*f*) Other Health Agencies

The above-mentioned points are discussed below.

Financial Plan for Health

Financial planning is an integral part of any National Health Policy and no health plan can be properly implemented without adequate financial support and assistance. There is no meaning in making ambitious Health plans without locating necessary financial sources for the achievement of its national goals. The National Health Policy should therefore depend upon reliable sources for funds and then only the programmes can be implemented giving full benefits to the people.

In a country like India where majority people are living in rural areas and where a lion's share of health expenditure is earmarked and spent for urban population and developed areas, top priority should be given for rural health in the Health budget so that the Health plans and programmes can be implemented with equality and justice. As a matter of fact there should be more sanctions for rural areas because of the poor socio-economic environment and malnutrition that prevails in such areas and also the majority population is in the rural areas.

The sources to which a Nation can look forward for funds mobilisation for its Health plans can be summarised as under :

(*a*) Nations's own exchequer—allotment on priority.

(*b*) Resources mobilisation from within the country through sharing of health services by co-operative sector, private sector and also by collecting health and medical taxes/fees from affluent population.

(*c*) Integrating National Health Policy with U.N. based and other Health Organisations like the World Health Organisations.

(*d*) Direct government to government co-operation for health finanacing and aids through bilateral arrangements.

(*e*) Aids from International Financing Agencies such as World Banks and other development banks.

Thus as proved by experience, finance required for a well though out and well planned Health Policy can be mobilised from the internal and external sources to support the Nation's own exchequer. Finance can also be made available if a World Health Fund is established by the developed countries in the world by diverting a portion of the money being sent on nuclear and other destructive purposes. Developing countries too can contribute a sizeable amount to this Fund out of their defence expenditure.

Care has to be taken to ensure that the money available is :

(*a*) properly utilised for implementing the health policies and the programmes of the nation and the benefit really reaches the people in each family.

(*b*) not misused, misappropriated or diverted by vested interests by way of money or material or otherwise.

(*c*) equally distributed to rural and urban areas without any favouritism.

(*d*) utilised with all sincerity, seriousness and discipline for the good health of the people.

In the matter of financing of health plans, the call of Director-General of the World Health Organisation will provide a new direction to the individual nation.

> "If health for all is to attained by the year 2000 AD, the next few years are critical for Member States and WHO as a whole. Member States will have to rethink and reshape their priorities and policies and undertake sounder financial planning for their strategies for Health for all, possibly with WHO Collaboration."

Considering the magnitude of the health problems of the people in India, the Government has been giving top priority for Health plans allotting as much fund as possible. However, there is need to integrate the entire medical and health approach and allot sufficient funds to support an integrated National Health Plan providing full health protection to the people of India by the turn of the century. There is also need for dynamism, monitoring, evaluation and auditing of the work done and the money spent and the short-falls should be remedied then and there.

It has to be once again emphasised that carefull and meticulous planning is necessary not only to mobilise the needed funds but also in spending it for implementing the various plans and programmes. Then and then alone, the people will be fully benefited by it.

Human Resource Development in Health Planning

Human resources planning, development and management is a vital factor for the successful implementation of a National Health Policy. There is, therefore, need for meticulous planning of Health manpower from the beginning itself taking into account the exact needs of the society. There should also be plans to develop the potential of the existing manpower resources for the purpose of better utilisation. There should not be any gap between the production of trained health personnel and their utilisation, which if existed in the form of excesses/shortages will bring serious consequences and loss to the nation.

Human resources development has been a neglected aspect in many countries and consequently there have been qualitative and quantitative imbalances in Health manpower. The problem of ill-balanced health manpower is becoming curious year after year. This is evident from the resolution passed recently by the Executive Board of the World Health Organisation in Geneva reading as :

> "While shortage of certain categories of health manpower is still a problem in many countries, an increasing number of member states have an over supply of certain categories of health professional such as Physicians and dentists, leading to their under-utilisation, un-employment and migration to other countries."
>
> The resolution further urged the member countries :
>
> "to reorient education and training of health manpower to respond fully to the local needs and to employ measure urgently, when actual imbalances exist or occur, to adjust the production of health manpower, in order to bring the supply and distribution into line with expected future demand for services, bearing in mind the country's ability to support such services."

The resolution was meant for debate in the 40th World Health Assembly in the context of "Promotion of balanced health manpower development".

The concern of WHO clearly reveals the fact that the problem has world wide significance.

The Conference on "Health Manpower Out of Balance : Conflicts and Prospects" held in Mexico had thrown further light on the problem. The statistics provided in the conference has revealed the frightening situation all over the world. It was stated that while 45,000 physicians are unemployed in Italy, it was 40,000 in India, 23,000 in Spain and 2,500 in Netherlands. The United States estimate an excess of 70,000 physicians in the year 1990. According to 1984 figures, Mexico has about 40,000 unemployed physicians, Bangladeshi 5,000, Pakistan 6,000 and Republic of Korea estimates their surplus at 26,000 by 2000 AD. In developing countries, the situation was very grave even as early as 1972, when they lost about 67,000 physicians by migration and the gain for the developed countries by migration was 1,18,000. In this context, the Mexico Conference as well as WHO has given a world wide alert.

Looking at the picture in India, we find that there are as many as 40,000 physicians surplus and unemployed. But a realistic and need-based look at the health picture of India would only reveal that there are many areas where health personnel are still wanted or in shortage, and there is maldistribution of doctors and if a re-distribution is made in a realistic manner giving due weightage to the rural areas, this surplus may perhaps disappear.

A clear picture emerges from the following demographic profile of Physicians in India published by the World Health Organisation in their journal.

Table 3.1

Demographic Profile of Physicians in India

Year	*No. of medical colleges*	*No. of physicians graduating*
1947	<20	<2,000
1986	>106	>13,000
Year		
	Ratio of population to physicians	
1951	1 : 6,000	
1985	1 : 3,000	
2000A.D	1 : 2,300 projected.	
	No. of physicians unemployed	
1986	40,000	

Another matter of serious national concern is the shortage of nurses and other essential persons in various categories. Although this is a common phenomenon all over the world large problem of migration of Indian nurses and other key professionals to other countries is like adding fuels to the fire to the problems of imbalanced health personnel. According to estimate, the shortage of nurses in India is about 35,000.

According to the studies conducted by the World Health Organisation and various other bodies, the reasons for the imbalanced manpower can be found in the following reasons :

(*a*) excess production of certain categories of medical personnel.

(*b*) under production of another categories of personnel.

(*c*) Improper utilisation, lack of incentives and encouraging environment leading to large scale migration.

(*d*) lack of health manpower planning taking into account the local needs.

The persistent increase in imbalanced manpower in the health field will not only jeopardise the Health policy and programmes of the nation but will also erode the economic base of the country. Some of the consequences may be summarised as under :

(*a*) uncontrolled production of medical professional by spending huge money and their non-utilisation and unemployment after education results in colossal economic waste to the nation. Their migration leads to the loss of money spent on them for education and training.

(*b*) such large scale production and unemployment brings down the standards of medical education and professional status.

(*c*) It retards the achievement of health goals and progress.

There is, therefore, imperative need for urgent action to change the entire situation through short-term and long-term plans implemented by each nation. These programmes should, *inter alia*, aim at the following objectives :

(*a*) Bringing all the Medical Colleges and other Training Institutions on a national grid to have effective control over inflow and outflow of medical personnel.

(*b*) Re-plan the existing distribution of health manpower keeping a balance between the rural and urban areas and employ all the existing surplus physicians for Health programmes of the Nation.

(*c*) Stop starting of new medical colleges, increasing strength in existing medical colleges till a clear picture about the need based requirement is arrived at through meticulous planning and assessment.

(*d*) Introducing new training Institutions to produce needed categories of health personnel like nurses to meet the short-fall and future requirements.

(*e*) Upgrade the medical education and training standards keeping in view the development in other parts and also the professional status of health personnel.

(*f*) Have a Master plan for production and distribution of health manpower with scope for their professional advancement.

The recommendations of the Conference held in Mexico in 1986 will only be a source of inspiration and guidance to the countries in the world where there is an existing or emerging problems of imbalanced Health manpower. The recommendations are :

(*a*) Honouring the internationally agreed upon Health for all concept through massive emphasis on primary health care.

(*b*) Each country should develop health manpower data banks to avoid the current over-production of physicians to the detriment of other more relevant health personnel.

(*c*) Health care and health manpower planning must be realistically based on a country's health budget.

(*d*) Changes in curriculcum content are needed for all health personnel schools in order to provide greater insight and knowledge of the pressing health problems of the region served.

(*e*) Production of certain categories of health manpower should be reduced by limiting the intake into training schools or restricting the numbers who graduate, and surplus manpower should be restrained so as to meet the needs more appropriately.

(*f*) Incentives and disincentives should be introduced to bring about a better re-distribution of health manpower.

(*g*) Some countries may have to postpone opening of new medical colleges or even consider closing existing one.

(*h*) Some countries might find it necessary to impose a compulsory retirement age of their physicians.

In order to make a Nation's health policy and administration more meaningful and useful to the common people in line with their actual needs, there is need for careful health manpower planning, manpower development, distribution and utilisation and then alone the goal of Health-for-all can be achieved in letter and spirit.

Medical Education, Training and Research

The importance of medical and training education and research can be capsuled in a golden saying. "It is in the medical education that the Health plans of a Nation begins and it is in the researches that the health plan survives." As a matter of fact, the medical and training Institutions supported and supplemented by the research organisation are the basic foundation of the health policy of the nation. It is precisely so because of the fact that it is the medical education and training that provides necessary input, infrastructure and manpower to meet the requirement of Health Planners. If there is any error, in the planning for medical and training education or for medical research, that will reflect on the health of the nation. If adequate care is not taken in training the medical and health personnel, that will jeopardise the health programmes of the nation. Similarly excess production of medical and health personnel, or shortage of such personnel or maldistribution of such personnel or inactiveness of such personnel will also erode the basic health policies of a nation.

India can be today proud of having about 16 permanent and reputed Medical Research Institutions and Centres where advanced medical research is being carried out under the guidance of the Indian Council of Medical Research. The areas of research include Family Planning, Nutrition, dreadful diseases like leprosy, TB, Cancer, mental health and other communicable and infectious diseases.

Extensive research is also being done on drugs including indigenous systems of medicines in specialised institutions. Thus it can be seen that we have made much headway in the field of medical research.

However, in order to fully and fruitfully support the Health Policy and Programmes of a nation, it has to be integrated to :

(*a*) Advanced medical research Institutions of the world

(*b*) medical colleges and training centres within the country to enable such Institutions to update their knowledge.

(*c*) national health plans for taking the new knowledge and advance of medical research to solve the health problems of the people.

The Medical Institutions and Research Organisations should be spread all over the country and they should make the medical colleges in the country of high standards. The number of medical colleges should be limited to the needs of the nation. In spite of all the advances, we have made, we are yet to catch momentum in medical research and an important missing element in this field is to put it in the words of our Hon'ble Prime Minister "Perhaps the greatest need today in our medical system is for a much higher dedication. We have to instil this enthusiasm. We have to build it into the system of education and training."

Thus the Medical Colleges, Training Institutions and Research Organisations should be a connecting link to the Health Policy of the Nation.

Hospitals and Treatment Centres

Medical and health services in India have made much headway since Independence. Today we have a large number of hospitals and treatment centres in the country which provides both general and specialised treatment to the people. Apart from the hospitals of the Central and State Governments, there are hospitals managed by Missionaries, hospitals of private nature and public hospitals.

But surprisingly and understandably, most the these well equipped hospitals are in urban areas and cities. And majority of the rural population in India have no easy excess to the specialised hospitals in cities and urban areas. They have to satisfy with what is provided to them at their residential areas. And we know that many of the hospitals in the rural areas are under-funded, under-staffed, under-equipped and over-stretched and there are several rural areas where proper health services are not available. In many cases, people are also not aware of such services within their reach. So much so, in the matter of rural health, we have to go miles to provide them with the facilities available in urban areas. There is need for a fresh look at these matters in order to :

(*a*) re-distribute the available medical services with a balance between rural and urban areas.

(*b*) provide all future approvals for hospital in rural areas till a balanced medical and health service is achieved.

(*c*) modernise all the hospitals and treatment centres in rural areas solving the existing problems of staff, equipment, funds and medicines.

(*d*) establish new hospitals, integrated survey. Education and Treatment centres in rural areas in collaboration with Research Institutions in India and abroad and also with UN Health Agencies like WHO.

So, the Health Policy of the nation should clearly lay down norms for establishing sufficient number of hospitals with equality and justice in rural areas, to maintain high standards and cleanliness in hospitals, to provide efficient and dynamic administration in all hospitals and treatment centres and above all to provide health and medical services to the people with a human touch and missionary zeal.

Drugs and Medicine

The National Health Policy should be necessarily linked to country's drug policy which in turn should produce all the drugs that are necessary for the speedy and result-oriented implementation of the health plans and programmes.

List of drugs : An exhaustive list of drugs and medicines that can be produced/imported into the country should be prepared in collaboration with UNI Aided Health Agencies like WHO and considering such list available in developed countries. These drugs should be, as a matter of policy made available to all the people through established trade channels.

Production/import :Production/import of approved drugs should only be allowed in the country. Import of sub-standard or inferior drugs banned in other countries should not be allowed to come into the country, even for free distribution. The production and distribution of drugs should be linked to the Health Policy of the Nation.

Quality and Standards : There is need for rigid quality control in the production of drugs. There should not be any drugs in India, which are not in conformity with the national standards approved by the Government as part of the National Health Policy. The Specifications and Standards finalised and approved by the Government should be as rigid as that of USSR, so that drugs harmful to the health of the people will circulate the market.

All Medical Practitioners should be brought under the national grid giving them centralised directions on drug policy in order to ensure that drugs are prescribed according to the guidelines in the Health Policy.

Drugs and medicines, as a matter of policy, should be made within the reach of all people in the country irrespective of whether they are in the rural areas of urban centres. All Government and other hospitals in rural areas should have sufficient stock of essential drugs needed for solving the health problems of the common man.

Other Health Agencies and Voluntary Organisations

The Voluntary Organisations, Missionaries, Health and Social Welfare Agencies and other similar bodies which have been playing a notable role in solving the health problems of the people should be brought into the Health Policy. The Health Plans of the nation should not only integrated their activities but also provide incentives and support for making their activities dynamic and result oriented. So, there is a need to bring together all these Agencies, both national and international working in the country, so that it will give a new direction to the health movement in the country. These organisations should be incorporated in the Resources and Infrastructure planning so that it will help better co-ordination.

3. COMPONENTS AND PROGRAMMES

The second and equally important part of a Health Policy is its components and programmes. It is through these components and programmes that the message of good health reaches the people. In order to get clear-cut results, an integrated approach should be taken into the plan so that it will co-ordinate the activities under the different components and programmes. The success of the implementation of the programmes and the amount of benefit that goes to the people would depend upon the sincerity and efficiency with which it is implemented. Each and every health personnel has an active role to play in this regard. What is all the more important and imperative for the successful implementation of the health plans and programmes is public awareness and involvement.

Primary Health Care

Experts has defined health as a state of complete physical, mental and social well being and not merely the absence of disease or infirmity. Every nation should therefore aim at highest attainable standard of health for each individual in the community. The individual will be able to realise the full potential of his life only if he is healthy. So much, so in developing countries in general and in India in particular, where the diseases and ill-health overtakes often the progress of science and technology, the concept of Primary Health Care has great significance. With a broad-based primary health programme, the health services can be made within the reach of all.

The Alma Ata Conference on Primary Health Care organised jointly by the World Health Organisation and the United Nations Children's Fund (UNICEF) in September 1978 has provided solid foundation for establishing Primary Health Care Centres in all countries. The Conference had made 22 specific Recommendations while finalising a ten-point Programme. In the Conference, Public Health Care was defined "as essential Health Care based on specifically sound and socially acceptable methods and technology made universally accessible to individuals and families in their community through their full participation and at cost the community and the country can afford to maintain at every stage of their development in the spirit of self-reliance and self-determination."

Primary Health Care include atleast health education, the promotion of proper nutrition, adequate safe drinking water, proper sanitation, maternal and child health care, Family Planning and Welfare, immunisation programme, prevention and control of endemic diseases, treatment of all common ailments and injuries, and the supply of essential drugs.

The achievement of the goal of the Primary Health Care as recommended by the World Health Organisation would mean :

(*a*) priority allocation of budgetary resources to Public Health Care.

(*b*) better distribution of existing resources.

(*c*) Improved management and administration of planning, implementing, monitoring and evaluating, health programmes to remedy the short-falls, to measure the health progress and to make Health Services within the reach of all.

The success of the system would depend upon the self effort, hard work and professional efficiency of all the people concerned, availability of sufficient drugs and infrastructure and the co-operation and involvement of the people. There is need for a Primary Health Care Centre in each village. So it can be seen that the Health Policy and Administration can be made effective and result-oriented at grassroot level only through the specially designed administrative strategy aimed at the efficient and people-oriented functioning of the Public Health Care Centres. This should be a primary component in the National Health Policy.

Health Education

Health education is a very important sub-component of the Primary Health Care. The sole objective of Health Education can be termed as making the individual and the community 'health conscious'. In this context, the words of Mahatma Gandhi reading as "we must first know enough of our body, our own house, our village and its surroundings, the crops that grow there and its history before going on to anything else. General knowledge broad-based on this primary knowledge alone can enrich our life," have great relevance today. Health education is preventive and promotive effort to drive away the illiteracy, superstition, ignorance and misunderstanding of the people and bring them close to the correct knowledge about the preventive, curative and rehabilitative aspects of various diseases.

The Government of India recognising the importance of Health education established the Central Health Education Bureau within the Directorate General of Health Services in 1956, which have been playing a notable role to achieve the objectives of such a programme. However, health education has still to move into the social, and economic aspects of rural life and the main hurdle appears to be non-co-operation of people in line with the requirement. Keeping in view the future needs, the Seventh Plan has given special attention to this aspect of Health. In order to achieve better results, there is need to adopt :

(*a*) the guidelines provided by International Health Organisations.

(*b*) a method to develop sufficient manpower and infra-structure resources.

(*c*) each family as a basic unit.

(*d*) Health education as a subject in all educational Institutions.

(*e*) modern methods to give maximum publicity and create an awareness among the people to enable effective and efficient involvement of the individual and the community.

It is, therefore, necessary that the Health Policy of the nation should give due weightage to the above aspects of Health Education and it should be included as an activity in the Primary Health Care centres.

Promotion of Nutrition

Food is the prime necessity of health and availability of safe and nutritious food can prevent and control many diseases. The present nutritional status of the under-privileged sections of people is far below. There is necessity to increase it above the present level so.

that poor people can be saved from malnutrition, and the consequences of malnutrition are many and varied. According to the former Director-General of ICMR (1980). Infant and child mortality rates are excessively high, although variable with an infant mortality rates of 55 per 1000 live births in Kerala and 160 per 1000 live births in the eastern parts of U.P. with a national average of around 130. A third of all deaths that occur in the country are among children below the age of four. It is the young and the poor that suffer most from the effects of malnutrition and under-development. Nutritional anaemia and Blinding are widely prevalent. In this context, the following activities will help a lot in this direction.

(*a*) Control of food adulteration and making safe food supply within the reach of all.

(*b*) Making people aware of the nutritious food items and encouraging cultivation of the same.

(*c*) Making diet therapy popular way of life in rural areas.

(*d*) Changing life styles and food habits for good health.

Health education has to move into the rural and under-developed areas as part of Health Policy and effective administrative strategies should be adopted to make it effective so that the majority poor and under-nourished people will be benefited.

Safe Water Supply and Sanitation

According to WHO estimates, 25 million people in developing countries die from water-born diseases every year. In India 80 per cent of the diseases are water-born. Safe water supply and sanitation has received world-wide attention and the United Nations has declared "International Drinking Water Decade 1981-1991." Describing the large amount of impurities in the water, it was reported that if the world's water was represented in one gallon bottle, the quality of fresh water would be only two teaspoons. Contaminated water is a major problem today and this can be averted to a great extent by providing proper sanitary facilities in rural areas. Again, education of people in this regard is a very important factor as without active public involvement and co-operation, nothing tangible can be achieved in this direction.

Health Polity and Administration should therefore give top most priority to providing safe water supply so that it will help to prevent major water-born diseases and death of millions of children and poor people.

Maternal and Child Health Care

In order to prevent maternal mortality, infant mortality and child deaths and to bring down their rate below or at the level of developed countries, special attention has to be given to this aspect of health. This would mean special programmes for the health care of the pregnant women, improved, timely and better maternal facilities and child care, family planning and welfare and immunisation of children. If there is an administrative strategy to provide improved maternity and child health care, this service can be integrated with the Primary Health Centres so that the majority of the rural people will be able to avail the facility at lesser cost/no cost and without much difficulty. All the pregnant women in the rural areas should be brought under the scheme and similarly all children should be immunised and saved from the major killers like measles, diphtheria, whooping cough, tetanus, polio and tuberculosis. Millions of children fall victims of these diseases and die every year in developing countries.

Population control and family welfare is a very important factor in the Health Policy of a nation. The present population of 100 crores being very high, it is necessary to promote Family Planning Programme on a two child basis and this programme can be effectively implemented through the Primary Health Centres. The administrative strategies adopted should be powerful enough to influence the people and take them into confidence so that successful results can be obtained. Rigid control of population growth is an essential factor for the successful implementation of a Health Policy. Having averted new births of 68.25 million since inception of Family Planning Programme, the nation is now on the move to achieve a crude birth rate of 21, crude death rate of 9, and infant mortality rate below 60 to 1000 children. It is possible to achieve the goal if our Health Plans are integrated with that of the International Health Agencies. A Political will and support and active involvement of people are also indispensable.

Prevention and Control of Endemic Diseases

It is possible to prevent, control and completely eradicated dreaded diseases, like Leprosy, Tuberculosis, Cancer, Malaria and such other diseases by a three cornered method as below :

(*a*) Education to remove superstition, social stigma and prejudices about the disease.

(*b*) Early detection and treatment of diseases to arrest further growth and cure the disease, and also rehabilitation programmes wherever necessary.

(*c*) Integrating the programmes with International Health Organisations.

Although, National Eradication Programme exists for Leprocy, Sexually Transmitted Diseases, tuberculosis, Malaria, Blindness, Goitre, Diarrhoea, etc., we have not been able to achieve the required results for a variety of reasons. The Programme have to be further strengthened with full public support and Survey, Education and Treatment, supported by necessary trained manpower and drugs should be established within the Public Health Care Unit in each village. It is felt that we will be able to get better results in this way. The work done by International Voluntary Agencies and Organisations within India in eradicating these diseases should be fully encouraged and their activities should also be made part of the National Eradication Programme.

Treatment for Common Ailments and Injuries

The Primary Health Care Centre should have all facility, trained personnel, equipment, drugs and other services required for the prompt treatment of all common ailments in rural areas and also injuries etc., so that rural people need not have to go far for receive treatment for such ailments and accidents.

Essential Drugs

As a matter of policy, all essential and needed drugs should be made available in the Primary Health Care Centres so that it will help timely treatment of poor people averting complication of diseases and death. This will also prevent death due to non-availability of essential drugs in rural areas. Proper administrative strategies should be developed in order to make available these drugs in time, store them properly and distribute the same without error or diversion to other areas by vested interests.

Public Health Administration

There is need for a National Organisational set up for all Primary Health Care Centres. All the Primary Health Centres in the country should be connected to the National grid through a properly developed administrative system. This will help a lot for better co-ordination and to create organisational effectiveness in providing health services to the people.

A National Health Policy for Children and Youth

Although the Primary Health Care Centre will have a general coverage of the health of the children and youth, there is need for a comprehensive National Policy in the Health Plans specially for children and youth for the following reasons:

(a) children and youth constitute about 40 per cent of the Nations population and without giving proper health protection to them, they will not able to grow in the right way to work for the nation building.

(b) Majority of the children, particularly in rural areas are exposed to malnutrition and dangerous diseases, and if they are allowed to grow in that way, that will bring a bad image for the nation, apart from losing their productive capacity.

So much, without a healthy, disciplined, educated and hard working youth, there will be no future for the nation. There is therefore need for a special policy within the National Health Policy for children and youth, which will *inter alia* aim at :

(*i*) comprehensive child health programme through the Primary Health Care Centres.

(*ii*) special nutritional programmes for children both in schools and other Institutions and also for children who are not covered by education.

(*iii*) Improving the school health programme to ensure that each and every child is benefited by such programmes.

(*iv*) special programmes for poor, destitute and handicapped children to mould them as good citizens.

(*v*) Broad-based physical education, training, sports and recreational activities to cover all children.

(*vi*) Programmes to cultivate good life styles in children keeping them away from habits like smoking, alcohol and drug even before attaining maturity.

The above-mentioned objectives should be made part and parcel of the National Health Policy so that all the child population of India will grow as healthy citizens to create a better future.

The National Health Policy should therefore give special attention to the Children and Youth so that their energy can be properly converted into national wealth. Apart from immunisation, education and treatment programmes, there is need for special programmes to provide nutritional services and physical health of the children and youth in rural areas.

Control of Smoking, Alcohol and Drug

The Medical Science has since fully recognised the grave dangers of the life styles supported by Smoking, Alcohol and drugs. In view of the rigid policy and control of these habits in developed countries, it is moving towards the developing countries in a big way, knowingly and unknowingly, eroding the health of the people, particularly the youth. The disappointments and depression prevailing among the people, make India a fertile land for these habits. Today millions of people, particularly, the young are victims of the habits of smoking, alcohol and drugs, and the nation is losing their energy and health.

In the case of smoking, alcohol and drug addiction, there is need for an international code as these items are moving through an international channel. The international code designed and aimed at controlling these habits fully should be incorporated in the National Health Policy, World Health Organisations and several other Conferences of experts have been studying the health problems arising out of these habits, and there are a number of effective recommendations and guidelines to the developed and developing nations. Some of the recommendations are making non-smoking a social habit, prohibition of all forms of tobacco promotion, discouraging tobacco exports, eradication of smoking in industries, and work places, bringing down the proportion of harmful elements like tar, nicotine, and carbon monoxide and banning smoking in public places. Research has since proved that use of tobacco in any form would mean a greater risk of getting cancer or other life threatening diseases.

Similarly, a number of Recommendations and guidelines exist in respect of alcohol and drugs. The drug addiction and alcohol has become a great menace to every nation in the world. There is, therefore, urgent need to recognise this in the National Health Policy and chalk out effective methods to control and eliminate these habits. The following points are important in this connection.

(*a*) Banning sale and use of cigarettes and alcohol to all those who are aged below 25.

(*b*) Legislation to control and limit the production and sale of these items to general public.

(*c*) Right rules to control the flow of drugs into the country and also the give deterrent punishment to those who indulge in drug transactions at national and international levels.

(*d*) Hospitals and Counsel centres for alcohol and drug addicts.

(*e*) Integrating national programmes on these matters with International health Agencies and Organisations.

(*f*) Working in co-operation with other countries in implementing the programmes aimed at controlling these habits.

(*g*) Parental care and control to prevent children and youth from entering into these habits.

(*h*) Wide publicity in all places bringing out the dangers of these habits.

In view of the magnitude of the problem, the Health Policy should frame special programmes to control these habits among the people of our country.

Rehabilitation of the Handicapped

In the world today about 450 million people are estimated to be handicapped. The problem of handicapped today is a major socio-economic problem in the world, particularly for developing countries. The causes of the handicap are listed as congenital disturbances, communicable diseases, non-communicable diseases, malnutrition, trauma and injury, alcohol and drug addiction and functional and psychological defects. Experts say 50 per cent of the disability can be prevented. Paradoxically, 80 per cent of the handicapped are in the developing countries, while 90 per cent of the total resources for the handicapped are spent in developed nations. The fact that most of the handicapped persons in the developing countries are depending population, and a good percentage of them are thrown out as discarded human beings. This situation is actually a great socio-economic problem to the nation.

There is, therefore, need to prevent disability as far as possible and to make the disabled partners of national development and integrate them with Society as normal citizens. The disabled children alone is about 140 million in the world, 80 per cent of whom live in the developing countries. The situation, therefore, calls for strengthening the national capabilities for prevention of impairment, and disability particularly through immunisation of children, special programmes for safe food and nutrition, prevention of accidents, safe water supply and provision for improved maternal and child health services, and improvement in the psycho-social environment in which the individual is living. The National Health Policy should therefore take into account, the serious socio-economic problems posed by the health problem of the handicapped and chalk out programmes to find a lasting solution to the problem.

Specialised Hospitals and Medical Centres

Indian can be proud of having specialised and reputed Medical Centres, both in the government and private sector, in important cities. However, at present, this is a restricted health service to certain categories of people living in the cities and urban areas. Majority poor people have no access to such services, since it is not affordable to them.

There is therefore need to increase such facilities in different parts of the country, particularly in rural areas determining a certain number of population to each such specialised hospitals and centres, so that such advanced medical and health facilities would be available to all the people of India with equality and justice. The Health Policy of a Nation should have programmes aimed at these objectives.

In a nutshell, Health Plans and Programmes should be based on meticulous planning and its implementation would be monitored, reviewed and improved periodically in order to give full benefit to the people.

4. ADMINISTRATIVE POLICY AND STRATEGIES

The successful implementation of the Health Policy would depend upon the Administrative policies and strategies adopted for its implementation. The first requirement of a comprehensive administrative policy would be 'uniformity' of methods, procedure and strategies adopted in implementing the Plans and Programmes throughout the country. This is essential to ensure 'equality and justice' at the TERMINATING point. Secondly, there is need for 'dynamism and quickness' in the administration of health services and this can be achieved only if the Health Policy keeps away the 'bureaucratic procedure and make it independent with sufficient delegation of powers and authority at different levels. This will not only help to implement time bound programmes within the time schedule with maximum benefits to the people. So much so, the Administrative machinery behind the National Health Policy should move with rapid speed to catch the momentum of the advance of Science, medicine and health technology.

Objectives

The general Objectives of an Administrative policy can be summarised as under :

(*a*) Planning, Training, Developing, distributing and controlling the utilisation of human resources on a need-based basis to make the health services within the reach of all.

(*b*) budget planning, controlling funds utilisation and expenditure to ensure that the earmarked amount is fully and fruitfully spend for the benefit of the people.

(*c*) providing necessary infrastructure for the Health services.

(*d*) Co-ordinating with Government and various other Organisations on all matters connected with health services.

(*e*) Monitoring, evaluating the short-term and long-term plans, to measure the progress made through Health indicators and to remedy the short falls and improve services.

(*f*) Other administrative services required for speedy and result-oriented implementation of the Health Programmes.

Methods and Procedures

Methods and Procedures which will ensure timely availability of medicine, establishing infrastructural facilities, proper utilisation of human resources and flow of health and medical technology etc. should be firmed up and introduced under the Administrative policy. Administrative machinery should ensure that the ingredients are available to all the Health Centres in time and without much difficulties.

Essential Qualities

In order to give a human touch to the health services, there is need for qualities like 'Social Consciousness', self-sacrificing mentality, self-discipline and sincerity, and above all a dynamic and determined approach, in the Administrative set up so that the health services will be able to mould a better and healthy society.

Organisational Set up

Central Health and Medical Authority : In order to get expected results out of the Health Plans and Programmes, there should be a nationally linked Health services. For this purpose, there should at the National level, a Central Health and Medical Authority under which there will be three divisions *viz.* the Health Authority, Medical Authority and Research Authority.

Health Authority : Health Authority is responsible to control and manage the Public Health Care and National Control Programmes up to the village level through the States/ District and Taluk level offices and centres.

Medical Authority : Under the Medical authority, there will be a full-fledged directorate for planning, training, developing, and controlling the utilisation of human resources for health services. They will also be responsible to keep the high standards of Medical profession and to decide the compensation payable to Health and Medical personnel. The medical Authority will also be the controlling authority for production/import, distribution, quality control and other matters related to drugs and medicine through a well planned Drug Policy..

Research Authority : The third and equally important division will be a Research authority which will have over-all control of Research activities in the country. This body will also co-ordinate with International Medical and Health Research Organisations in order to give a international outlook and standard to our research activities. As a matter of policy, we should plan our own researches in large scale, apart from adopting what is coming in from outside world. For this purpose, the research activities of all the Central, State and Private Medical Research Institutions should be brought under one authority, who will provide common guidelines and control to these Institutions. There is need for a fresh look at the Medical and Health Research in India so that it can move forward in line with the development elsewhere in the world.

Computerised Control

As a matter of administrative strategy, the entire Medical and Health activities in the country should be controlled through Computerised information, which in turn will increase the efficiency and effectiveness of the administrative system.

Audit

There is also need for audit of work, audit of achievements, audit of expenditure, audit of manpower utilisation etc. at various levels in the country and finally by the Central Medical and Health authority, which will help to attain perfection and better control of the activities in the country.

General Management

General management of health services at all levels should be modernised and humanised. Leadership qualities, training and development programmes, refresher courses, better service conditions, supervisory effectiveness, systems and controls at various levels etc. should be made part and parcel of the Health and Medical Services in the country. There is also need for over-all organisational effectiveness in the Health services so that it will become administratively efficient, effective and result-oriented.

Involvement of Public and Other Agencies

The Administrative policy behind the Health Plans should bring the public and voluntary and health organisations close to the implementation process. This is necessary not only to understand the health problems better but also to inject a sense of urgency, enthusiasm and dynamism in the activities which is concerned with the health of people.

5. SUGGESTIONS AND RECOMMENDATIONS

Summarising the discussions in the foregoing paragraphs the following suggestions are offered :

(*a*) Establishing village level Primary Health Care Centres integrating all health activities making each family a unit.

(*b*) Priority financial allocation and mobilising international Aids.

(*c*) Meticulous human resources planning; development and need-based utilisation.

(*d*) Integrating the health services with International Organisations.

(*e*) Use of advanced medical science and health technology in rural areas.

(*f*) Rigid control of production, import, quality and distribution of drugs in line with the requirements of the people.

(*g*) Active involvement of public and voluntary organisations.

(*h*) Monitoring, evaluation, and Audit of health activities at National level.

(*i*) Creation of world health fund for the benefit of developing countries.

(*j*) Broad-based administrative policies and strategies.

The above suggestions are arrived at in the context of India and developing countries.

6. CONCLUSION

In conclusion it can be seen that the goal of Health all can be achieved only by :

(*a*) establishing full-fledged Primary Health Care Centres in all villages to look after all the health and medical needs of the people taking each family as an unit, for the purpose of survey, education, treatment and rehabilitation, as the case may be.

(*b*) Reorganising the present health and medical services in order to make it people-oriented, need based and result-oriented.

(*c*) The ultimate control of all the Health services will be exercised at the Central authority level, from where needed administrative delegation of authority will be given downwards till the village level to supervise, manage, monitor, audit and control the entire Health and Medical activities. There will be periodic evaluation of the services rendered by the Central authority.

(*d*) Giving more importance to research, professional ethics and standards and working with dedication in line with the latest development.

Above all, what is necessary and imperative is the full co-operation and participation of public and voluntary organisations, timely availability of drugs and trained health personnel on a need-based basis.

4

Policy-Making for Health Care Administration

A. Nature and Jurisdiction

Nature and Significance

Policies may be thought of as the main system which provides the framework for the accomplishment of intended objectives. Formulation of policies involves making explicit, the various assumptions which are made with respect to the basic premises and the priorities of needs and allocating the finances accordingly. Besides, policies are intended to spell out the parameters in the context of which organisational decisions are to be made. Policy is very essential in administration, for it gives a concrete shape to the political and social objectives which the government lays down in the form of laws, rules, regulations, etc. Davis states : "A policy is basically a statement either expressed or implied of those principles and rules that are set up by executive leadership as guides and constraints for the organisation's thought and action. Its principal purpose is to enable executive leadership to relate properly the organisation's work to its objectives."

Policies may be looked upon as general guides to action. They may be verbal, written or implied. They set the overall boundaries for action by individuals or groups in an organisational setting. They indicate the framework within which executives may make decisions for the performance of organisational action. According to Ishwar Dayal,

> Policy prescribes the aims, the objectives, the targets that would be used to achieve the objectives. Operationally, the policy statement, in this sense, must specify the expected results, the measures for achieving them and mechanism or method with which the results are expected to be achieved... Policy formulation refers to that aspect of administration which is concerned with defining the objective and determining the choice of action. Decision-making refers to the process by which this policy is determined.[1]

It may be mentioned that public policies may be written or unwritten, explicit or implicit. Important policies of the government are often clearly expressed in a written form. Public policies are mostly formally adopted by governmental authorities. There are, however, public policies embodied only in a set of practices, conventions and precedents.

According to Koontz and O'Donnell, written policy is preferable, as : "It builds on proved decisions of the past conserving executive energy of new decisions : it creates an atmosphere in which individual actions may be taken with confidence; it speeds administration by reducing repetition to routine; it supports consistency of endeavour across a large group through the years; it stabilises the enterprise; it frees the top management so that more creative considerations can be given to the problem of today and the new programme of tomorrow."

In order to appreciate policy-formulating process in government including health administration, it is desirable to acquaint ourselves with Dror's optimal model of policy.

"Dror's model consists of three stages :

1. *Meta-policy making*. This involves :
   (a) Processing relevant values,
   (b Processing facts or realities,
   (c) Actual problems, and
   (d) the resources.
2. *Policy-making itself*. This involves,
   (a) Sub-allocating resources,
   (b) Deciding operational goals and targets,
   (c) Examining related values through cost-benefit analysis.
3. *Post-Policy making*. It is a process of analysis and examination from feedack to make the necessary changes in execution as well as future policy formulation."

Essentials of Public Policy Formulation

Policy formulation in India at the Union and State levels, has improved considerably since independence. Governments have developed a good infrastructure for the policy-formulation. We can still improve upon policy-making in Governments at various levels if we keep the following facts and suggestions in mind.

1. *Need for an Effective Management Information System (MIS)*. At present, the availability of data is quite sufficient at Union and State levels. There has grown a large number of statistical and other organisations which generate plenty of information on the various aspects of the policy to be formulated. However, the information system has not been designed scientifically. In most of the cases, desired information is not available while the information not required is available. Therefore, there is a need for the departments of the governments to

design MIS according to their requirements. This would go a long way in the formulation of effective policy.

2. *Need for consultative and advisory bodies.* There are a large number of consultative and advisory bodies in various departments of the Government of India (530) Advisory Committees). There has been a haphazard growth of these bodies. There is a need to examine the functioning of these bodies so that they can play an effective role in policy-making.

3. *Need of co-ordination among inter-related department.* At present there is no effective machinery which can bring coordination among the related departments. For example, in order to frame effective social policy, there is a need of coordination among all the social services departments e.g. Health Education, Social Welfare etc.

4. *Need for induction of modern management methods.* Governmental recognition and induction of modern management tools in the policy-formulating apparatus is necessary to ensure the reliability and feasibility of the proposed policy. We may not use these techniques blindly but should evaluate the usefulness of the sophistication of these tools and utilise whatever is relevant and possible.

5. *Need for training the personnel.* We must take urgent and right steps for training the necessary manpower in the art and science of policy-making. We must make conscious effort to fit the experts and administrators to the task of policy formulation so that they may not depend on the usual hit and miss method of administration.

6. *Need for vision on the part of the policy-makers.* Policy-makers must not only understand their problems but also know how their work fits in the overall scheme of things. This requires wider knowledge and wide vision on the part of the personnel engaged in policy-making. The policy-maker must know how his policy will affect the total development. He must know the capability of the machinery that is available to implement the policy. Thus the administrator has to be trained to fit into the new role of the policy-maker.

7. *Need for participation of beneficiaries.* At present, there is not much involvement of the beneficiaries in the formulation and implementation of the policies. Community Development Programmes and Panchayati Raj institutions have not made much headway because of the lack of involvement of the people. Consultation with and involvement of the beneficiaries of the programme is essential and needs to be built consciously into the policy-formulation and implementation machinery.

8. *Need to monitor implementation of policies.* It is often said that the policies, programmes and even projects of the government are well conceived but a determined implementation of all these by the administration is conspicuously lacking. The country faces the crisis of 'policy implementation, and not so much

its 'policy-formulation.' Hence the key to achieve the pre-determined objective may lie in the successful implementation of the projects. The problems of implementation arise out of weakness at all levels of the implementing machinery starting with the government departments at the Centre and the States, through to the various non-secretarial organisations, autonomous corporation, boards and other authorities down to the organisations, in the field at the project, district or village level. Government in the recent past has shown a desire to solve the problems of implementation. This requires a continuous and consistent interest of the policy-makers to see that the policies framed are properly implemented. If we examine the administrative machinery of the Union and State Governments, we find a number of weaknesses, e.g.,

(a) Non-existence of action programmes

(b) Absence of well designed monitoring and evaluation system

(c) Lack of dedicated and capable administrative leadership

(d) Defective organisational structures

(e) Non-existence of state level committees to watch implementation.

Definition of Health Policy

The aim of health policy is to secure a fundamental change in health status of the people to help break the circle of poverty encircling the masses in the developing world and liberate the population to secure the change that they have chosen and in which they participate. It includes the decisions on medical education, health facilities , health coverage, medical research, choice of systems of medicine etc. It also includes the decision as regards the relative role of the government, the private and voluntary agencies in the promotion of health care. The health policy must be made with relevance to the time dimension. It can be a long-term policy, e.g. provision of comprehensive health care to all by the year 2000, or a medium-term e.g., providing elementary care to all by 1990, or immediate i.e., covering half the population by 1985 and so on. In the developing world, there is no comprehensive health policy encompassing all the components affecting the health status of the people. There are piece-meal policy decisions about a particular aspect of health care administration. Besides, there is no continuity in the formulation of health policy because of the change of political leadership. Ministry of Health and Family Welfare and the State Health Departments must come out with a Health Policy which can provide a decent health care to all especially the people living in rural areas, urban slums and the tribal areas.

The objectives of the policy of health care delivery system are described under :

1. To provide universal coverage and enable the whole population to have access to the type of services best suited to their state of health, richness or disablement.

2. To provide comprehensive, preventive, curative and rehabilitative health services for whoever requires them, without financial or other bars and making the best possible use of the available scientific and technological knowledge.

3. To reduce the cost of treatment, giving priority to primary care and services of a preventive and ambulatory type and reserving hospital treatment for those who need it. The hospital standard should correspond to the average standard of living of the population covered.

4. To decentralise health care through a system of levels of care designed so that each person enters the system through the level best equipped to provide the form of treatment most suited to his individual needs and that all services, from, the primary up to the specialised level, are accessible to whoever needs them through an information and referral system.

5 To organise the "health team," composed of professional, technical and auxiliary staff in various discipline who assume responsibility for the health of the community, acting individually at different levels but with their activities coordinated through an effective system of communication and supervision.

Relationship Between Policy Making and Planning

Planning and policy-making are inter-related. Policy determines the principle for action and planning provides the instrument for the application of policy and review. Policy decisions are needed in the planning process and in defining its goals and limitations (Fig. 4.1). Therefore, planners who ignore the policy only jeopardize the good results of their endeavours. On the other hand a planning process has various possible feedback effects on policy. For example :

(a) it requires explicit policy statements, thus bringing certain subjects to the political arena;

(b) it should reflect the rationale of the policies, show how they can be implemented, and indicate their financial and other implications;

(c) it provides the policy-making with instruments for dialogue, coordination, mobilisation of resources; and continuity of action;

(d) its impact on the national situation should influence future policy-making.

The Executive Board of WHO has stated (Health for All, Series No. 2, p.14) :

"National policies, strategies and plans of action form a continuum and there are no sharp dividing lines between them. . .

"A national health policy is an expression of goals for improving the health situation, the priorities among those goals, and the main directions for attaining them. A national strategy, which should be based on the national health policy, includes the broad lines of action required in all sectors involved to give effect to that policy. A national plan of action is a broad inter-sectoral master plan for attaining the national health goals through implementations of this strategy. It indicates what has to be done, who has to do it, during what time frame and with what resources. It is a framework leading to more detailed programming, budgeting, implementation and evaluation."

RELATIONSHIPS BETWEEN POLICY AND PLAN

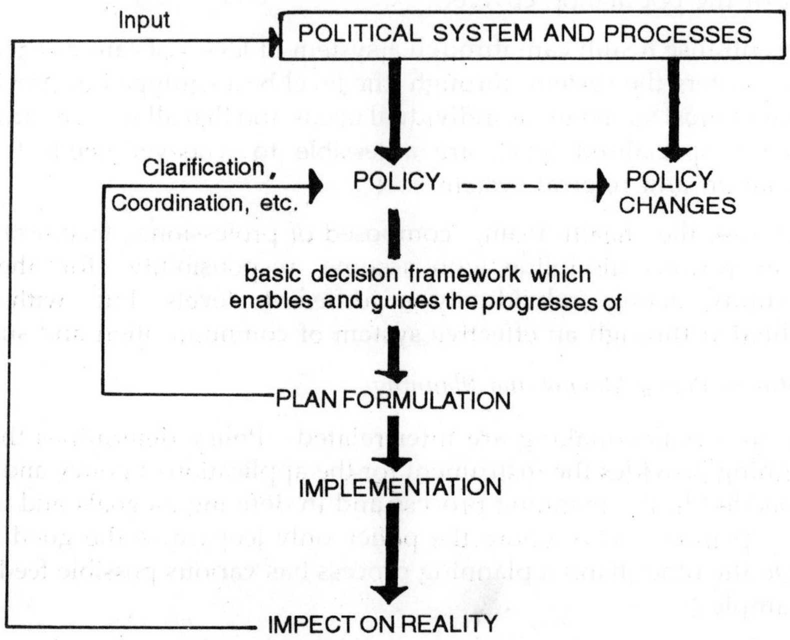

Fig. 4.1

Source: WHO Chronicle, Vol. 31, No. 11.

Relationship Between Policy-Making and Decision-Making

Policy-making and planning involve decisions. Decision-making is the core of policy formulation and planning. Man has been performing the act of taking decisions ever since he became a social animal but a scientific study of these actions is of a very recent origin. During World War II, some studies led to the theory of decisions. Todays, the process of decision-making has become the essence of any productive activity. It is an act of intelligence, will and precision. B. Governay suggests that there are a minimum of four elements which when put together result in a decision :

(a) There must be choice.

(b) The choice must be conscious.

(c) The choice must be oriented by various purposes.

(d) The choice must lead to an action.

It is essential to understand the meaning and art of decision-making to formulate scientific and sound health policies. Webster's dictionary defines *decision-making* as 'the art of determining in one's own mind upon an opinion or courses of actions.' According to W. Brooke Groves, "Decision-making is the selection from two or more reasonable possibilities of a course that will, at the time and under the circumstances, provide the suitable solution of the problem at hand."

It is essential for the policy-makers to keep in mind the five steps mentioned below while taking decisions.

1. *Problem identification or recognition of the existence of a problem or problems.*

In this step, the decision-maker must separate the relevant from the irrelevant; the material from the immaterial: the important from the unimportant based upon clear thinking and open-mindedness. The old proverb that "a problem defined is a problem half-solved" is more than true in this situation.

2. *Problem analysis or determining the What, Why, When, Where, How and Who of a problem.*

It involves classification, analysis and evaluation of data.

3. *Determining the possible alternatives or structuring of resources to solve problems.*

This is a difficult step in decision-making. The decision-maker should keep in mind all logical solutions to the problem and not only those which tend to share his preconceived or pet solutions.

4. *Evaluate the impact of alternatives or forecasting to the impact of alternative if implemented.*

The decision-maker now takes into account each alternative solution to the problem and weighs it in terms of the parameters within which the decision must be made. In effect, the policy-maker is here forecasting the impact of certain alternatives if it is implemented. The impact may be analysed for :

Suitability—Will it solve the problem completely or partially, permanently or temporarily?

Feasibility—Will it work? How much will it cost? Can we afford it?

Acceptability—Is it acceptable to those involved and responsible?

5. *Selection of an alternative or commitment of resources to a course of action.*

This is the final stage of the decision-making process. All the alternatives except the one chosen are cut off. That decision may be adopted which would give the greatest results with the least effort. In other words we accept that course of action which would give highest ratio between the expected gains and the anticipated risk.

The best approach to make decisions is the *Integrative Approach* which combines the rational and humanistic, the economic and social, authoritarian and the autonomous in such a way that all members of the work group feel involved. This approach is most successful when decisions are made by those who do the work at the scene of action rather than by those occupying an executive office, a long way from the firing line. Rational, ethical, economic and social considerations must be considered concurrently at the limit of decision-making.

Thus we see that decision-making is an important constituent of the process of policy-making and planning as the decisions weave individual choices into a web of relationships which constitute a policy. According to Herbert A. Simon, decision-making comprises three principal phases : (i) finding occasions for making a decision; (ii) finding possible courses of action ; and (iii) choosing among courses of action. The first phase has been described as *intelligence* activity, second phase as *design* activity, and the third phase as *choice* activity. This analysis of the process of decision-making has special reference for the policy-makers and planners in the Government as they are to ensure that the policies based on such decisions are not only correct and just but must also appear to be correct and just to the people at large.

Jurisdiction of Policy-Making

The first important question arises about the jurisdiction of policy-making. Let us take the case of India. The Constitution of India has established a federal set-up in India.

The three lists are enumerated in the VII Schedule of the Indian Constitution as List-I (Union List), List-II (State list) and List III (Concurrent List). The Parliament alone has the prerogative to legislate in respect of subjects in List-I. State legislatures have the exclusive right except under certain conditions, to make laws regarding matters in List II and in regard to List-III Parliament and legislatures of the States both may make laws, the functions of the States being restricted within the framework of functions assumed by the Centre. Further, all the residuary powers of legislation are vested in Parliament that is, Parliament has the exclusive powers to legislate on any matter not enumerated in the Concurrent List or State List. Parliamentary legislation on a subject in the State List is permissible under Articlea 249, 250 and 252.

Under Article 249, if the Council of States, declares by two-thirds majority vote that it is necessary or expedient in the national interest that Parliament should make laws in respect of matters enumerated in the State List, Parliament can legislate on the matter, subject to the limitation that the law so made, remains in operation during the period when the resolution of the Council of States remains in force; this period cannot exceed one year on each occasion, although it is permissible to extend its operation year by year by successive resolutions. After a lapse of six months from the termination of operation of such a resolution the Parliamentary Law so passed will cease to be in force.

Under Article 250 of the Constitution, Parliament can legislate on any subject in the State List for the whole or any part of India while a proclamation of Emergency is in operation, the maximum operational period for such law being the period for which the emergency lasts and six months beyond.

A third type of parliamentary legislation on subjects included in the State List is provided for under Article 252. If the legislatures of two or more States pass a resolution suggesting parliamentary legislation on any matter included in the State List, then it is lawful for Parliament to make laws regulating that matter and such laws can be extended to any other State as and when the legislature of that State passes a resolution to the same effect; an amendment or repeal of such a law can be done only by Parliament, the initiative for promoting legislation of this kind for its amendment or repeal has, however been left in the hands of the State, the intention being that when the conditions necessitating such law cease to exist or become modified, it should be possible for the States to ask for appropriate action and for Parliament to carry out the necessary legislative changes.

Besides, Articles 256, 257, 339(2), 350 A, 353(a) and 360(3) empower the Union to give directions to the States for policy-formulation.

It is not easy to determine in certain cases whether the functions implies under specific items in each List have a direct or indirect bearing on health. We can show the items as direct when it forms a clear-cut health functions and indirect when it influences the promotion of health indirectly.

The items bearing direct or indirect relationship with health under the three Lists are listed as follows:

	Direct		*Indirect*
UNION LIST			
20.	Pilgrimage to places outside India (Health functions form the most important part).	24.	Shipping and navigation on inland water-ways, declared by Parliament by Law to be national watereways as regards mechani-cally propelled vessels; the rule of the roads on such waterways.
28.	Post quarantine, including hospitals connected therewith; Seamen's and marine hospitals.		(In so far as regulation of health requirements and control of infection on such vessels are concerned. A similar relation to health exists in other items.
66.	Coordination and determination of standards in institutions for higher education or research and scientific technical institutions.	27.	Ports declared by or under law made by Parliament or existing law to be major ports, including their delimitation, and the constitution and powers of port authorities therein.
81	Inter-State migration; Inter-State quarantine.	29.	Airways, aircraft and air navigation; provision of aerodromes; provision for aeronautical education and training and regulation of such education and training provided by States and other agencies; regulation and organisation or air traffic and of aerodromes.
		30.	Carriage of passengers and goods by railways, sea or by air or by national waterways in mechanically propelled vessels.

(Contd.)

Direct		*Indirect*	
		51.	Establishment of standards of quality for goods to be exported out of India or transported from one State to another (e.g. control of adulteration).
		52.	Industries, the control of which by the Union is declared by Parliament by law to be expedient in the public interest (e.g. occupational health).
		55.	Regulation of labour and safety in mines and oil-fields.
		56.	Regulation and development of inter-state rivers and river-valleys to the extent to which such regulation and development under the control of the Union is declared by Parliament by law to be expedient in the public interest.
		65.	Union institutions for : (a) Professional, vocational or technical training, including the training of police officers ; or (b) The promotion of special studies or research.
STATE LIST			
6.	Public health and sanitation; hospitals and dispensaries.	5.	Local Government that is, the constitution and powers of municipal corporation, improvement trusts, district boards, mining settlement authorities for the purpose of local self-government of village administration.
7.	Pilgrimage, other than pilgrimages to places outside India.	8.	Intoxicating liquors, that is, the production, manufacture, possession, transport purchase and sale of intoxicating liquors.
		9.	Relief of the disabled and unemployable.
		10.	Burials and burials grounds; cremation grounds.
		11.	Education including universities subject to the provisions of entries 63 and 66 of List-I and entry 25 of List-III.
		28.	Markets and fairs.

(Contd.)

Direct		*Indirect*
CONCURRENT LIST		
16. Lunacy and mental deficiency including places for the reception or treatment of lunatics and mental deficiencies.	20.	Economic and social planning.
18. Adulteration of food-stuffs and other goods.	23.	Social security and social insurance; employment and unemployment.
19. Drugs and poisons subject to the provisions of entry to opium.	30.	Vital statistics including registration of births and deaths.
26. Legal, medical and other professions.	31.	Ports other than those declared by or under law made by Parliament or existing law to be major ports.
29. Prevention of the spread, from one State to another infectious or contagious diseases or pests affecting men, animals and plants.		

Under Article 263, the Central Council of Health was created in 1952 and Central Family Planning Council in 1965 to encourage co-operation between the Union and the States in the promotion of health. We have discussed, the role of these agencies in detail at the end of the chapter.

B. Policy-Formulation—Agencies

The agencies responsible for policy-formulation within the Union and State Governments in their respective jurisdictions are not easy to locate. The main and more important organs concerning policy-formulation are the legislature. Cabinet and the concerned ministry e.g. Ministry of Health and Family Welfare. There are many other agencies which guide the legislation and executive in the formulation of policy, e.g., Planning Commission, National Development Council, Medical Council of India, Indian Council of Medical Research, public services in the ministries at the secretariat level and within attached offices, autonomous organisations and subordinate offices, advisory and consultative bodies, committees and commissions appointed from time to time, pressure groups, political parties, professional associations, international organisations, press, Central Council of Health and Family Welfare. Besides, there are advisory committees at all levels of administration which guide in the formulation of the policy at that level. We can explain the process of health policy formulation with the help of systems approach (Fig. 4.2.) explained below :

MODEL OF THE POLITICAL SYSTEM

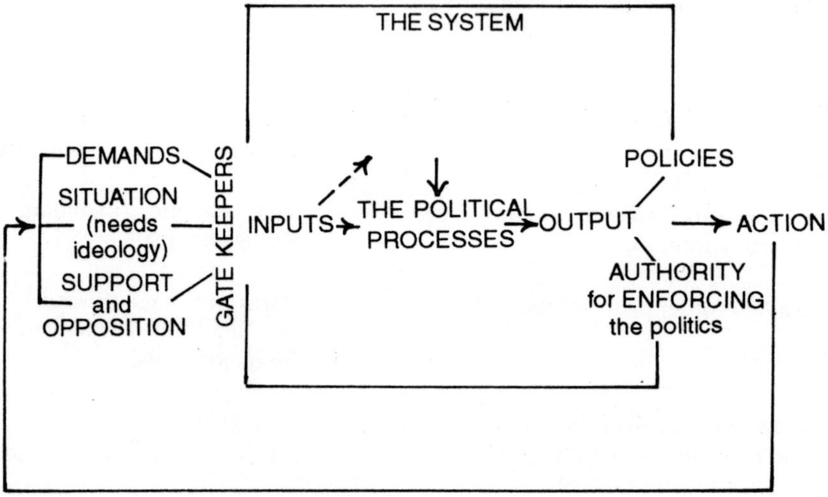

Fig.: 4.2

Source: WHO 77674

The inputs are :

Situation (needs and ideology) includes the health needs of the people and the prevailing value. Demands presented in the system include the support and opposition to the system and to its different 'actors' and outputs.

The demands are supported or opposed by gatekeepers i.e., by agencies already enumerated. Actors, endowed with power and influence are to take final decision i.e., to determine outputs (policies). Authority is mainly applied through the administrative cadre. Health planners and administrators can play an effective role in the formulation of effective policies provided they guide the actors scientifically.[3] Let us discuss the role of important agencies institutions in health policy-making.

Role of the Cabinet

Article 53 of the Constitution lays down that the executive powers of the Union are vested in the President. He has a Council of Ministers to aid and advise him in the exercise of his functions. The President has to act on the advice of the Council of Ministers. It is thus clear that the Indian Constitution vests the President with vast powers but Constitutional experts are of the view that in practice, the President can, and should, set only in accordance with the advice of the Cabinet in the interest of smooth administration and conventions of

Parliamentary democracy. The Council of Ministers consists of four categories of ministers –cabinet ministers, ministers of state, deputy ministers and parliamentary secretaries. The real power to take decisions at the executive level vest in the Cabinet. Sir John Marriot refers to it as "The pivot round which the whole political machinery revolves." In the words of Ramsay Muir, "The Cabinet is the Steering Wheel of the ship of the State." While Sir Ivor Jennings considers it as "The Core of Government."

The same situation prevails at the state level where the governor is a constitutional head (except under emergency) and the council of ministers is the real executive authority.

The volume of work with the Council of Ministers at the Union and the State levels is so large and the problems are so complicated that it is impossible for any number of Ministers to deal with all the matters themselves. The civil servants provide all the information and analysis for the guidance of the ministers and the cabinet. The channel through which a minister must operate is the secretariat. The secretariat acts as an institutionalised memory to enable the Government to examine the feasibility of the proposed policy. As mentioned in the Report of the Administrative Enquiry Committee, Government of Bombay, 1948 (para 91), "the existence of a secretariat in the government organisation arises from the need for separating questions of policy from current administration so that the latter is entirely handed over to a separate agency which enjoys a certain amount of freedom in the field of execution." The effective contribution below the minister and the secretary is that of subject-matter joint secretaries who carry full responsibility in their own sectors.

Role of the Administration in Policy-Formulation

One of the most significant developments in the theory and practice of public administration since the post-war period is the increasing role that the administrative arm of government plays in public policy making. There are two schools of thought in regard to the role of administration in policy-formulation. The first one is of the view that policy-making is exclusively a political function while the administration is concerned only with the implementation of the policy. Thus, they believe in the dichotomy of policy-making and administration. In the words of Woodrow Wilson,

> The field of administration is the field of business. It is removed from the hurry and strife of politics.[4]

According to the second school of thought, politics-administration dichotomy is not possible and that administration cannot be completely separated from policy-formulation. Luther Gullick was one of the first exponents of this view. To quote Paul H. Appleby :

> Administrators are continually laying down rules for the future and administrators are continually determining what the law is, what it means in the terms of action, what the rights of parties are with respect both to transactions in process and transactions in prospect. Administrators always participate in another way in the making of policy for the future; they formulate recommendations for the legislation, and this is a part of the function of the policy making.[5]

Thus public officials are today carrying on both policy-making and policy-implementation. In recent years, administration especially in developing countries has become increasingly involved in politics in the sense of policy-making. There are a number of reasons for it. Let us mention some of these :

(i) In order to take policy decisions on complicated and technical matters, the political leaders have rely heavily on civil servants to provide them with knowledgeable advice.

(ii) In complicated situations, policy-making and policy execution are inter-related and influence each other. Various operational decisions taken during implementation, often have significant policy-implications.

(iii) Policies are generally subject to various interpretations. In such cases the administrators responsible for the implementation of policy can use their own discretion in its interpretation.

In a sense, public administrators always have an advisory role in policy-making. In the Indian political system, based on the British model it is recognised that the senior administrators must render advice to their ministers on policy matters, although the ministers concerned, sometimes with their cabinet colleagues, are responsible for any policy decision. The new policy role for public administrators have been suggested by the advocates of 'Policy Sciences.' It includes the building up of an administrative machinery capable of providing sophisticated aids to high-level policy-making and using policy analysis based on modern management technology. This represents a rational approach to policy-making. Its main assumption is that in the policy area it is possible to evaluate various policy alternatives and transform such evaluations into a scale of values so that the policy-makers can compare relative merits of the policies and take decisions on as rational basis as possible. In order to enable the administrative arm to perform this new function, it is important to enhance its capability in policy analysis. A UN publication states :

> On the assumption that the public administrators or government servants do accept the basic values and the general direction of the political system, the public administrators, in their dual capacity as those who give expert advice on policy issues and those who implement policies, have the following functions to perform in connection with policy-making (especially at the higher levels).

(a) Assuming that certain basic values are given in the form of national goals or mega policies, administrators must clearly understand the nature and significance of these basic values. They should assist policy-makers to avoid ambiguities and unclear points as far as possible, so that any vagueness or ambiguity is the result only of deliberate considerations. They should know who is to give interpretation of the exact meanings of the unclear elements—the court, the legislature, the executive or the government servants. If it is the government servants, who are to interpret their meaning, then they must define the boundary of their discretion in such matters;

(b) It is the duty of public administrators to advice political leaders on the feasibility of various policies, including mega policies. Such advice should be given before a decision is taken on a policy, and it should include the technical, economic, administrative and perhaps also political feasibility of a proposed policy or various policy alternatives. When the problem is one relating to military hardware, then the question of technical feasibility is of primary importance. When the problem is one of the production or allocation, then economic feasibility is often the central issue. In all cases, public administrators should examine the administrative feasibility of a policy. They should assist policy-makers to avoid adopting policies which do not appear feasible unless it is the specific wish of the policy-makers to adopt such policies;

(c) If a policy is adopted in general terms, it is often the responsibility of the public administrators to translate the general policy into operational targets or operational goals. Where costs and benefits constitute important considerations, administrators should analyse the probable costs and benefits of each way of achieving either the general objectives or the operational goals translated from the original objectives. Such analysis facilitates the choice of the alternatives;

(d) While administrators today must adopt a scientific approach and utilise a rationality model as far as possible, they must recongnise that for certain policies, cost and benefit (or rationality or optimisation) do not enter into the picture. For example, the policy analysis work done by the modern management team on the choice of the third London airport late in 1960's was an excellent piece of professional work utilising the rationality model. But the optimum solution on the basis of cost-benefit analysis was finally rejected by the British government for non-technical and non-economic reasons. The public administrators must also recognise that they themselves, in their formulation of advice on policy questions must from time to time make use of intuition where necessary; he who cannot make judgement without assistance from a calculating machine or fails to use the wisdom he has gained through experience, cannot be a good administrator, either as an adviser on policy-making or as one who implements policy;

(e) In view of the multiplicity and complexity or both objectives and policies, public administrators should pay special attention to the questions of coordination of policies and policy instruments or harmonisation at the operational level of policies. The administrators, in rendering advice on a policy, must not limit their vision solely to that particular policy. They should examine it in relation to other policies to see if any inconsistencies or contradictions exist, and analyse whether it complements and supplements other policies to produce better results. Special attention should be paid to environmental acts, including those outside the country, since government policies in the modern world should take external factors fully into consideration. The coordination of internal policies with external policies is a necessary condition of successful public policy-making.[6]

Rule of the Specially Constituted Expert Committees

It is always good to appoint expert committees for policy decisions. The eminent persons from different specialisation may be appointed to constitute a committee. Such specialists and representatives can supply to the Government authentic and valuable information on which the details of the measures may be constructed. They can even suggest the probable implications of such policy-decisions. The committees provide the means of access to the Government of all the interests involved in policy decisions.

"A Government" says Professor Laski, "which embarks on a policy must offer the means of judging that policy. The opinion it has elicited by organised inquiry is fundamental to that end. The evidence it has collected, the facts at its disposal, can never be refused to its subjects if it is to build its opinion in the reasoned judgement of its citizens."

The democratic and scientific technique of administration demands the presence of permanent and continuous organs of consultation before decisions are reached by the Government.

"We think", reported Lord Haldane's Committee on the Machinery of Government, "that the more they (committees) are regarded as an integral part of the normal organisation of a department, the more will ministers be enabled to command the confidence of Parliament and the public in their administration of the services which seem likely in an increasing degree to affect the lives of large sections of the community."

Every ministry appoints from time to time committees including expert committees to advise the Government on a particular issue or a number of issues. The views of these committees have an important influence on the formulation of policies. When the advice of these bodies is accepted by the Government, it may take the form of a policy either through the legislative enactment or executive orders. Let us now discuss the role of some of the important committees appointed by the government of India to look into the issues of health care administration.

BHORE COMMITTEE, 1946

The Government of India appointed this committee in 1943 to survey the then existing health conditions and health organisations in the country and to make recommendations for the future development.

The health of the nation (British India), as it stood in 1946, was reviewed by the Health Survey and Development Committee (Bhore Committee). The Committee reviewed the nation's health under :

1. Public Health
2. Medical Relief
3. Professional Education
4. Medical Research
5. International Health

The report of the Bhore Committee was published in 1946 on the eve of India's Independence, and the proposals for the health programmes were made to provide, among others, the following :

(a) No individual shall fail to secure adequate medical care because of inability to pay for it.

(b) In view of the complexity of modern medical practice, the health services should provide, when fully developed, all the consultant, Laboratory and institutional facilities necessary for proper diagnosis and treatment.

(c) The health problem must from the beginning lay special emphasis on preventive work.

(d) The need is urgent for providing medical relief and preventive health care to the vast rural population of the country.

(e) The health service should be placed as close to the people as possible in order to ensure the maximum benefit to the community to be served.

(f) It is essential to secure the active cooperation of the people in the development of the health programme.

(g) The report in this long-term programme recommended a primary health unit for a population of 20,000, a secondary unit for a population of 6,00,000 and a district headquarters organisation for a population of three million. The committee in its short-term programme recommended a primary unit for a population of 40,000, a secondary unit for a population of one and half million, and a district headquarters organisation for a population of three million.

(h) Recommended a three-month training in preventive and social medicine to prepare social physicians who would guide the people to a healthier and happier life.

This report continues still to be an important document in the field of health care administration.

MUDALIAR COMMITTEE, 1962

In 1959, the Government of India instituted a "Health Survey and Planning Committee" called the Mudaliar Committee to survey the progress made in the field of health since submission of the Bhore Committee's Report and to make recommendations for future development and expansion of health services.

The Mudaliar Committee found the quality of services provided by the primary health centres inadequate and stressed the need to strengthen the existing primary health centres before new centres are created. It also stressed the need to strengthen sub-division and district hospitals so that these could effectively function as referral centres. The main recommendations of the Mudaliar Committee were :

(a) Consolidation of advances, efforts and achievement made in the first two five-year plans in the field of health.

(b) Equipping district hospitals with specialist services.

(c) Need of regionalisation of health services i.e., setting up of regional structures between the State and District headquarters.

(d) Each primary health centre should serve not more than 40,000 people.

(e) The quality of care provided by the primary health centre needs improvement.

(f) Integration of medical and health services should be achieved as already suggested by the Bhore Committee.

(g) Constitution of an All-India Health Service on the pattern of Indian Administrative Services.

CHADAH COMMITTEE, 1963

This committee was set up by the Government of India in 1963 under the Chairmanship of Dr. M.S. Chadah, the Director General of Health Services, to study the arrangements for the maintenance phase of the National Malaria Eradication Programme. The Committee recommended that :

(a) The vigilance operation of the National Malaria Eradication Programmes should be the responsibility of the general health services i.e., primary health centres at the block level.

(b) Vigilance operations through monthly home visits should be implemented through basic health workers. The norm of one basic health worker per 10,000 population was recommended.

(c) The basic health workers should look after additional duties of collection of vital statistics and family planning, in addition to malaria vigilance. Three to four such workers may be supervised by a Family Planning Health Assistant.

(d) The general health services at the district level should undertake the responsibility for the maintenance phase.

MUKERJI COMMITTEE, 1965

The Committee was appointed by the Government of India to review the strategy for the family planning programme. The major recommendations of the committee were :

(a) There should be separate staff family planning programme and the family planning assistants should look after family planning work exclusively.

(b) The basic health workers should not be utilised for the family planning programme.

(c) The Malaria Eradication activities should be separated from the family planning, so that the latter can concentrate on family planning programme.

MUKERJI COMMITTEE, 1966

The States were experiencing difficulties to shoulder the whole burden of maintenance phase of malaria and other mass programmes like family planning, smallpox, leprosy, trachoma, etc., due to paucity of funds. A committee was constituted under the Chairmanship of Sh. B. Mukerji, the then Union Secretary, Health, to work out the details of the 'Basic Health Service' which should be provided at the block level and some consequential strengthening required at higher levels of administration.

The Committee recommended the following additional staff for the various agencies administering health services in the country :

I. *Primary Health Centre*

1.	Basic Health worker	...	1 for 10,000 population
2.	Health Inspector	...	1 for every four basic health workers
3.	Clerk	...	1
4.	Laboratory Technician	...	1

II. *District Health Organisation*

1.	Up-gradation of the post of Administrative Officer sanctioned under the Family Planning Programme.		
2.	Health Supervisor	...	1 for every 10 primary health centres subject to a maximum of one per district.
3.	Public Health Engineer	...	1 or 2 or 3 districts.
4.	Sanitary Supervisor	...	1

III. *District Hospital*

1.	Administrative Officer	...	1

IV. *Urban Areas*

1.	Basic Health Workers	...	1 for 15,000 population
2.	Health Inspector	...	1 for 5 basic health workers.

JUNGALWALLA COMMITTEE, 1967

The Committee on 'Integration of Health Services' was appointed in 1967 under the Chairmanship of Dr. N. Jungalwalla, the then Director of National Institute of Health, Administration and Education, New Delhi, to examine the various problems including those of service conditions. The major recommendations made by the Committee were :

(a) Integration of organisations and personnel in the field of health from the highest to the lowest level in the service through :

1. Unified cadre
2. Common seniority
3. Recognition of extra qualifications
4. Equal pay for equal work
5. Special pay for specialised work
6. No private practice but good service conditions.

The Committee did not spell out steps and programme for the integration recommended by it and left the matter to the States to work out the set-up. It, however, defined the integrated health service as :

(a) Service with a unified approach for all problems instead of segmented approach for different problems.

(b) Medical care of sick and conventional public health programmes functioning under a single administrator and operating in a unified manner at all levels of hierarchy with due priority for each programme obtaining at point of time.

KARTAR SINGH COMMITTEE, 1973

The Committee on 'Multipurpose workers under Health and Family Planning' was constituted by the Government of India in 1973 under the Chairmanship of Shri Kartar Singh, the then Additional Secretary, Health, Government of India. The Committee's terms of reference were to study and make recommendations on :

1. the structure for integrated service at the periphery and supervisory level;
2. the feasibility of having multipurpose, bi-purpose workers in the field;
3. the training requirements for such workers; and
4. the utilisation of mobile service units setup under family planning programme for integrated medical, public health and family planning services operating in the field.

The main recommendations of the Committee were :

(a) The present Auxiliary Nurse Midwives be replaced by newly designated 'Female Health Workers' and the present day Basic Health Workers, Malaria Eradication Assistants and Family Planning Health Assistants to be replaced by 'Male Health Workers.'

(b) The programme for having multipurpose workers should be first introduced in areas where malaria is in maintenance phase and smallpox has been controlled and later to other areas as malaria passes into maintenance phase or smallpox controlled.

(c) For proper coverage there should be one primary health centre for a population of 50,000.

(d) Each primary health centre, should be divided into 16 sub-centres, each having a population of about 3,000-3,500 depending upon the topography and means of communication.

(e) Each sub-centre should be staffed by a team of one male and one female health worker.

(f) There should be a male health supervisor to supervise the work of 3-4 male health workers and a female health supervisor to supervise the work of 4 female health workers.

(g) The present day lady health visitors to be designated as female health supervisors.

(h) The doctor incharge of a primary health centre should have the overall charge of all the supervisors and health workers in his area.

SHRIVASTAVA GROUP REPORT, 1975

The Shrivastava Group also known as "Group on Medical Education and Support Manpower" was appointed by the Government of India in 1974 under the Chairmanship of Dr. J.B. Shrivastava, the then Director General of Health Services, Government of India. The terms of reference of the group were :

(a) To devise a suitable curriculum for training a cadre of Health Assistants conversant with basic medical aid preventive and nutritional services, family welfare, maternity and child welfare activities so that they can serve as a link between the qualified medical practitioners and multipurpose workers, thus forming an effective team to deliver health care, family welfare and nutritional services to the people.

(b) Keeping in view the recommendations made by earlier Committees on Medical Education, specially the Medical Education Committee (1968) and Medical Education Conference (1970) to suggest suitable ways and means for implementation of these recommendations and to suggest steps for improving the existing medical educational processes so as to provide due emphasis on the problems particularly relevant to national requirements; and

(c) To make any other suggestions to realise the above objectives and matters incident thereto.

After carefully examining various reports and papers relevant to the subject including the recommendations of as many as 12 conferences and committees held earlier, the major recommendations of the group were :

(a) A nationwide network of efficient and effective services suitable for our conditions, limitations, and potentialities should be evolved.

(b) Steps should be taken to create bands of para-professional or semi-professional health workers from the community itself to provide simple protective, preventive and curative services which are needed by the community.

(c) Between the community and the primary health centre, there should be two cadres—health workers and health assistants. (1) Health workers should be trained and equipped to give simple specified remedies for day-to-day illness. (2) Health assistants would work as intermediaries between the health workers and the Primary Health Centre. The health assistants should be located at the sub-centres. Like the health workers, they should also be trained and equipped to give specific remedies for simple day-to-day health problems. While they will have a supervisory role over the health workers, they would also function as health worker in their own areas and carry out the same duties and responsibilities, but at a higher level of technical competence.

(d) The Primary Health Centre should be provided with an additional doctor and a nurse to look after the maternal and child health services.

(e) The possibility of utilising the service of senior doctors at the medical college, regional, district or taluka hospitals for brief periods at primary health centre should be explored.

(f) The Primary Health Centre as well as taluka, tehsil, district, regional and medical college hospitals should each develop living and direct links with the community around them, as well as with one another within a total referral services complex.

(g) The Government of India should constitute under an Act of Parliament a Medical and Health Education Commission for coordination and maintaining standards in medical and health education on the pattern of University Grants Commission.

The recommendations of the various committees on health have been accepted by the Government and most of them have been implemented. But the fact remains that, however commendable the recommendations of the committees/groups may be, these will be of no avail if we do not have proper administrative machinery to put them into effect.

We have examined recommendations of various committees constituted from time to time. No one can deny the utility of these committees. We may keep the following facts and suggestions in mind while constituting such committees :

1. The membership of the committee should not be too big otherwise their deliberations cannot be fruitful.

2. We may not appoint such eminent persons who are extremely busy as such members circulate from one committee to another, seldom knowing about the business of any one Committee. Professor Wheare suggests, "The best advice is often to be obtained from persons of less eminence, still so little in demand that they are able to master fully one branch of knowledge or activity." We must ensure that only such members may be appointed on these committees who are not only competent but can also devote sufficient time. Shriram Maheshwari in his paper on Advisory Committees in the Central Government (India) suggests that "while appointing persons on these committees, the primary consideration should be their qualifications, experience and probity."

3. It is always better to associate an expert from public administration who can help the committee in designing the administrative structure required to implement the policy decisions. Most of the policy-decisions produce no result for lack of proper administrative apparatus.

4. The committees must submit their report within the specified time, otherwise, their recommendations may not yield good results as the circumstances may change after some time and the recommendations may not hold good to suit the changed socio-economic environment.

5. The Government must give top priority to examine the feasibility and utility of these recommendations so that these recommendations (if accepted) may be duly processed through the formal machinery of Government and converted into policy decisions.

6. The university teachers in their respective areas may be appointed to serve on these committees. They can provide valuable material. This would encourage useful and meaningful relationship between the Government and the universities. Prof. W.A. Robson in his article "India Revisited " (published in *The Political Quarterly* Oct-Dec., 1960, p. 436) rightly says, "University professors are seldom, if ever, invited to serve on advisory committees of other public bodies where their specialised knowledge and highly trained minds could be valuable. It is perhaps desirable for teachers not to take too active a part in political controversy in the public forum, but it is short-sighted to refuse to make use of their special qualifications outside the lecture room."

Role of Health Legislation

Besides the committees which are appointed from time to time, the Union Ministry of Health and Family Welfare pilots draft legislation in the legislature. These laws assist in the formulation and execution of national health policy. These laws also empower health authorities to implement health policies. The first health legislation dates back to the year 1825 when the Quarantine Act was passed. During the 19th century, the following health legislations were enacted :

i. The Indian Penal Code, 1866.

ii. The Bengal Births and Deaths Regulation Act, 1873.

iii. The Bengal Vaccination Act, 1880.

iv. The First Indian Factories Act, 1881.

v. The Bengal Municipal Act, 1884.

vi. The Local self-Government Act, 1885.

vii. The Medical Act, 1886.

viii. The Birth, Death and Marriage Regulation Act, 1896.

ix. The Epidemic Disease Act, 1897.

x. Lepers Act, 1898.

During the 20th century (before independence) the following legislations were enacted :

(i) Medical Drugs Act, 1916.

(ii) Red Cross Society Act, 1922.

(iii) Medical Council Act, 1933.

At the time of independence, the following Acts were passed :

(i) Indian Medical Council Act (Amendment), 1947.

(ii) Pharmacy Council Act, 1948.

(iii) Dentist Act, 1948.

Since the first Lok Sabha the following laws relating to health have been enacted which are classified as below :

1. *Laws Related to Drugs, Food Adulteration and Cosmetics*

(a) Drugs and Magic Remedies (Objectionable Advertisement) Act, 1954, 1963.

(b) Prevention of Food Adulteration Act, 1954, 1964 (Amendment); 1971.

(c) Drugs Act, 1955.

(d) Opium Laws, 1957.

(e) Poisons Act, 1958.

(f) Drugs (Amendment) Act, 1960, 1962.

(g) Drugs and Cosmetics (Amendment) Act, 1964; 1972 (Amendment).

(h) Medicinal and Toilet Preparation (Amendment) Act, 1961.

2. *Medical Education*

(a) Dentists (Amendment) Act, 1955; 1972.

(b) Indian Medical Council Act (Amendment), 1956,1958, 1964.

(c) Indian Nursing Council (Amendment) Act, 1957.

(d) Pharmacy (Amendment) Act, 1959.

(e) Indian Medicine Central Council Act, 1970.

(f) All India Institute of Medical Sciences Act, 1956.

(g) P.G.I.M.E.R., Chandigarh, Act, 1956.

(h) Homoeopathy Central Council Act, 1975.

3. *Maternity*

(a) Maternity Benefit Act, 1961 (Amendment), 1972.

(b) Medical Termination of Pregnancy Act, 1971.

4. *Miscellaneous*

(a) Registration of Births and Deaths Act, 1969.

(b) St. John Ambulance Association Act, 1956.

(c) Indian Red Cross Society (Amendment) Act, 1956.

(d) Countess of Dufferin Fund Act, 1957.

Public health laws provide the working tools to health administrators to enable them to safeguard the communities from health hazards and to promote health. Such a legislation would help in the demarcation of functions at various levels—Union, State, Local and would bring about a uniformity of procedure and action. The health laws in India, today are scattered in piece-meal enactments. Some of them have become outmoded while some need change in contents because of the environmental changes. The present corpus of health legislation is inadequate. Regulations are lacking in many vital subjects. The model Public Health Act, 1955, divided into 4 parts and 57 chapters was circulated among the States but so far the States have not come forward to adopt this legislation. There is an urgent need to enact and approve this legislation as it would provide guidance to the policy-makers, planners and health administrators.

Role of the Committees of the Parliament/State Legislature

Besides, there are Committees of Parliament which help the Government in policy-formulation by examining the operations of the current policies in the country. Special mention may be made of the two financial committees—Estimates Committee and Public Accounts Committee.

Estimates Committee. It consists of 30 members. Its functions are :

(a) to report what economies, improvements in organisation, efficiency or administrative reform, consistent with the policy underlying the estimates, may be effected;

(b) to suggest alternative policies in order to bring about efficiency and economy in administration;

(c) to examine whether the money is well laid-out within the limits of the policy implied in the estimates; and

(d) to suggest the form in which the estimates shall be presented to Parliament.

The following important reports of the Estimates Committee have analysed the various health and family welfare programmes.

Fifth Lok Sabha	*Sixth Lok Sabha*
13, 33, 57, 83, 102	6, 11, 26

The exhaustive and objective studies made by the committees always indicate new directions which the Government can pursue for a better utilisation of the resources. The implementation of its suggestions provide alternatives to the existing conditions and in that process it offers a choice to the decision makers. The existence of this choice makes decisions more scientific and more realistic too.*

* The comments of the Estimate Committee have been used at different places. It is difficult to examine these reports.

Public Accounts Committee. It consists of 22 members—15 from Lok Sabha and 7 from Rajya Sabha. The duty of the Committee as embodied in the Rule of Procedure and Conduct of Business, is to satisfy :

(a) that the moneys shown in the accounts as having been disbursed were legally available for and applicable to the service or purpose to which they have been applied.

(b) that the expenditure conforms to the authority which governs it, and

(c) that every reappropriation has been made in this behalf under rules framed by the competent authority.

Let me mention some of the latest reports of Public Accounts Committee relating to health :

Fifth Lok Sabha	*Sixth Lok Sabha*
18, 21, 34, 40, 42, 67	5, 35, 49, 93, 103
72, 75, 84, 101, 107, 124,	
138, 152, 197	

Public Accounts Committee has been able to influence the future health policy to a great extent through its recommendations.

Role of the Ministry of Health and Family Welfare and the Formulating of Draft National Health Policy

We have examined the role of other agencies under the Ministry. The main responsibility is of the Ministry itself. We do not have the requisite machinery and expertise to develop scientific health policy to provide health care to all by the year 2000. Our health policies have always appeared to be ambitious and spectacular but in terms of benefiting the rural masses, these have so far fallen far short of expectations. The best test of efficiency of any health policy is the improvement its brings about in the areas of preventive, promotive and curative health services. Indeed, judged by these simple yardsticks of literacy, life expectancy and infant mortality, India comes low down in the physical quality of life index (POLI) with some areas of the country competing for the bottom most position in the world. Among the elements relating to the development of administration, public policy-making is the most important and yet perhaps the least developed.

A statement on the "National Health Policy" was laid on the Table of both the Houses of Parliament on the second November 1982.[8] The National Health Policy was discussed at length in both Houses and was approved by the Rajya Sabha on fourth August 1983, and the Lok Sabha on 22nd December, 1983. (Refer Appendix I for the Statement on National Health Policy). The Policy lays stress on the preventive, promotive, public health and rehabilitative aspects of health care and points to the need of establishing comprehensive, primary health care services to reach the population in the remotest areas of the country, the need to view health and human development as a vital component of overall integrated national socio-economic development, decentralised system of health care delivery with the maximum community and individual self-reliance and participation. The policy also lays stress on ensuring adequate nutrition, safe drinking water supply and improved sanitation for all segments of the population. The policy sets out specific goals to be achieved by 1985, 1990, 1995 and 2000 A.D. in pursuance of the national commitment for the attainment of the goal of Health For All by 2000 A.D.[9]

C. Suggestions to Improve Policy-Making

Before this draft policy is adopted, it is suggested that the general administrators and health experts should keep in mind the genuine health needs of the people and motivate the political actors to formulate balanced health policy based on scientific methods. The health administrators must keep the following facts in mind to frame effective, efficient and relevant health policies. (See fig. 4.3)

Policies Should be Made in Consonance with the Objectives

By goal or objective is meant the end towards which action is directed. Since a policy is a guidance for action, it is reasonable to expect that a policy indicates the direction towards which action is guided, either explicitly or implicitly. For this reason, students of policy sciences often define public policies as a programme of goals and objectives.

Absence of Contradictions and Inconsistencies

It is necessary for public administrators to help in making policies purposeful and goal-oriented, and to assist in defining goals and objectives clearly, in making them concrete and also quantifiable if possible and in removing, to the extent possible, any contradictions and inconsistencies.

Temporal Dimensions

The modern world is rapidly changing. So, our policies must not remain constant but should change with the change in times. A UN report suggests the following three points :

(a) It is a well-known fact that a public policy, in order to be effective, must not be too little or too late;

(b) Time sequence is an essential part of a successful policy. An effective policy should comprise not only what a government should do but also when to do one thing after another. Timings is often an essential factor for the success or failure of a policy; and

(c) Synchronisation is another timing element. Something, for example, what is required is not only that action '2' should follow action '1', but also that action '3' should be taken at the same time as action '4'.[10]

Feasibility, Probability and Possibility

Policies which are not based on the technical, economic, administrative and perhaps also proposed political feasibility should be avoided unless it is the specific wish of the policy-makers to adopt such policies. It is important to note that feasibility, probability and possibility are all relative terms. If the policy-makers have reason to believe that what they plan will change the circumstances in favour of the planned objectives, then they are justified in the planning for what may appear to be 'Improbable' or even 'Impossible' to the experts who assume that the circumstances will remain constant. For the developing countries, estimated by experts on feasibility, probability and possibility are often poorly informed guess-work, in part owing to lack of sufficient or decisive evidence and in part owing to a high degree or uncertainty. In a UN document which warns against 'paper planning' and blind commitments to the blatantly impossible, it is stated :

> From the previous extremes of seeking the impossible, the planners may go so far in emphasising the possible that they will think of short-run feasibility. In this effort, they will often be encouraged by economists who have become accustomed to fighting utopia with myopia, that is with 'hard nosed' calculations of small benefits that might be obtained quickly. The result can easily be that instead of planning for the impossible, they will focus upon most possible and feasible of all, namely, the inevitable. This is the fallacy of epiphenomenal planning. Here the main advantage is that the planners can take credit for any minor progress that might have taken place.

Relevant Forecasts and Projections

According to a UN report "Forecasting and projections are important for public policy-making mainly for two reasons. First, as just indicated, policy is a guidance for action that lies necessarily in the future. Therefore, no rational approach to policy-making is possible without some basis for making assumptions about the future. Forecasting and projection can assist policy-makers in this respect. Secondly, public policies should be used, if at all possible, to avoid crisis rather than to meet crisis situations. Unless a government is capable of making useful forecasts and projections, it is not in a position to avoid crisis and may have to devote most of its resources to crisis management. At the same time, a government which is under constant pressure from immediate crisis may not be able to devote its attention and resources to the future in order to prevent the recurrence of crisis. This is a vicious circle which a government should break, and it can succeed in doing so only by assigning suitable priority to forecasting the future."

Appropriate Administrative Machinery

Within the central policy cluster there should also be special arrangement for ensuring that appropriate administrative machinery is established for :

(a) policy and plan implementation

(b) reporting and feedback

(c) evaluation and control

(d) the adjustment and revision of policies, plans and programmes.[11]

This would ensure effective relationship between policy formulation and policy implementation.

Understanding the Implications of Policy

Policies must be interpreted and explained, to all members of the organisation. What people do not understand they cannot use correctly and are likely to distrust. Therefore, there is a need to explain it to all persons to whom it applies.

Environmental Considerations

Policy is based on actual information or factual data which can be collected from a number of sources by applying different methods. But, before the data can be changed into a policy, many factors have to be taken into considerations e.g., policies must be made in accordance with the provisions of the constitution and the laws enacted by the legislature; these must also be made in accordance with the social, political, cultural, economic and ethical environment prevailing in the country; these must also be linked with the agencies interested in the same policy to have maximum utility and effectiveness; these must also be made in accordance with the opinion of the public otherwise they (the people) would not cooperate with the government in their execution.

FIVE DIMENSIONS OF NATIONAL HEALTH POLICY

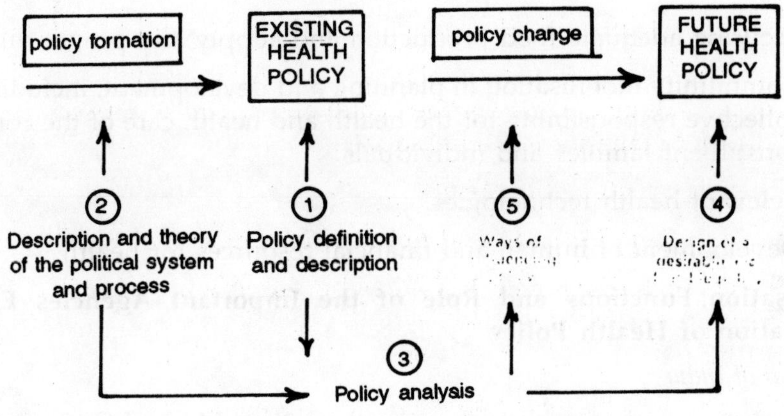

Fig.: 5.3

Dr. Karan Singh has rightly said that, " If the nation wants a first class health care service with special emphasis on nutrition and child health and the combating of communicable diseases, it will have to readjust its priorities so that adequate inputs are made available during the current and subsequent periods.[12]

Perhaps never before the need to reassess our priorities was as great as it is today. The formulation of realistic and scientific health policy based upon our realistic assessment and understanding of our health needs and problems and approaches to deal with them will go a long way towards better planning of health services,, however, meagre may be our resources.

While reviewing the national health policies the following issues need considerations:

1. Geographical coverage of the population with at least all the essential components of primary health care and the corresponding referral system.
2. A system of financing health care ensuring that all strata of society have an equal opportunity to avail themselves of such care.
3. Coverage of particular population groups, such as mothers and children, working women, school children, workers and the elderly, and any particular risk group.
4. Preferential allocation of health resources to under-privileged population groups.
5. Improvement of the human environment by progressively providing safe drinking-water to the whole population, building up waste disposal system and ensuring clean air.
6. Improvement of housing and basic sanitation.
7. Securing adequate food production and supply and proper nutrition.
8. Community mobilisation in planning and development, including promotion of collective responsibility for the health and health care of the community and its constituent families and individuals.
9. Relevant health technologies.
10. Development of human and financial resources for health.

D. Organisation, Functions and Role of the Important Agencies Engaged in the Formulation of Health Policy

Medical Council of India

It is a statutory body established under the Indian Medical Council Act, 1956, and is responsible for the maintenance of informal standards of medical education in the country. The Council prescribes minimum standards of medical education and also the standards of requirements of a Medical College for the award of medical degrees.

Under its functions, one can mention the following :

(a) to prescribe standards for post-graduate medical education for the universities;
(b) to acquire information regarding courses of study and examinations;
(c) to make representation to the Union Government in regard to the recognition of medical qualifications;
(d) to inspect medical colleges and suggest methods of improving the efficiency of training;
(e) by an amendment in 1964, the Council was given powers to prevent quackery;
(f) to maintain the Indian Medical Register.

The total number of doctors borne on the Indian Medical Register as on 31 December 1982 was 2,95,099. The Council also issues 'Good Standing Certificates' to the doctors who desire to seek registration with the General Medical Council of UK and other Commonwealth countries. The number of such certificates issued upto 31.3.82 was 17,847.

Besides Medical Council there are three other councils — The Indian Nursing Council (Indian Nursing Act, 1947), Dental Council of India (Dentist Act, 1948), and the Pharmacy Council of India (Pharmacy Act, 1948). These councils have powers and functions similar to those of the Medical Council of India in their respective jurisdiction.

National Board of Examinations

The National Board of Examinations has been set up as a registered society under Societies Registration Act, 1960, with effect from March 1, 1982. The main objective of the Board is to conduct national level examination at Postgraduate level in the disciplines of modern medicine and other allied sciences on the lines of the foreign qualifications like FRCS and MRCP etc. Earlier the functions of this Board had been entrusted to the National Academy of Medical Sciences and the Board conducted the examination for the Membership of National Academy of Medical Sciences (MNAMS) qualifications. The MNAMS qualifications granted by the National Board of Examinations is recognised by the Medical Council of India as equivalent to post-graduate qualifications in different specialities of modern medical sciences. With the establishment of the Board as a separate entity, the Board will award its own qualifications to be known as 'Diplomate of National Board'. The qualifications of this Board, namely, Diplomate of National Board Examinations have been recognised and included in the First Schedule to the Indian Medical Council Act, 1956. Besides, a research cell has been established in the National Board of Examinations.

It is suggested that the Medical Council of India, Dental Council of India, Pharmacy Council of India, Nursing Council of India may be merged with the UGC (University Grants Commission) having its separate identity. In this way medical education can be viewed as a part of the total spectrum of education and not an isolated phenomena.

However, under the provisions of the existing Indian Medical Council Act, there are certain inherent limitations on the powers of the Council in respect of enforcement of standard of medical education. The Medical Council of India lacks the authority and power to enforce standards in individual colleges. In order to remove these deficiencies, the Government is at present actively considering a proposal to amend the Medical Council of India Act. Some of the proposed amendments are as follows :

(a) No new undergraduate or post-graduate medical course shall be started in any institution without prior approval of the Council.

(b) Recognition/de-recognition of medical qualifications will be institution-wise and not university-wise.

(c) The Council will be entrusted with powers to recognise/de-recognise the medical qualifications. The Central Government will only act as an Appellate Authority.

Indian Council of Medical Research (ICMR)

Medical research enables us to plan our defensive and offensive action against diseases by augmenting our knowledge of their basic causative and propagative factors. Till 1947, there was not much emphasis on medical research in the country. The Bhore Committee was very critical of the prevailing research facilities in medical colleges and universities. Organised medical research in the country depended mainly on researches through central and provincial laboratories and the Indian Research Fund Association (IRFA).

The Indian Council of Medical Research came into existence in 1950 as the Central Medical Research Organisation recommended by the Bhore Committee, by taking the place of the IRFA (Indian Research Fund Association). The objectives of the Council are to prosecute, coordinate and assist research in communicable diseases, to finance enquiries and research projects, to exchange information with other institutions similarly engaged and interested, to prepare and publish reports of research work, papers and periodicals, and to grant fellowships. The Council maintains, besides a number of semi-permanent units, 18 permanent research institutes and centres. The Council Governing Body is presided over by the Minister for Health and Family Welfare. It has a Scientific Advisory Board under the chairmanship of the Director-General of Health Services and other members representing experts in scientific fields, directors of research institutes etc.

The objectives of ICMR are as follows :

(a) The prosecution and assistance of research, propagation of knowledge and experimental measures generally in connection with the causation, mode of spread and prevention of diseases.

(b) To intimate, aid, develop and coordinate medical, scientific research in India and to promote and assist institutions for the study of diseases, their prevention, causation and remedy.

(c) To finance enquiries and researches.

(d) To exchange information with other institutions, associations and scientists interested in the same projects.

(e) To prepare, print and publish any paper or periodical in furtherance of the objects of the Council and to contribute to any such periodical.

(f) To grant fellowships, scholarships, etc., for training research workers and to offer prizes in order to encourage research pursuits.

(g) To serve as an apex body for the planning, organisation, implementation and coordination of medical research in the country. In the past, foreign support for bio-medical research has been forthcoming from WHO, Ford Foundation, Swedish Foundation, PL-480, etc. The practice of foreign agencies directly contacting Indian scientists and formulating and supporting research programmes led to undesirable consequences as it resulted in duplication of efforts and neglect of priority areas. The Ministry of Health has decided that all proposals for foreign support must be supported through ICMR.

The ICMR (Indian Council of Medical Research) has been following two broad directions in the field of research : (i) *applied* research for solution of outstanding current problems in the field of medicine, public health and allied subjects; (ii) *fundamental* research in these areas.

Five-year plans have provided financial support for these activities. It can be visualised from the finances invested in research projects. The finances have increased from 12 lakhs in 1947 to 1,763 lakhs in 1983-84 i.e., an increase of about 140 times. In addition, State Medical Research Committees, Medical Research Organisation of the Armed Forces and collaborated research with other scientific agencies of the country like Indian Council of Scientific and Industrial Research and Indian Council of Social Sciences Research are also contributing to these efforts.

During 1983-84, the total number of projects was 712 as against 600 during 1982-83. The continuing schemes included those in the field of communicable diseases like malaria, cholera, TB, filariasis and leprosy etc. In addition to the *ad hoc* research schemes, the Council has a fellowship scheme to attract medical graduates in this field of medical research. During 1983-84, 619 fellows were working under this scheme.

Central Council of Health

The Central Council of Health was established under the provisions of Article 263, by a Presidential Order in August 1952, in pursuance of the decisions of the Health Ministers' Conference held in August 1950. The Council consists of the Union Health Minister as Chairman and Health Ministers of all States as its members.

Organisation of the Council : The Council shall consist of :

(a) (i) The Union Minister for Health and Family Planning. (Chairman)

(ii) The Ministers of State in the Ministry of Health and Family Planning. (Members)

(iii) The Ministers in-charge of the Ministries of Health in the State.

(b) Experts and technical advisers to the Central Government and State Governments shall not be members of the Council and shall not have any right to vote when a decision is taken by it but shall, if so required by the Council, be in attendance at its meetings.

(c) The Council shall have a secretarial staff consisting of a Secretary and such officers and servants as the Chairman may, with the approval of the Central Government, think fit to appoint.

Procedure of the Council : The Council shall in its conduct of business observe the following procedures, namely :

(a) The Council shall meet at least once every year;

(b) It shall meet at such time and place as the Chairman may decide;

(c) Five members (including the Chairman) shall form quorum for a meeting of the Council;

(d) The Chairman and, in his absence, such members as may be designated by him on his behalf, from among the members shall preside at a meeting;

(e) All questions which may come before the Council at a meeting shall be decided by the majority of votes of the members (including the Chairman) present at the meeting;

(f) In case of any equality of votes the person presiding shall have second or casting vote; and

(g) The Council shall observe in the conduct of its business such other procedures as it may, with the approval of the Central Government, lay down from time to time.

Functions of the Council : The Council has a wide field of functioning.

(i) To consider and recommend broad lines in regard to matters concerning health in all its aspects much as the provisions of remedial and preventive care, environmental hygiene, nutrition, health, education and the promotion of facilities for training and research.

(ii) To make proposals for legislation in fields of activity relating to medical and public health matters, laying down the pattern of development for the country as a whole.

(iii) To examine the whole field of possible cooperation on a wide basis in regard to inter-state quarantine during times of festivals, outbreaks of epidemic diseases and serious calamities, such as earthquakes and famines, to draw up a common programme of action.

(iv) To make recommendations to the Central Government regarding distribution of available grants-in-aids for health purposes, to the states and to review periodically the work accomplished in different areas through the utilisation of these grants-in aid.

(v) To establish any organisation or organisations invested with appropriate functions for promoting and maintaining cooperation between the Central and State Health Administration.

The Council met for the first time at Hyderabad in January 1953. Till the end of the First-Five-Year Plan it concentrated on a number of issues, some of the important issues are mentioned below :

1. Integration of the general health programmes and development programmes.
2. Control TB and malaria.
3. Devising uniform standard of education in medicine.
4. Enactment of a Comprehensive Public Health Act and legislation against use of tobacco by juveniles.
5. Training of para-medical and MCH workers.
6. Establishment of Central and State Health Education Bureaus.
7. Promotion and coordination of research in states.

8. Inclusion of public health engineering under the purview of Central and State Health Departments.

During the Second Plan Period (1957-62) the emphasis was laid on :

1. Family Planning Programme.
2. Expansion of post-graduate education facilities.
3. Re-organisation of Primary Health Centres.
4. Appointment of Review Committee to look into the Equality of Medical Education and Central Medical Stores Organisation.
5. Protection to workers from radiation, etc.
6. Toilets and cosmetics.
7. Amendment of Food Adulteration Act, 1954.
8. Leprosy Control Act.
9. To curb unregistered people from practicing medicine.

During the Third Plan Period (1962-67) the deliberation of the Council related to the following areas :

1. National Health Programme.
2. Centrally sponsored and Centrally assisted programmes.
3. Family Health Centres.
4. Family Planning.
5. Drugs Control.
6. Medical Education.
7. Health Education.
8. Water Supply and Sanitation.
9. Medical Care.
10. Mental Health Services.
11. Health-Intelligence.

From 1968-73, the Council has been able to meet only once in two years. The major areas of their deliberations were : Primary Health Centres, Management of Health Information System, National Health Programme, Food Adulteration and Medical Care.

The meeting of the Central Council of Health held in New Delhi on 5, 6 and 7 April 1974, was the first joint meeting alongwith the Central Family Planning Council. The major areas as deliberated by this joint meeting were as under :

1. Minimum needs programmes in the area of health and family planning.
2. Integration of family planning, health and nutrition programmes, including training for multipurpose workers.

3. Prevention of food and drug adulteration.
4. Control of communicable diseases.
5. Family welfare planning programme.
6. Indigenous system and homoeopathy.
7. Monitoring and evaluation.

Further meeting upto 1983 went on dealing with these programmes.

A conference meeting of the Health Ministers of the State/Union Territories was held on June 1982.

A joint meeting of the Central Councils of Health and Family Welfare was held in New Delhi on 29-31 January 1978. The entire gamut of new policies and programmes relating to rural health scheme and progress thereof, under both Health and Family Welfare, were discussed in detail and useful recommendations evolved.

The 5th Joint meeting of the Central Councils was held in New Delhi on 6-8 October 1978. The important matters discussed were rural health services, multipurpose workers scheme covering all districts by 1982-83 stepping up of training of traditional birth attendants, evolution of methods to attract medical and para-medical personnel to rural areas, strengthening of PHCs and sub-centres, national medical education policy, banning of private practice by doctors and the adoption of a health policy in line with the Alma-Ata Declaration to provide health care to all by the year 2000. The Sixth Joint Conference of the Councils was held on 27, 28, and 29 April 1979, at New Delhi. It concentrated on the following issues — Family Welfare Programmes, Alma-Ata Declaration, Rural Health Programme and Integration of Medical and Health Services, National Medical and Health Education Policy, Centrally sponsored schemes proposed to be transferred to State sector, National Health Policy, Indian system of Medicine and Homoeopathy, Amendment of Rule 65 (15) of the Drugs and Cosmetic Rules and Section 42 of the Pharmacy Act, Prohibition Policy *vis-a-vis* the Drugs and Cosmetics Act, private practice by government doctors, budget for health sector and water sanitation. Seventh deliberated the same issues. Eighth Joint Conference of the Central Councils of Health and Family Welfare :

The Eighth Joint Conference of the Central Council of Health and the Central Family Welfare Council was held from 18th to 20th August, 1982, at New Delhi, under the chairmanship of Shri B. Shankaranand, Union Minister for Health and Family Welfare.

(a) The conference reviewed the implementation and progress of the Family Welfare Programme and National Programmes for the control of leprosy, TB and blindness, which are included in the new 20-Point Programme. It also considered all aspects of the functioning of the educational institutions imparting education in I.S.M. and homoeopathy and other major issues concerning these systems of medicine. It reiterated that at the national level the responsibility of ensuring supply of safe drinking water and sanitation to the population should rest with the Ministry of Health and Family Welfare and that the Public Health Engineering Departments, which look after these aspects in the States, should be under the charge of their Health Ministers.

(b) Considering the importance attached to various health and family welfare programmes, particularly those which are included in the 20-Point Programme, their implementation and effort made by this Ministry, the Conference made the following recommendations/suggestions :

(i) The State/Union Territory Governments were urged to treat Voluntary Organisations at all levels—B.H.C., District, State—as equal partners in joint national ventures to enable them to take active part in the Family Welfare Programme.

(ii) It urged the need for involving private medical practitioners of all systems of medicine in all appropriate aspects of the Family Planning and MCH Programme.

(iii) Family Welfare Programme should not be considered as the one to be implemented by the Health Sector in isolation but in view of its importance and the priority assigned to it, a multi-sectoral approach should be adopted and concerted efforts by all other sectors should be made and a machinery for coordinating these be set up.

(iv) The State/Union Territory Governments should energise the effective implementation of the national programmes to control leprosy, TB and blindness, which are included in the new 20-Point Programme.

(v) The State Governments were urged to establish separate food cells at the State level, with properly qualified and experienced officers for co-ordinating, guiding and supervising the activities of the various authorities entrusted with the enforcement of the food laws.

(vi) The States were urged to strengthen their Drug Control Organisations so that they can play a more effective role in combating drug adulteration.

(vii) The perspective plans for tribal areas be drawn up by the States and the deficiencies be made up by the end of the Seventh Plan. The districts with 20 per cent or more population of Scheduled Castes at Panchayat level be taken up first for providing the required facilities. Suitable machinery for monitoring, evaluating and reviewing the programmes for Scheduled Tribes/ Scheduled Castes be created and a task force be constituted in each State/ Union Territory to review the progress.

(viii) Steps should be taken by the State/Union Territory Governments and the Central Government to educate and motivate people for promoting blood donation on a voluntary basis.

(ix) Mental Health must form an integral part of the total health programme and it should be included in all the national policies and programmes in the fields of health, education and social welfare.

(x) The States were urged to reorganise the existing system of collection, compilation and dissemination of health information at various levels for effective monitoring of the programme.

(xi) Health education activities on National Malaria Eradication Programme should be intensified through all available methods.

The Ninth Joint Conference of the Council was held from 7th to 9th July, 1983. Among other important matters, implementation and progress of Family Welfare Programme, National Control of Leprosy, TB and Blindness which form part of the revised 20-Point Programme of the Prime Minister, were reviewed.

Conferences of Health Secretaries of States/Union Territories

With a view to ensuring expeditious and effective implementation of the various health and family welfare programme, particularly those included in the new 20-Point Programme, two conferences of the Health Secretaries of all the States/ Union Territories were convened.

A. *February 1982*—At this conference the focus was on the following :

1. Family Welfare Programme, Family Planning Performance, M.C.H. including Dais' Training Programme, Health Guides Scheme.
2. Progress of schemes under the Minimum Needs Programme.
3. Reorientation of Medical Education Scheme, utilisation of Mobile Clinics.
4. National Malaria Eradication Programme.
5. National Programme for Control of Leprosy and Blindness.
6. Central and centrally sponsored schemes under the Indian Systems of Medicine and Homoeopathy.

B. *January 1983*—At this conference the focus was on the following :

1. Family welfare Programme.
2. Primary Health Care including Minimum Needs Programme.
3. National Programme for Control of Leprosy.
4. National Programme for Control of Blindness.
5. National Programme for Control of TB.
6. National Malaria Eradication Programme.
7. Drugs Control.

The conference facilitated a first hand appraisal of the implementation of the various programmes, besides enabling identification of gaps in the implementation, their filling up and evolution of future strategies.

The Central Council of Health and Family Welfare has been serving a useful role in bringing about informal coordination among the various States and Centre. Health is a state subject and as we know that disease knows no barriers, therefore, there is a need of concerted effort on the part of all the State Health Administrations. Besides, the Council has been highlighting and reviewing the important health challenges facing the country. There has been a gradual evolution of the status and functions of the Council since its establishment in 1952. Its deliberations have provided a common platform to the Centre and the States and also given a new orientation to their relations, symbolic of a healthy development of democratic procedures and traditions. The Council has however, not succeeded in co-ordinating India's health agencies to the extent desirable. In fact, federal and State health agencies have grown into exclusive entities and there is little co-operation among them.

The Council has not been given the task of allocating grants-in-aid to the State Governments. Its effectiveness as an instrument for giving a definite direction to the health policies of the country has therefore, been found to be limited in the matter of implementation of its decisions although collectively taken by the Council. It needs to be given more powers to make it effective. It is also suggested that its recommendations must be given priority consideration by the health administration at Union and State levels. The deliberations of the meeting can be more productive and useful if the specialists in the various fields under discussion are invited to take part in the discussion.

References

1. Ishwar Dayal, "Organisation for Public Policy in Government," a paper submitted to the Seventeenth Conference of the *Indian Institute* of Public Administration, 30 October 1973.
2. Aguilar Montoya C., Medical Officer, Division of Strengthening of Health Services,WHO, Geneva, "Health Goals and the Political Will; Definitions and Problems of National Health Policy" in *WHO Chronicle*, Vol. 31, No. 11. (November 1977), pp. 41-42.
3. WHO, *WHO Chronicle*, November 1977, pp. 441-48.
4. Quoted in Waldo, *Ideas and Issues in Public Administration*, p. 71.
5. Apple by, Paul H., *Policy and Administration*, p. 71.
6. UN, *Development Administration: Current Approaches and Trends in Public Administration, National Development*, New York, 1975, pp. 56-58.
7. *The Indian Express*, New Delhi, 22 April 1977.
8. *The Tribune*, Chandigarh, November 3, 1982.
9. *Ibid.*
10. UN, "The Administration of Economic Development Planning: Principles and Fallacies" (ST/TAD/M/32), Paras 44 and 45.
11. UN, "Administration and National Development Planning," Report of a meeting of experts (ST/TAD/M/27).
12. *Population, Poverty and the Future of India*, by Dr. Karan Singh, p. 89 (Quoted from his speech as "Investment in Man", National Institute of Family Planning, New Delhi, September 1975.

5

Challenges of Health and Health Care Administration

A. Environmental Challenges

Challenge of Poverty

Poverty and low standard of living loom large in the developing world which constitutes 66 per cent of the world population while in terms of GNP it constitutes only 12.5 per cent of the total GNP of the world.[1] The widespread poverty and the depressed standards of living among such large number of people pose a very serious threat to development, peace as well as human creativeness. It is a fact that poverty breeds poverty and poverty of opportunity perpetuates it. The problems of poverty have complex political, social, cultural and environmental roots. Among the developing countries, Eastern Asia and the Pacific is comparatively more poverty stricken. A recent UN report mentioned, "Widespread mass poverty remains the most serious and difficult problem in the region. It was estimated that in 1969, for a number of developing countries in the region which together accounted for nearly a quarter of the world's population, almost 40 per cent of the people were poor (with a per capita income below 50 per year). This proportion was higher than that which obtained in either Latin America or Africa."[2] The same is true today.

The major concern of the developing countries and areas of the region is mass poverty. Johann Peter Frank had rightly said that the people's misery is the mother of all diseases. Let us review the economic scene in four countries of this region.

The analysis of Table 5.1 reveals the prevalence of mass poverty. The per capita figures provide a shocking contrast with an estimated per capita income in the USA of $10,630 and in Switzerland of $13,920 a year in 1979. Again, a further analysis of the GNP per capita statistics reveals that an overwhelming majority of the people are not only poor but are absolutely poor. The World Bank has defined absolute poverty as an income per capita of less than 75 dollars a year. In India, according to UN estimates, two-thirds of the people live in absolute poverty.

The gross national product per capita for the countries of the Region can be seen in the table below, along with the indices of food production, in respect of both total and per capita production. (Refer Table-5.1).

Table: 5.1

Country	*GNP per capita, (1979 US$)*	*Index of food production 1978 (Base 1969-71 = 100)* Total	Per capita
Bangladesh	100	109	93
Burma	160	119	98
India	190	124	102
Indonesia	380	122	99
Nepal	130	110	91
Sri Lanka	230	139	117
Thailand	590	158	122

As regards GNP, Thailand and Indonesia are the two countries with the highest figures, these being US $380 per year respectively. Bangladesh has the lowest figure of US $ 100 per year. With respect of food production some interesting observations may be made. For example, while in all countries total food production increased in 1978 compared to the base period of 1969-71, per capita food production increased only in Sri Lanka and Thailand, and only marginally in India. In the other countries the production of food per capita in 1978 was, in fact, below the level of 1969-71. This indicates that while food production has certainly increased over the period of about 7 to 9 years, a comparatively higher rate of population growth has meant less per head in general.

Table 5.2

Country	*GNP (per capita dollars)*	*Population with income below $ 50 percentages of total population*	*Population with income below $ 75 percentages of total population*
Bangladesh	100	—	—
India	190	45	67
Sri Lanka	230	33	64
Thailand	590	27	44

A World Bank Annual Report (1978) sums up the position in the South Asian Region in these words :

> "Although resolute development efforts have led to significant improvement in the production structure and quality of labour force, economic growth has been sluggish, in most years barely exceeding the rate of population growth. For many of the inhabitants

of this most populous region of the world, conditions have improved only slowly, and some 300 million people have continued to live in extreme poverty and, as a result, are still deprived of adequate food, clean water, and other basic necessities. In the last three years, however, economic growth has generally been somewhat ahead of population growth in the countries of the region with the exception of Pakistan and Nepal."[3]

In the countries of South-East Asia, however, the socio-economic conditions tend to be comparatively better than in the countries of South Asia on the whole. The comparatively well-to-do countries in the economic sense are Indonesia, Malaysia, South Korea, Singapore, which are maintaining a growth rate of 6 per cent GNP. The Philippines and Thailand have also shown a satisfactory record of economic development, by and large. But Burma, the Republic of Vietnam, Laos and Cambodia are poverty-stricken.

According to Dr. H. Mahler : "Social justice demands that the greatest attention be paid to the underprivileged, so that they are able to extricate themselves from the poverty equilibrium in which they are trapped."

Changes of Population Explosion

The problem of rapid population growth and the attendant demographic changes continue to be a grave challenge. Indeed, in view of the 'staggering size of the population and the appalling potential for further increase' the world's population problem is in large part that of the region[4]

The population covered by the WHO South-East Asia Region constitutes almost one-fourth of the world population :

WHO Region	*Population around 1980 (in million)*	*Per Cent*
African	356	8
America	611	14
Eastern Mediterranean	268	6
European	834	19
South-East Asia	1053	24
Western Pacific	1309	29
Total :	4431	100

The land areas covered by the territories of these ten* countries amounts to about 8.5 million square kilometres—a mere 6 per cent of the *World's land surface area*. The gross density of population per sq. km. of 124 for the South-East Asia Region thus compares very unfavourably with the global average of about 31.

* Bhutan became a Member of the Organisation on 8 March, 1982. Information on this country is not included.

CHALLENGES OF HEALTH AND HEALTH CARE ADMINISTRATION

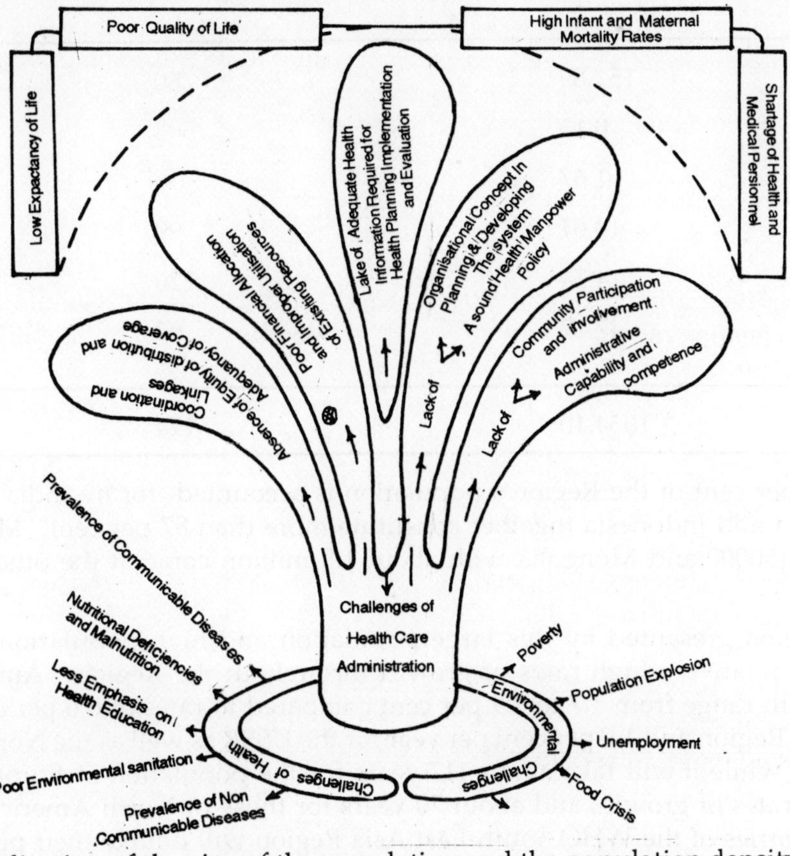

An indication of the size of the population and the population density for each country in the Region in 1980 is shown below:

Country	*Population 1980 (in million)*	*Approximate Population Density (persons/sq. km.)*
1	2	3
Bangladesh	87.66	618
Burma	35.30	53
DPR Korea	17.91	
India	663.60	198

Contd..

1	2	3
Indonesia	151.89	80
Maldives	0.15	503
Mongolia	1.67	1.1
Nepal	14.01	99
Sri Lanka	14.74	226
Thailand	47.17	92
Total :	1034.10	124

Sixty-five per cent of the Region's population is accounted for by India alone, while Bangladesh, India and Indonesia together constitute more than 87 per cent. Maldives with a population of 150000 and Mongolia with about 1.5 million come at the other end of the scale.

The problems presented by this large population and high population density are compounded by relatively high rates of growth throughout the Region. Annual rates of population growth range from 1.7 to 2.9 per cent compared to rates of 0.6 per cent per year for the European Region and 1.0 per cent per year for the USSR as well as the North American continent. Thus, while it will take about 117 years for the population of Europe to double itself at Current rates of growth, and about 70 years for those of North America and USSR, the Member countries of the WHO South-East Asia Region will double their populations in periods from 24 to 41 years.

Country	*Annual rate of growth (per cent)*
Bangladesh	2.4
Burma	2.3
DPR Korea	2.1
India	2.1
Indonesia	2.3
Maldives	2.8
Mongolia	2.9
Nepal	2.2
Sri Lanka	1.7
Thailand	2.4

Projections illustrating population growth to the year 2000 in the countries of the Region are shown in the table below. These were prepared by the United Nations on the basis of likely demographic trends in view of current trends, population age structures, expected social and economic development, government policies and prevailing public attitudes towards population issues. On these assumptions the total population of the Member countries of the Region will increase from the 1975 level of 946.9 million to 1615.6 million by the year 2000, i.e. a 70 per cent increase over 15 years (Refer Table 5.2)

Table: 5.2
POPULATION, 1950-2000 A.D.
WHO SHOUTH-EAST ASIA REGION

	Population (in thousands)*		
Year	*Urban*	*Rural*	*Total*
1950	78650	455774	534424
1960	104366	545559	649925
1970	149014	678841	827855
1975	178258	752897	931155
1980	217100	831541	1048641
1985	267779	909551	1177330
1990	332360	980572	1312932
1995	413095	1041915	1455010
2000	510942	1077797	1588739

The population of the countries of the Region is predominantly rural and comparatively young. Thus, in all countries except Mongolia, more than 75 per cent of the population live in rural areas. The rural proportion of population ranged from 49 per cent (Mongolia) to 96 per cent (Nepal). A trend of gradually increasing urbanisation is discernible in all the countries.

Children under 15 years of age constitute between 39 and 47 per cent of the total population. This percentage has either slightly increased or remained stable in the different countries in recent years. Sri Lanka provides an exception with a slowly declining trend.

Challenge of Unemployment

Although there are difficulties in estimating the extent of unemployment in most developing countries, the problem in Asia is acknowledged as one of massive proportions despite some success in achieving higher rates of economic growth.[5]

* Excluding Democratic People's Republic of Korea.

There is widespread unemployment and underemployment in these countries. In India, according to an assessment made by the Committee on Unemployment (1973), the number of unemployed persons in 1980 was 20.7 million. In the Philippines, it was reported in 1980 that 7.2 per cent of the labour force (out of the total of 15.2 million) were wholly unemployed while 13.5 per cent were underemployed.

In Sri Lanka, 18 per cent of the labour force was reported unemployed in 1980. Unemployment rates are even higher among young people. The unemployment rate is frequently higher in urban areas as compared to rural areas.[6]

Challenge of Food Crisis

There is a grave deterioration and grim future prospects of the world food and nutrition situation with inevitable repercussion on health. President Sanjeeva Reddy while inaugurating the Golden Jubilee Symposium of the Indian Council of Agricultural Research (ICAR) and the First Global Convention of the International Federation of Agricultural Research Systems for Development (IFARD) remarked that "there has been a virtual stagnation in crop yields in many developing countries" and warned the audience about the dangerous implications of the 'dichotomy' between affluent nations where food is no problem and the developing countries where 'God is bread'.[7] Agricultural experts give this warning : "In less than a decade world food supplies must be increased by at least one third to avert widespread families."[8]

Professor Lord Ritchie-Calder (Scotland) has rightly said :

> "In the semantics of today there are gradations of hunger : famine, starvation, undernourishment and malnutrition. On missions for WHO and the other specialised agencies of the UN I have seen many of them... I have seen acute famine in South East Asia, Africa and Latin America."[9]

This position seriously affected the children.

> "They were malnourished to the extent that they were physically, mentally and temperamentally crippled. In less developed countries that generation at risk has numbered tens of millions."[10]

All these factors have adversely affected the health situation in the developing countries.

Challenge of Illiteracy

All the people of the region have not so far been able to get elementary education, e.g. illiteracy rates are very high as can be seen from the Table 5.3 given below :

LEVELS OF EDUCATION IN FOUR SELECTED COUNTRIES

Country	*Percentage of illiteracy*
Bangladesh	75.7
India	71.5
Sri Lanka	21.5
Thailand	30.0

The conditions are worse in Bangladesh and India while the position is better in Sri Lanka and Thailand. Without higher literacy rates, it is difficult to provide good health care. It has been rightly said by the Education Commission that the destiny of a nation is shaped in her classrooms. The future of a nation depends upon the quantity and quality of students coming out of schools and colleges. Illiteracy is a great obstruction in the path of development, and education is the backbone of democracy. The Director General of UNESCO has described illiteracy as :

> "The most monstrous of all the many instances of wasted human potential—which still at the present time keeps more than one-third of the human race in a state of hopelessness, below the level of modern civilisation."

Thus, it is imperative to increase the literacy rate to bring about all-round development. Education helps an individual to develop his potential to the full, to increase his productivity and to become a useful and responsible member of the society.

Dr. Amin El Gamal, Under-Secretary of Health, Egypt, in his article "An Attainable Target" in *World Health* (November, 79) states that "the degree of literacy in any country can be shown to relate directly to that country's health status."

B. Challenges of Public Health

We shall now discuss the health situation in the developing countries with the help of some indicators,[11] with special reference to four countries of the South-East Asia Region:[12] Bangladesh, India, Sri Lanka and Thailand. This will help us in understanding and analysing the problems of health care administration.

Low Expectation of Life at Birth

A vast number of people are dying because of low standards of health in the developing world. The life expectancy at birth has increased marginally during the last two decades. In these countries over the years, as seen from Table 5.4 the life expectancy at birth has registered an increase in India from 41.9 (male) and 40.6 (female) in 1960 to 52.6 and 51.6

respectively in 1978. There has been marginally in the expectation of life at birth from 1960 to this date in Sri Lanka and Thailand. There has been reverse trends in Bangladesh, i.e., expectation of life at birth has gone down from 54.3 (male) and 47.4 (female) in 1960 to 45.8 and 46.6 respectively in 1974. It indicates the poor progress of health facilities. The corresponding figure for Europe and North America has been 71.

Table:5.4

EXPECTATION OF LIFE AT BIRTH IN THE FOUR SELECTED COUNTRIES

Country		*1960*	*1970*	*Latest Information*	*Available Reference data*
Bangladesh	Male	54.3	—	45.8	1974
	Female	47.4	—	46.6	
India	Male	41.9	47.1	52.6	1976-81
	Female	40.6	45.6	51.6	
Sri Lanka	Male	61.9	—	68.0	1981
	Female	61.4	—	68.0	
Thailand	Male	53.6	62.8	57.6	1980
	Female	58.7	68.9	61.0	

Source : WHO; SEARO

High Infant and Maternal Mortality Rates

During the last three decades, maternal and childhood mortality rates have been steadily decreasing in most parts of the world. In the South-East Asia the progress has been slow. As seen from Table 5.5 infant mortality rate in India has come down marginally from 125 (1970) to 122 (1978), in Sri Lanka from 56.8 (1960) to 37.1 (1978), in Thailand from 48.9 to 13.3 while in Bangladesh from 149 (1970) to 140 (1980). This is a clear indication of unsatisfactory maternal and child health services, mentioned by a joint WHO-UNICEF study:

"In the less developed regions the infant mortality rate was 140 per 1000 life births, dramatically higher than the rate of 27 per 1000 in the more developed region, there was an enormous variation among countries from an estimated maximum of about 200 to a minimum of 9.6 per 1000. If developing countries could bring their infant mortality rates down to the average rate of the developed, some 11 million infant lives could be saved each year...While on average the infant mortality rate is 10-20 times higher in developing than in the developed countries, the average mortality rate between the ages of one and four years is 30.50 times higher."[13]

Table 5.5

INFANT (IM) AND MATERNAL MORTALITY RATE (MM) IN THE FOUR SELECTED COUNTRIES

Country		*1960*	*1970*	*Latest information*	*Available reference data*
Bangladesh	IM	—	149	140	1980
	MM	—	25	30	1980
India	Registration of Infant death is poor. No reliable All India figures are available. Prior to 1969-70, the registered infant death rate varied, from 28 in Andaman and Nicobar Islands to 136 in Pondicherry in 1961 and from 27 in Kerala to 106 in Pondicherry in 1965. Same is true of MM. In 1980, IM and MM in India are 125 and 5-8 respectively.				
Sri Lanka	IM	56.8	50.3	37.1	1978
	MM	3.0	1.2	0.8	1978
Thailand	IM	48.9	25.5	13.3	1980
	MM	4.2	2.3	1.2	1980

Source : WHO - SEARO.

Shortage of Health and Medical Personnel

The doctor-population ratio is accepted as a general but rough indicator of the development level of health services. If we examine the figures given in the following Table 5.6 we find that the increase in medical personnel has merely kept pace with the increase in population.

In the table 5.6, this information is summarised and presented, for comparative purposes, in terms of doctors and hospital beds per 10000 population.

Table 5.6

	Number per 10000 population			
Country	*Doctors*	*Nurses*	*Hospital Beds*	*Health Centres*
1	2	3	4	5
Bangladesh	1.2	0.3	2.4	0.03
Burma	2.1	2.3	8.2	0.48

Contd..

1	2	3	4	5
India	2.8	2.1	7.1	0.84
Indonesia	0.8	1.3	6.5	0.75
Maldives	0.5	0.5	3.5	1.04
Mongolia	21.3	0.4	106.3	9.00
Nepal	0.3	0.3	1.9	0.44
Sri Lanka	1.4	4.6	29.4	0.97
Thailand	1.4	3.5	13.3	1.05

Let us also mention in the context of Doctors per 10,000 in various regions of the world to understand the gravity of the situation.

Let us see the situation in this regard in other regions.

World Average	*Number of doctors per 10,000 in various regions*
Africa	8
Americas	1.36
Asia	10.76
Europe	2.84
USSR	14.85
Oceania	12.8

The general inference to be drawn from these figures is that the medical personnel in Africa and Asia has not kept pace with the needs of the people. The difference within the regions is very high.

The situation is more critical than it would appear since the great proportion of medical personnel in this region are located in urban centres, and the rural population receives correspondingly less service from the professional staff. Then, there is loss to the region through the migration of trained health personnel. What can be done? The only alternative is to prepare health personnel of a lower category at a quicker rate to meet the basic needs of the rural people. The *Ceylon Medical Journal* has reported that in any formal education programme, depth of understanding must yield place to breadth of knowledge.[14]

Health Expenditure vis-a-vis Total Expenditure

The health expenditure in countries (see Table 5.7) has been very low and has been decreasing over the years, e.g., the present health expenditure in Bangladesh, India, Sri Lanka and Thailand has been 5.5, 2.1, 6.09 and 6.07 per cent of the total budget which is very low. Most of the countries invest about 40 per cent of their total budget for health. The developing countries must invest more money in social services to obtain lasting results.

Table 5.7

Health Expenditure as per cent of Total Expenditure in the Four Selected Countries.

Countries	*1960*	*1970*	*Latest information*	*Available reference data*
Bangladesh	—	—	5.5	1980
India	3.0	2.11	2.1	1980
Sri Lanka	8.7	7.5	6.09	1980
Thailand	2.8	4.9	6.07	1980

Source : WHO - SEARO.

We have reviewed some of the statistics to indicate the present low-level of health in this region. Let us now review the specific health challenges.

Prevalence of Communicable Diseases

Communicable diseases continue to constitute the regions's major public health problem. In spite of increased efforts to control malaria, the morbidity and mortality due to the disease appear to be on the increase in most of the countries. The region is free from small-pox . However, tuberculosis, cholera and diarrhoeal diseases have been the cause of concern. Besides, sexually transmitted diseases pose a serious challenge to the region. Let us discuss in detail in the context of cholera.

Despite annual variations in the number of countries reporting cholera and in the number of cases notified to WHO, the global cholera situation has not changed substantially during the last ten years. Cholera is still present in many countries in an endemic form with serious outbreaks periodically. In 1980, there was a noticeable decline in the number of cases in Asia with 19108 reported compared with 35397 in 1979; the number of countries reporting cholera dropped from 21 in 1979 to 15 in 1980. This decline is mainly caused by the absence of notifications from Bangladesh and by the decrease in Indonesia from 18817 cases in 1979 to 5541 cases in 1980. In the South-East Asia region the number of cases reported were : Burma — 1018; India — 5960; Indonesia — 5541; Thailand — 4331; Sri Lanka — 33; and Nepal — just one case. The total number of cases in the region is 16884 against the total of 19108 for Asia and the world total of 36815. Cholera incidence reported in three successive years in the region was as follows :

Table 5.8

	1979	*1980*	*1981*
Bangladesh	2154	Nil	Nil
Burma	874	1018	28
India	2912	5960	4659
Indonesia	18817	5541	5857
Nepal	22	1	24
Sri Lanka	46	33	547
Thailand	1739	4331	39
Total	26564	16884	11154

For the region as a whole, there has been a decline in the reported cases over the three years, but individual countries did not conform to this pattern. While 1981 was the year of lowest incidence of reported cholera for Burma and Thailand, it was of medium incidence for India and Indonesia, and of highest incidence for Sri Lanka and Nepal.

Communicable diseases were mainly responsible for high mortality and morbidity and an immediate need of the region is the control and eradication of these diseases.

Nutritional Deficiencies and Malnutrition

Malnutrition, which is a more serious scourge than hunger, is, to a certain extent, caused by ignorance and faulty food habits, though largely it may be due to depressing poverty. According to Dr. Mahler :

> "Malnutrition is both one of the consequences of social injustice and one of the factors contributing to its maintenance. It bears hardest on small children, contributing to the massive death toll among the young, and together with other adverse environmental factors, it interferes with the growth and development of the survivals. It reduces their capacity to learn during childhood and to earn during adulthood. The inevitable result is a downwards spiral in which poor malnourished parents produce malnourished children who in turn will become poor and malnourished parents."[15]

Malnutrition is responsible for five main diseases—anaemia, endemic goitre, kwashiorkor, marasmus and erophthalmia. Thus even when the general demands for food are met, this does not mean that nutritional needs are satisfied.

Nutritional deficiencies, especially in proteins, are likely to persist for a long time to come. However, in order to raise general standards of health, productivity of labour and general equality of life, improved nutrition is indispensable. It is especially important to child health. It is estimated that 70 per cent of children in developing countries are suffering from malnutrition. It needs immediate attention of the policy makers.

> "Nutrition of underdeveloped countries can no longer be viewed as a narrow task aimed at providing the human body with right quantities and qualities of carbohydrates, proteins and micronutrients. In these countries it must be regarded as synonymous with modernisation, an important wind of change of social and economic development. Technological change in poor countries must have central concern with nutrition."[16]

It has been estimated that at the beginning of this decade, about 30 million people, 30 per cent of the population of the region did not have a sufficient protein energy supply.[17]

J.M.Bengoa, [18] Chief Medical Officer, Nutrition, WHO stated :

> "At a conservative estimate, there are at least 100 million undernourished children in the world mostly in the developing countries. While some of them die from the malnutrition, a vastly greater proportion suffer from physical and possible mental retardation and are highly susceptible to infectious disease."

The estimated number of children aged 0-4 years suffering from severe or moderate protein calorie malnutrition (PCM) in these regions of the world are given below in Table 5.9.

Table 5.9

NUMBER OF CHILDREN (0-4 YEARS) SUFFERING FROM SEVERE & MODERATE PCM IN THE DIFFERENT REGIONS OF THE WORLD

Region	*Severe PCM*	*Moderate PCM*	*Total*
Latin America	700 000	9 000 000	9 700 000
Africa	2 700 000	16 000 000	18 700 000
Asia	9 000 000	64 000 000	70 000 000
	9 400 000	89 000 000	98 400 000

Less Emphasis on Health Education

High morbidity and high mortality particularly among children result from low priority accorded to health education. Many diseases can be averted if proper education is given to the people. Without the understanding active cooperation and involvement of all members of the community and a knowledge and motivation on their part of how to obtain the most from the health services provided, whether preventive or curative, much of the time, money and effort invested in these services can be lost.[19]

Poor Environmental Sanitation[20]

Poor environmental sanitation in the region is responsible for a number of diseases. We must ensure healthy environment for healthy living. Exposure to infection in the region comes mainly from lack of safe water and sewerage disposal facilities in most of the areas. The condition in regard to these services is very serious. Let us review the situation with the help of the Table 5.10.

Safe water supply should normally include treated surface water and untreated but uncontaminated water from protected boreholes, springs and wells. Other sources of doubtful quality should be considered unsafe and not included in the estimate of coverage. Percentage figures of coverage are available, giving population served by completed water systems separately for urban and rural areas from the International Drinking Water Supply and Sanitation Decade (IDWSSD). Facilities for hygienic waste disposal are considered adequate if they effectively prevent contact with or access to excreta by humans, animals and insects. Population coverage data are available from the IDWSSD data for hygienic waste disposal facilities. These data for each country are summarised and given in the table below. They refer to the year 1981.

Table 5.10

STATUS OF WATER SUPPLY AND SEWERAGE DISPOSAL (1981)

Country	*Percentage of population covered by*			
	Water supply		*Sanitation*	
	Urban	*Rural*	*Urban*	*Rural*
Bangladesh	26	40	22	1
Burma	38	15	38	15
DPR Korea	100	100	100	100
India	75	31	27	1
Nepal	83	7	16	1
Sri Lanka	75	18	75	63
Thailand	65	64	64	41

Source: WHO:SEARO—Bulletin of Regional Health Information, 1981.

The above figures reveal that the situation of safe water supply for drinking is quite inadequate. Rural areas received less service than urban areas. Facilities for safe public sewerage disposal are seriously inadequate, while in rural areas facilities tend to be absent altogether.

Prevalence of Non-Communicable Diseases

Non-communicable diseases are not considered priority problems in the region except in Democratic People's Republic of Korea. Cardiovascular diseases, cancer, drug addiction, mental diseases and radiological hazards are emerging as significant health problems.

UNICEF, WHO study has nicely analysed the health problems in developing countries. It was stated :

> "The principal causes of morbidity in the developing world are malnutrition, vector borne diseases, gastro intestinal diseases, and respiratory diseases themselves the result of poverty, squalor and ignorance. To them must be added the disease of mothers related to deprivation, unregulated fertility, and exhaustion, with their effects on the unborn and new born child. These conditions are linked with social problems such as over work among women, unemployment among the young, population growth and urbanisation; and their solution calls for an integrated effort in which the health services have a major role to play."[21]

C. Challenges of Health Care Administration

We have examined the present health situation in the developing countries which is quite discouraging though hope-inspiring. There is a great potential in the developing countries to solve all the present and emerging health problems. This needs resolute determination to solve health problems based on proper planning. Health services have become more complex as the result of technological, social and economic advances. In order to reap the benefits of modernisation, recent UN report has indicated that in both developed and developing countries, "a growing awareness has emerged for the need of a more efficient administration, management and delivery of health care services, which will have to be more adapted to local conditions."[22]

We shall discuss the challenges of health administration which need the attention of policy-makers, planners and health administrators, to provide adequate and effective health care to all at the earliest. This calls for strengthening the administration and management of the national health services.

> "Effective administration and management call for more intensive preparation and training of senior medical and non-medical administrative personnel, whose functions must be considered in the wider context of the national public administration and not just in the mere limited sphere of public health administration. The major share of national budgets in the future will most certainly go to the departments that develop and use the best systems of planning, performance and programmes— accountability."[23]

Let us now review some of the inadequacies of health administration which need immediate attention to provide decent health care to all.

The health care administration has been functioning with the following shortcoming:

(a) The inability of the health care system to make available the services required to meet the demands of those most in need, who are usually too poor or too geographically or socially remote to benefit from such facilities.

(b) Wide differences in resources distribution and service and a multiplicity of institutions which are unrelated and not functioning as a system.

(c) The placing of emphasis on medical rather than overall health care. The curative aspect of care has been stressed with insufficient priority to promotive, preventive and rehabilitative care. This has resulted in a fragmentation of the care provided to the individual.

(d) Training of health personnel directed primarily towards medical and institutional care, and largely irrelevant to the tasks and functions required outside institutional setting.

(e) The education and training of health professionals in such a manner as to accentuate the social distance between health professionals and the population, resulting in an inability on the part of the providers of health services to identify with the consumers.

(f) A lack of recognition as well as a rejection of useful, traditional healing practices.

(g) An inadequate assessment of other community resources, imposing unnecessary limitations on the scope of action of health services and often preventing them from approaching major community needs in an effective manner.

(h) The people have rarely been given the opportunity to play an active role in deciding the types of activities they want and have not participated in the actual services they receive. Community interest and resources have too often been inadequately expressed and activated because there has been a failure to recognise that people will be most interested in and responsive to activities related to their own priority concerns.

We have discussed in detail some of these problems in the various chapters that would follow. We shall concentrate here only on some of the challenges of health care administration.

Lack of Coordination and Linkages

Coordination means bringing about consistent and harmonious action of persons and programmes with each other towards a common goal. The coordination is lacking in the field of health care administration resulting in poor delivery of health services. Professor Mofide (Iran) has rightly indicated the prevailing atmosphere when he states : " In the majority of countries with some or all of these problems (environmental) pollution, uncontrolled population growth; nutritional deficiencies; the high risk of disease; shortages and maldistribution of trained staff; and insufficient financial, material and physical resources, there exists also a fragmentation of responsibilities for the delivery of health care, with overlapping, conflicting, and competing organisations within the health system and widely scattered funding mechanisms with little control over costs. Health services authorities give only token recognition to those segments of the services that are not under their direct executive or financial control, and often plan only for that part of the national budget that is said to be their responsibility. The state of affairs is unjustified and harmful."[24]

Resources for the health care delivery are limited in the developing world. An effective health approach and strategy requires the coordinated efforts of sectors and agencies that can contribute directly or indirectly to the promotion of health care. Such coordinated efforts would promote health services that will be more efficiently and effective from both standpoint of the providers and that of the beneficiaries. The need of coordination is so great that according to Findlay, "It expresses the principles of organisation in toto; nothing less."[25]

The first essential requisite to achieve coordination is to develop meaningful linkages with sectors of social and economic development which can influence the promotion of health care, e.g., agriculture, public works, housing, communication, education, etc.

The second step is to pool the efforts of all health agencies at all levels in a system to achieve maximum output—public and private; national and international; curative and promotive; peripheral, intermediate and central; western medicine and traditional medicine. This would avoid the dangers of dysfunctional attitudes.

Third, there is the need of welding different aspects of health services into a total health package, e.g., integration of maternal and child care, family planning, prevention of communicable diseases, health education, environmental sanitation.

Coordination and linkages on a systematic, rather than on ad hoc basis will definitely reduce costly duplications of efforts and lead to increased health coverage of the needy population and neglected area, while making the optimum use of the resources. Most of the countries in their reply to the WHO admitted that the lack of coordination in health care delivery system is a serious challenge. To quote WHO :

> "The consensus of opinion is that the most important managerial problems are foreseen in the continued reduction of the imbalance of the system and the lack of integration in the distribution of care with the existence of parallel systems with different objectives. Fragmentation and division of responsibility between the different levels of care have led tó a lack of effective communication between the health and social welfare agencies... As there are several agencies providing medical care there is overlapping and duplication of activities... The major managerial problems... is to recognise the various components of this system in a way that reflects complementarily, eliminates duplication, and minimises waste of resources."[26]

This problem becomes more acute in a federal country like India where health is a State subject. It becomes important to coordinate the health programmes at the national level. The dilution of health standards in one State may affect adversely the whole country. There is a need, therefore, to give more powers to the central authority by making health a Concurrent subject. One of the health experts went to say: "The present health situation in developing countries, especially India, is in a chaotic condition as no scientific and realistic attempt is visible to coordinate the available inputs to produce maximum output. We can locate a large area without any health care facilities while in some areas, every third shop or house is providing medical care."[27]

How can we achieve effective coordination ? According to Dr. White, its achievement may require.

> "The most delicate insights, the most mature wisdom, and perception of a truly artistic quality."[28]

It has to be achieved through formal as well as informal methods.

The effective co-ordination and linkages would automatically result from effective planning, policy-making, manpower planning.[29] After planning and policy making, the effective instrument to achieve coordination is to design a sound organisation. Dr. While says :

> "An organisation characterised by clear lines of authority, adequate powers, well-understood allocation of functions, absence of overlapping and duplication of effort and proper delegation of work in itself reduce the necessities of coordination."[30]

Besides, if the organisational boundaries are properly demarcated, there would be little scope of confusion and misunderstanding and coordination would naturally flow from this inherent structure.

The coordination among different agencies, however, can be obtained through mutual consultation or information. This mutual consultation should be encouraged through setting up of inter-departmental agency/committees for joint planning, joint decision-making and joint action in areas concerning more than one agency. While achieving coordination, we may keep the cost factor in mind. Such inter or intra agencies can serve a useful purpose when the members come duly prepared with a sense of urgency and commitment. According to Key, "a session of an inter-departmental committee tends to be a place where departmental representatives come well prepared to defend their positions and leave more convinced than before of the correctness of their attitudes."[31]

We are to take care that the benefits achieved through coordination would surpass the expenditure incurred to obtain coordination.

Besides formal methods, we should adopt informal methods which are as effective as the formal ones, e.g., the Central Council of Health and the Central Council of Family Welfare (India) uses the informal method to achieve coordination among the different States and between the Union Government and the State Governments. "It is the most powerful cement in the whole executive structure."[32]

We must encourage such informal methods at all levels of Government.

We must try to achieve coordination to obtain coherency in all the agencies dealing directly or indirectly with health care, all the systems of medicines, all the persons responsible for health care (team work) and at all the levels through well designed formal and informal organisation with minimum costs to fulfil the goal — the betterment of the health of mankind irrespective of the status and location and to obtain optimum benefit from available and potential resources.

Lack of Equity of Distribution and Adequacy of Coverage in Relationship to Need

According to David Morely : "Three quarters of our population are rural, yet three quarters of our medical resources are spent in the towns where three quarters of our doctors live. Three quarters of the people die from diseases which could be prevented at low cost and yet three quarters of medical budgets are spent on curative services."

The large population of the people living in rural areas are not being provided even rudimentary health care in this age of modern medicine. The benefits of modern medicine are available only to the chosen few living in metropolitan cities, e.g., 10-20 per cent of the people are consuming 80 per cent of the resources invested in health care in India. What has happened during the last three decades is not in tune with the spirits of the Constitution of India. The Government must serve the millions of people who suffer from chronic poverty, ignorance, disease and inequality of opportunity. The Government must fulfil the aspirations of the people enshrined in the Constitution Austin summed up the Constitution of India in the following words :

> "The Indian Constitution is first and foremost a social document. The majority of its provisions are either directly aimed at furthering the goals of the social revolution or attempt to foster this revolution by establishing the conditions necessary for its achievement. Yet despite the permeation of the entire constitution by the aim of national renaissance the core of commitment to the social revolution lies in part III and IV, in the Fundamental Rights and in the Directive Principles of State Policy. They are the conscience of the Constitution."[33]

Have we lived up to the expectations and aspirations of the people ? The answer is plain and simple: certainly not. What can we do in future ? We can devise technology and organisation objectives and structure that would benefit the largest number of the people and if possible to the last person as desired by Mahatma Gandhi. What is required is change of ideology, philosophy and priorities in favour of the poor people, i.e., any device to improve health care should ensure improvement in the health status of the whole population. This may be possible if our planning in future takes care of the following :

(a) We should attend to the needs of the largest groups rather than meet the demands of a particular group or section of society. We can ascertain the need of the target groups through epidemiological studies.

(b) We may provide that health care to the people through the technology that may reach all. We may not invest in highly sophisticated technology only to be used by the few. The dilemma can be best described as an attempt to ride two horses galloping in different directions. On the one hand is maintenance of the high standard of medical excellence taught in the West. The other is the problem of providing health care for the millions of poor who cannot possibly provide an economic support base for our Western styled health systems. There is no particular merit in promoting the health level of medical services when the direct result is medical care costed beyond the reach of four-fifths of the population.[34]

The Government of India is presently thinking of reviving short-term LSMF (Licentiate of the State Medical Faculty) to provide health care to the rural population in 580,000 villages. The Tribune Editorial has rightly mentioned :

> "The Medical Council of India's opposition to the short-term medical course and the doubling of Licentiate Doctors as half baked seems strangle in view of the fact that in three decades we have failed to remove dichotomy of 85 per cent of the health resources being utilised for the benefit of less than 15 per cent of the country's population. On the contrary, the revival of the licentiate cadre may lessen the burden of the MBBS doctors, especially, general practitioners."[35]

Thus, we want train more and more health personnel of lower categories who can serve the people at large and restrict the few specialities only for referral services.

The United Nations in its 1974 Report on the world social situation reported :

> "Despite the generally greater availability of resources, most governments are faced with difficult choices, because of the recognised need to provide the best possible personnel health care to the rapidly growing population, on the one hand, and because of limitation created by the increase in costs, on the other. Even the most affluent countries have started encountering growing financial difficulties in responding to the health demands of their people. Governments are now paying closer attention to the amount they spend on health services and the value they get in return. They are considering new financing arrangements in the health care field with the objective of reducing the rate of cost escalation and enabling health authorities to achieve flexibility in determining priorities and in pursuing the most efficient and effective approaches to health care."[36]

Kenneth Hill is surprised to notice the opposition of the health experts in the use of Auxiliaries. He says, "Although the use of intermediary personnel is on the increase, resistance to their recognition continues and this is often even stronger in developing countries than it is elsewhere. It is hard to understand the rationale of such opposition. It is true that there is a remote danger of people with less advanced training developing inflated ideas of there own capabilities, but such people can only be relatively few and they will be found at the fringe."

All this would be possible if the principles of socialism are put into practice. This would encourage political, economic and social democracy. Nehru, in his presidential address at the Lucknow session of AICC in April, 1936, expressed his deep faith in the success of socialism. "I am convinced". He said, "that the only key to the solution of world's problems and that of India's problems lies in socialism and when I use this word, I do so, not in vague humanitarian way but in the scientific-economic sense. Socialism, however, is something more than an economic doctrine, it is a philosophy of life...I see no way of ending poverty, the vast unemployment, the degradation and subjection of Indian people except through socialism."

If socialism is established in the real sense in the developing world, the entrenched disparities would go away benefiting the poor. This would automatically solve the problems in the field of health care administration as well.

Poor Financial Allocation to the Health Care Delivery and Improper Utilisation of Existing Resources

The developing countries give low priority in the allocation of resources to the health care of their people. We can see from the table given earlier that the expenditure has been very low. The health expenditure to the total expenditure has been very low in South-East Asian Countries, i.e., 1.6 per cent in Indonesia, 2.1 per cent in India, 3.8 per cent in Bangladesh, Mongolia has been spending 10 per cent for the health care of its people. There is a need to raise the health allocations to improve the quality of life. Dr. White has rightly said that, "Nothing can be done without the expenditure of money...Available financial resources set a maximum limit on administrative activity as a whole and on each of its separate parts."[37]

A sound state of finance is of paramount importance to the political health of a nation... The soundness of public finance depends both upon the right policy and good organisation, but a great deal upon the latter.[38] The scarcity of resources affect all aspects of the health delivery system. There is a need to step up the health allocations to the minimum of 10 per cent of the total budget.

Secondly, there is maldistribution of health resources. Most of the health budgets (about 80 per cent) are being spent only on a few people (20 per cent). This deprives the people living in rural areas and urban slums. A WHO study group on the Financing of Health Services which met in Geneva from 21 to 25 November, 1977, mentioned the following characteristics which reflect the situation in, the developing countries.[39]

(a) Disproportionate concentration of expenditure on health services in urban areas compared with expenditure in rural areas.

(b) Heavy concentration of expenditure on secondary and territory care services compared with expenditure on primary care services.

(c) Heavy concentration of expenditure on curatives services compared with expenditure on preventive services.

We can correct this imbalances through the innovative health policies developed in tune with the needs of the country rather than based on any foreign model.[40]

The third serious problem in this area is of inefficient use of expenditure and non-utilisation of actual and potential resources judiciously and properly. In the developing countries, huge resources are being wasted because of the selection of inappropriate technology,[41] inefficient management,[42] and unsatisfactory control mechanisms.

> "It is necessary that public revenue should be raised is an equitable manner and spent economically so that the tax-payers may get full value for his money."[43]

The objects of financial control are to ensure —(i) that no wastage of resources occurs; (ii) that public money is not misused; and (iii) that intended results are obtained with the money spent. We can exploit the potential resources through careful planning and management. The traditional system of medicine can be of immense value to provide health care at a very low cost provided this is properly tapped by the designers of health services. It was reported in a recent UN Survey (1976) that, there adverse trends are despite the higher percentage of government expenditure being devoted to health, compared with 1960s and the fact that ratio of population to the numbers of beds and of medical personnel have moved favourably. Essentially, the continuance of poor health standards is indicative of a less-than-optimal use of resources available. Some aspects of this are the emphasis on curative, as opposed to preventive techniques embodies in the existing hospital systems, the inadequate development of indigenous medicine systems on which there is a continued reliance and the limited coverage of available medical facilities particularly in rural areas.[44]

In a paper presented by M.Siegel, Assistant Director-General, Department of Administration and Finance, WHO, Geneva, to the Advisory Group on Nursing Administration (16 December (1957) rightly remarked :

> "If the resources for health work, in trained persons and in finances, were unlimited, the need for constant attention to these factors would not be so great. But the limitation in the number of trained personnel and the lack of adequate financial resources are major obstacles to greatly improved health in the world today. We must, therefore, husband our resources carefully to accomplish as much as possible with what we have available."

The fourth serious challenge in this field is the rising cost of health services beyond the reach of most of the people inhabiting the developing societies. It is very difficult to afford the costly urban-based hospitals using highly sophisticated technology. A huge amount is being spent on costly buildings and equipment which the developing countries cannot afford. The only services which can meet the health needs of the people are low-cost services which should be efficient and effective. This is possible if we use methods and equipment appropriate to the socio-economic environment existing in a country, e.g., the people can contribute voluntary labour to maintain health services. This would reduce the cost. We must take decisions and think of alternative solutions to provide health care to the people as financing and decision-making are complementary functions. The health administrator should encourage the low-cost service programmes beneficial to the larger section of the community.

The fifth problem in this connection is the lack of coordination among different agencies financing health care services. This may result in wasteful duplication of efforts. Besides, many health services may not get the desired financial allocation because of this wastage. The situation can be improved through proper coordination among such agencies.

Lack of Adequate Information Required for Health Planning, Implementation and Evaluation

Information is the life-blood of an organisation. According to R.R. Duersch, "it is a system which provides management with the information it requires to monitor progress, measure performance, detect trends, evaluate alternatives, make decision and to take corrective action"[45]

There is no centralised department in the health organisation to collect, analyse, interpret, store and retrieve information. Confusion between 'Statistical data' and 'information' still prevail, with the result that many statistical services fail to provide public health administrators with the information they need for sound decision-making, planning and evaluation. In most of the health organisations, the data collected from the field is either not of the required type or is not presented in a form or in time to be really useful to health administrators. Besides, the data is collected without a clear understanding about the use that such information will have. The routine collection of data which is neither reliable nor timely serves no purpose. These defects can be weeded out if we can design a Scientific Health Information System or Management Information System (MIS). MIS is an analytical tool which facilitate more informal and better decision to be made and it helps to identify problem areas and to take timely remedial measures. It is in no case a substitution for management decision but it is management's most important tool for decision-making. *As Morton puts it* :

> "Good management information system is no cure for bad management. Bad information always leads to bad management, but good information does not in itself ensure good management.Information is only a tool of management. The ability to put information to work is what determines a successful manager."[46]

Four basic processes involved in an information system are — the collection of data, storing of data, processing of data and transmission of information. The term *data* is used to denote the input into the information system while *information* is the output. MIS should be designed to ensure smooth and proper flow of information into the desired channels. The information must be made available to the management at the required time and in right quantity and quality. It is also to be borne in mind that supplying unnecessary or unwanted information is also a sign of inefficiency of the system. To quote a UNICEF Report :

> "Information Services should be recast according to the priorities of the health system and should be aimed strictly at problem solving."[47]

Lack of Organisation Concept in Planning and Developing the System

The absence of a clear national health policy in most of the countries has created an environment in which fragmented health services have sprung up haphazardly. There is a need of a balanced health policy. Besides, the health planning though picking up, has yet to be adopted in the right earnest. The planning of health services and their expansion requires special skills and knowledge which must be cultivated among the personnel responsible for planning. Proper identification of the health needs and priorities of the general population, is essential for the development of a comprehensive national health plan.[48]

Lack of a Sound Health Manpower Policy[49]

A sound health manpower policy is the main requirement for the development of any functionally effective health care system. Most of the countries in the developing world have never formulated or implemented such a policy.

> "The most crucial factor for the improvement of the world health situation... is undoubtedly the development of health manpower that is properly attuned to the health problems of the people and suitably trained to respond to health programme and service need."[50]

We must find the method to achieve greater productivity, efficiency and cost-effectiveness in health manpower utilisation. No society, especially the developing, can long justify investing years of education and training in individuals who later on perform rudimentary duties that could be achieved satisfactorily by people trained in half that time. The critical decisions in health manpower planning concern the kinds of personnel required, the type and adequacy of education and training and financial resources necessary to produce them, their relationship to each other in the health team, and where and how they would practise.

Lack of Community Participation and Involvement

Merlie Fainsod remarks : " The most favourable setting for progress in development administration exists where a politically influential and dynamic modernising elite strongly desires development and can successfully project this attitude into both the bureaucracy and the population at large "[51]

Many well-intentioned and technically sound programmes aimed at solving health problems have been frustrated by a lack of popular acceptance and community participation. "It has been observed that such programmes are either not actively associated or passively ignored because they do not 'belong' to the population they are designed to help; they are rather seen by the population as imposed external programmes that belong to the government and consequently deserve and require little, if any, of the population's attention, action, or other response" We must be clear that health cannot be imposed; it can only be acquired. This requires participation based on enlightenment of the beneficiaries.

Dr. Madiou Toure, Director Hygiene and Health Protection, Ministry of Public Health, Republic of Senegal, in his article, "The Health Revolution", in World Health (November, 1979) has rightly said: "The medicine of tomorrow will be shaped by the people for the people, because the people themselves will determine their own condition, their own destiny."

Lack of Administrative Capability and Competence

Administrative capability is *sine qua non* for the success of any programme. It is a major and crucial factor in the success or failure of development programmes. It is the scarcest of all resources in the developing world. The general administrator is fit only for the maintenance of law and order and he is not suitably equipped to deal with the problems of development and welfare economics.

According to K.N. Rao : "Unlike advanced countries there is no pool of experienced and well informed leaders of thought available as potential leaders for ministerial positions which greatly handicaps their assuming policy making and decision-making responsibilities in the Government. This results in overdependence on the Secretaries who are non-technical general administrators."

The technical experts must be given training in public health administration to make them competent in the art of health planning and administration.

Highly Centralised : Need of Decentralisation

The national health system, within whose structure the services required to deliver care to the urban, suburban and rural family nucleus must be organised, is a mechanism of such administrative complexity that it cannot possibly be run on a centralised basis. Hence the need to decentralise the administrative process. This decentralisation should include the extensive delegation of functions from the higher to the intermediate and local echelons, so as to produce effective decentralisation in staff and management, budgetary control, application of laws and regulations and if possible, financing as well. A consequence of this will be the need to provide administrative facilities at the regional level. An important factor supplementing the mechanisms of decentralisation should be the participation of the community and of the health professional in the administration of the regional and local services.

In most countries there is a marked trend in the opposite direction, i.e., towards centralisation of authority, and it is not always easy to convince the powers that be of the need to decentralise the health services. There are nevertheless many reasons that justify decentralisation. One that has already been mentioned is the extent of the facilities needed to provide comprehensive preventive, curative and rehabilitative services to the whole population of a country. This requires a large multidisciplinary staff which must deliver an enormous variety of services involving different technologies to a population composed of millions of individuals of widely differing cultural levels and with different health needs. The administrative machinery required to operate this gigantic service is so complex that its management cannot be centralised furthermore, if planning and evaluation of these services is to be conducted locally, it is essential that the implementation of the health activities also be directed at the local level, with the effective participation of the suppliers and consumers of health services.

D. Meeting the Challenges

On the basis of our discussion and analysis the following suggestions are given in brief to revitalise the health care delivery system, to meet the challenges and fulfil the basic health needs of the people.

(i) Need of will and determination on the part of the political elite, to accept innovative measures to meet the population's health needs and priorities.

(ii) Identification and implementation of a clear and comprehensive National Health Policy.

(iii) Need of decentralised planning involving the participation of the target communities.

(iv) Mobilisation of existing and untapped resources— community, government (local and national), bilateral, multilateral and non-governmental to provide adequate health care for all.

(v) Establishment of appropriate administrative structures with necessary competence and capability and devolution of authority and responsibility for the implementation and development of the programme in a team spirit and a well designed information system to help in planning, implementation and evaluation.

(vi) Manpower development for national health needs.

(vii) Strengthening existing rural establishment and graded extension of national administrative structures to provide adequate and accessible referral, supervisory, logistical and other supporting services to ensure the judicious use of health services.

(viii) More allocation of financial resources based on the principles of equitable distribution and maximum utility.

(ix) Encouraging integration and coordination.

(x) Reorientation of Medical Education to suit the needs of the community.

(xi) Designing health technology to suit the environment and making the best use of existing technology of traditional system of medicine.

(xii) Improving research and development capacity to solve health problems.

(xiii) Devising measures to promote the use of simple, standardised equipment and drugs, placing reliance on available local resources whenever possible to foster self-reliance.

(xiv) The preventive health measures are crucial for sustained improvement and must be intensified to attain :

(a) Total coverage of the entire urban and rural population in the country with assured potable drinking water supply and sewerage;

(b) The disposal of urban wastes should also be given a high priority to ensure clean environment;

(c) For improving the environmental sanitation and hygiene, high priority must be given to town and country planning, provision of better working and living conditions, removal of congestion through the increased tempo of housing and construction, slum clearance and prevention of water and air pollution;

(d) The nutritional status of the population must be raised and total prevention of food adulteration and drugs control should be achieved through rigorous controls;

(e) Health education should be an integral part of all health programmes.

It is hoped that the implementation of these suggestions would ensure wider and more evenly distributed health care based on social justice, greater involvement and satisfaction of the beneficiaries and more efficient and more economical health services.

References

1. Lester B. Pearson, *Partners in Development*, London, 1969,p. 24.
2. UN 1974 *Report on the World Social Situation*, New York, 1975, p. 80.
3. World Bank, *Annual Report*, 1978, Washington D.C., p. 55.
4. UN, E/Conf. 60/CBP/13, p.14.
5. UN Employment Strategies and Poverty reduction policies of developing countries: Problems and issues in the light of experience in developmental planning, Journal of Development Planning No. 5, p. 20 (F. 72.11 A. 13)
6. UN, E, 73.11 F.1, p.19 (Economic Survey of Asia and the Far East, 1972).
7. *The Tribune*, Chandigarh, 4 September 1979.
8. UN, Commission for Social Development, *Report on the 23rd Session* (12 February - 2 March, 1973), New York, 1973, pp. 39-41.
9. WHO, *World Health, September* 1974, p. 4.
10. *Ibid*.
11. See the basis information-relating to Health.
12. South-East Asia here means the countries covered by the South-East Asia Regional Office of WHO, New Delhi (Members : 10).
13. UNICEF, *Health and Basic Services : Keys to Development*, p. 33.
14. The *Ceylon Medical Journal*, Vol. 16, No. 3, September 1971, pp. 125-28.
15. WHO, *World Health*, May, 1977, p. 3.
16. Ashok Mitra, Toward a National Nutritional Policy — Presidential Address to XII Annual Meeting of Nutrition Society of India, 3-4 March, 1979 (P.G.I.M.E.R., Chandigarh).
17. UN, E/Conf : 65/3, p. 66.
18. WHO, *WHO Chronicle*, 1974, Vol,. 28, No. 1, pp. 3-7.
19. For details see the Chapter on Administration of Health Education.
20. For details see Chapter on Administration of Environmental Health Programmes.
21. UNICEF, *Health and Basic Service, Key to Development*, pp. 33-34.
22. UN, 1974 *Report on the World Social Situation*, New York, 1975, p. 218.
23. WHO, WHO Office Records, No. 226, 1975, p. 113
24. WHO, World Health Papers, 55, p. 83.
25. R.M. Findlay, *Art of Administration*, Edinburgh, Oliver, 1952, p. 48.
26. WHO, *Public Health Papers*, 55, p. 61.
27. Based on personal discussions.
28. L.D. White; *Introduction to the Study of Public Administration*, Macmillan pp. 213-14.
29. For details refer to the respective Chapters.
30. L.D. White, *op. cit.*, p. 214.
31. V.O. Key, Politics and Administration in While (Ed.), *The Future of Government in the United States*, p. 155.
32. S.E. Finer, *Primer of Public Administration*, London, 1950, p. 68.

33. Granville Austin, *The Indian Constitution : Cornerstone of a Nation*, Clarendon Press, Oxford 1966, p. 50.

34. Christian Medical Commission : "An Exercise in the Development of Health Care Priorities", Geneva, 1974 (unpublished document – CMC/47/6) p. 1.

35. *The Tribune*, Chandigarh, 10 August, 1979.

36. UN, *1974 Report on the World Social Situation*, New York, 1975, p. 219.

37. L.D. White : *Introduction to the Study of Public Administration*, Macmillan, N.Y., p. 201.

38. Gyan Chand, *The Financial System of India*, p. 1.

39. WHO; *Technical Report Series*, 925, p.18.

40. Refer to the Chapter on 'Health Policy'.

41. Refer to J.H. Bryant, *Health and the Developing World*, Ithaca, N.Y. Cornell University Press, 1969.

42. WHO, *Modern Management Methods and the Organisation of Services, Geneva,* WHO, 1974 (Public Health Papers, No. 55).

43. P.K. Wattal, *Parliamentary Financial Control in India*.

44. UN (ESCAP), *Economic and Social Survey of Asia and the Pacific*, 1976, Bangkok, April, 1977, p.18.

45. Raymond J. Coleman and M.J. Rilley (Ed.), Management Dimensions, Holden —Day, INC, San Francisco, California, p. 5.

46. Morton F. Meltzer, *The Information Centre: Management Hidden Asset*, American Management Association, New York, 1967, pp. 136-137.

47. UNICEF, *Health and Basic Services : Keys to Development*, p. 50.

48. For details, refer to the Chapter on 'Health Planning'.

49. For details, see the Chapter on Health Manpower Planning and Development.

50. *WHO Chronicle*, 31 : 123-126 (1977) "Health Challenges for 1978-83".

6

Nature and Scope of Health Care Administration

A. Meaning and Significance of Health and Factors Influencing it

Significance of Health

Good health is a prerequisite to human productivity and the "development" process. It is essential to economic and technological development. A healthy community is the infrastructure upon which to build an economically viable society. The progress of society greatly depends on the quality of its people. Unhealthy people can hardly be expected to make any valid contribution towards developmental programmes. Health is man's greatest possession, for it lays a solid foundation for his happiness. Charaka, the renowned Ayurvedic physician is known to have said : "Health was vital for ethical, artistic, material and spiritual development of man."

Buddha has said that of all the gains, the gains of health are the highest and the best. Health is not only basic to leading a happy life for an individual but it is also necessary for all productive activities in the society. Who would deny that a soldier who is not keeping good health cannot be expected to defend the frontiers of his country even when he is provided with the latest sophisticated weapons? Similarly, who would deny that an unhealthy farmer with the best possible technological know-how would not succeed in producing the best that can be expected to him? Obviously what is true of an unhealthy soldier or an unhealthy farmer is also true of other categories of workers. Thus, no industry can expect the optimum output if it does not employ healthy workers or does not make and provide adequate facilities for proper maintenance of their health. Undoubtedly, professional efficiency, good health productivity are inter-related. Yet, health cannot be bestowed upon people if they themselves do not make any effort to maintain a proper balance between their external and internal environments.

Whatever one may say, a disease-stricken society can hardly hope to extricate itself from the clutches of poverty and ignorance that keep it backward and underdeveloped in many areas of life. A nation can become truly healthy only when it succeeds in overcoming all these deficiencies stemming from cultural, social, economic and other causes. A nation that is ill-fed can hardly afford to exhibit efficiency in any field. In fact, an epidemic or endemic disease in any part of the world can pose a potential danger to all mankind and even a challenge to modern science. The Planning Commission has stressed the vital importance of public health in the enrichment of community life. It has been stated :

> "Health is fundamental to the national progress in any sphere. In terms of resources for economic development, nothing can be considered of higher importance than the health of the people which is a measure of their energy and capacity as well as of the potential man-hours for productive work in relation to the total number of persons maintained by the nation. For the efficiency of industry and of agriculture, the health of the worker is an essential consideration."

In his address to 31st Session of WHO Regional Committee for South-East Asia held at Ulan Botor, Mongolia (22-28 Aug., 1978), Dr. Nyam-Osor, Minister of Public Health, Mongolia read a passage from a poem by Dashdorjin Natragdorj, which glorifies "Health." It is being reproduced below.[1]

> "Happiness, happiness, happiness
>
> It may be of different origin on this earth
>
> But the happiness of being healthy
>
> Is the real happiness."

Thus, there can be no two opinions that health is basic to national progress and in terms of resources for economic development nothing could be of greater significance than the health of the people. To quote Herophilas, C., 300 B.C.

> "When health is absent
>
> Wisdom cannot reveal itself
>
> Art cannot manifest
>
> Strength cannot fight,
>
> Wealth becomes useless
>
> And Intelligence cannot be applied."

As such, good health must be a primary objective of national development programmes. It is a precursor to improving the quality of life for a major portion of mankind.

Meaning of Health

Health is viewed differently by different people all over the world. The World Health Organisation defined health as "a state of complete physical, mental, and social well-being and not merely an absence or disease of infirmity."

Thus, good health is a synthesis of physical, mental and social well-being. As stated in the First Five Year Plan,

> "Health is a positive state of well-being in which harmonious development of mental and physical capacities of the individuals lead to the enjoyment of a rich and full life...It implies adjustment of the individuals to his total environment—physical and social."[2]

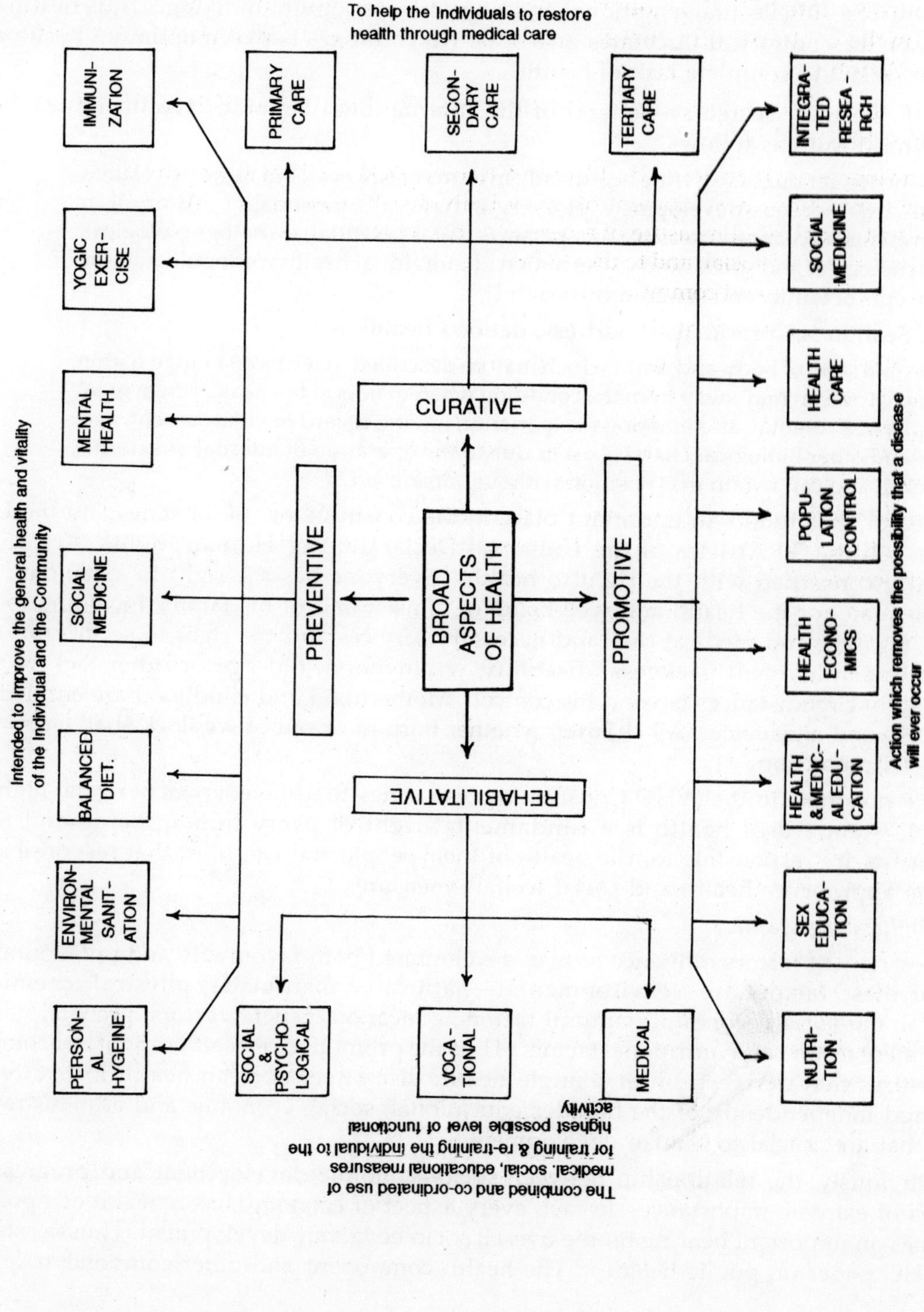
To help the Individuals to restore health through medical care
Intended to Improve the general health and vitality of the Individual and the Community
Action which removes the possibility that a disease will ever occur
The combined and co-ordinated use of medical, social, educational measures for training & re-training the individual to the highest possible level of functional activity
BROAD ASPECTS OF HEALTH
PREVENTIVE
CURATIVE
PROMOTIVE
REHABILITATIVE
IMMUNI-ZATION
YOGIC EXER-CISE
MENTAL HEALTH
SOCIAL MEDICINE
BALANCED DIET.
ENVIRON-MENTAL SANIT-ATION
PERSON-AL HYGEINE
PRIMARY CARE
SECON-DARY CARE
TERTIARY CARE
INTEGRA-TED RESEA-RCH
SOCIAL MEDICINE
HEALTH CARE
POPU-LATION CONTROL
HEALTH ECONO-MICS
HEALTH & MEDIC-AL EDU-CATION
SEX EDUCA-TION
NUTRI-TION
SOCIAL & PSYCHO-LOGICAL
VOCA-TIONAL
MEDICAL

Some people even define it as a condition under which an individual is able to mobilise all his resources—intellectual, emotional and physical—for optimum living. Thus health is not static; on the contrary, it fluctuates on a scale which ranges between optimum health as defined by WHO to complete lack of health.

Dr. E. Berthet, Secretary-General of the International Union of Health Education, Paris, defines health as follows :

> "We no longer ought to define health only in terms of sickness, but rather in relation to the harmonious development of every individual's personality. After all, it represents a balanced measure of a person's total potential—whether biological, psychological and social; and to the notion of individual health we should add the concepts of family and community health."[3]

S.C.Seal, in his presidential address, defined health as :

> "flexible state of body and mind which may be described in terms of a range within which a person may sway from the condition wherein he is at the peak of enjoyment of physical, mental and emotional experience, having regard to environment, age, sex and other biological characteristics due to the operation of internal or external stimuli and can regain that position without outside aid."[4]

"Health" has found an important place in the constitutions of all states and the UN agencies. Of the 30 Articles of the Universal Declaration of Human Rights, Art. 25 is particularly concerned with the right to health. Everyone has the right to a standard of living adequate for the health and well-being of himself and of his family, including food, clothing, housing and medical care and necessary services and the right to security in the event of unemployment, sickness, disability, widowhood, old age or other lack of the livelihood, in circumstances beyond his control. Motherhood and childhood are entitled to special care and assistance. All children whether born in or out of wedlock shall enjoy the same social protection.

The preamble to the WHO Constitution also states that the enjoyment of the highest attainable standard of health is a fundamental right of every human being and that governments are responsible for the health of their people and can fulfil that responsibility by taking appropriate health and social welfare measures.

Factors Influencing Health

A variety of factors influence human development both favourably and unfavourably. Some of these factors are : environmental—natural or man-made; physical, chemical, biological and social; economic, cultural factors; education, genetic factors; prenatal health development factors and nutritional factors. Thus the promotion of health cannot be achieved by measures that derive from any single health discipline, nor can health measures be considered independently of the broader educational, social, economic and administrative factors that are crucial to human development.

Obviously, the relationship between socio-economic development and progress of health is of extreme importance. In fact, every aspect of economy has a health component which has an important bearing on the overall socio-economic development. Thus, as stated in a WHO paper on public health : "The health component and other components of the total system necessarily interact. Health not only affects the remainder of the socio-economic complex but is also affected by it, sometimes unfavourably."[5]

Because of this intimate relationship, it has been mentioned in the First Five-Year Plan. "If this subject is regarded in the proper light as one which is concerned with everything affecting the health of the community, it must be admitted to be the biggest and the most important problem of India."[6]

Socio-economic development consists of various components related to the productive shares of activities. Health programmes cannot be related unilaterally to either the economic or the social spheres as they influence both and are influenced by both.

There, obviously, is a need for a unified integrated approach to public health, i.e., to combine services for nutrition improvement, communicable disease-control, better maternal and child-health and family-welfare. Thus, conventional linear planning and the execution of separate programmes cannot meet the needs of human development. As stated by T.Adeoye Lambo in his article "Total Health" in *World Health*.

> " It is now apparent that a more balanced consideration of the biological, social and cultural aspects of health is needed. Life is a process and not a substance — a living system based upon the primacy of continuity and inter-relatedness, throughout the universe...If man and his family are to remain in empathy with the emerging necessities in the developing milieu, an adequate design of inter-disciplinary tools will have to be made to assist in this task of providing a total health package."[7]

In general, the factors influencing health could be classified into three broad categories : hereditary, environmental and personal. Similarly, the various conditions which play a vital role in determining one's health status can be put under three major areas, viz., mental health, spiritual health and physical health.

Principles for Health Care Administrators

The Health Care administrators need to be aware of certain basic principles for the formulation of health policies. Some of the principles are stated below :

(a) Health opportunities need not be related to the purchasing power of the people.

(b) While planning Public Health Programmes for the benefit of the whole community, care should be taken to see that medical facilities are accessible to the poor people inhabiting the rural areas, urban slums and tribal areas.

(c) Investment on preventive as well as curative health programmes and activities should be considered as beneficial. However, the priority may be given to the preventive health care as we know that prevention is better than cure.

(d) Doctors should be trained to act as social physicians as well to promote healthy and happier life.

(e) Health should not be considered in isolation from other socio-economic factors.

(f) Health consciousness should be fostered through health education and by providing opportunities for the participation of the individuals in the health programme.

(g) Sound Health Administrative structures may be designed for the implementation of the health policy.

(h) All the systems if medicine must be encouraged to provide decent health to the people in a coordinated fashion.

(i) Utilise community resources and encourage local participation to promote self help programmes at the village level.

(j) Ensure basic health services available accessible and acceptable to the people.

Meaning of Health Administration

We have already defined the term 'Health'. Let us define the term 'Administration'. Administration is at the centre of all human affairs. Its principal aspect are formulation of policy and its implementation for the attainment in an optimum manner of stated ends in the shape of services or products. Administration is an activity which demands correct analysis and accurate orientation. According to Simon "In its broadest sense, administration can be defined as the activities of groups cooperating to accomplish common goals."[8] In the words of Marx :

> "Administration is determined action taken in the pursuit of a conscious purpose. It is the systematic ordering of affairs and the calculated use of resources aimed at making those things happen which one wants to happen — and forestalling everything to the contrary"[9]

In simple words, administration may be defined as the management of affairs with the use of well thought-out principles and practices and rationalised techniques to achieve certain objectives. Pfiffner and Presthus define administration as "the organisation and direction of human and material resources to achieve desired ends."[10]

Administration consists of a structure or an organisation of various institutions essential for its functioning; the processes, procedures and interaction of various constituents; and the techniques and skills of human relation. It is the management of human affairs concerned with the needs of carrying out specific objectives. Administration is involved in all fields of human endeavour where there is a planned effort. It is a force which lays down the objectives which an organization and its management are to strive for and the broad policies under which to operate. Administration provides the means whereby the most effective use can be made of the knowledge and skills of those giving the service. It is a way of conceptual thinking for attaining pre-determined goals through group efforts.

Now let us define the term 'Health Administration'. It is a branch of Public Administration which deals with matters relating to the promotion of health, preventive services, medical care, rehabilitation, the delivery of health services, the development of health manpower and the medical education and training. The purpose of Public Health Administration is to provide total health services to the people with economy and efficiency. Health Administration must use the knowledge of health economics to achieve economy. Three French teachers of Health Economics (Professor P. Bonamour, F. Guyot and D. Jolly) defined health Economics as :

> "that branch of knowledge which seeks to optimise medical action, that is, to study ways of spreading the available resources so as to ensure the best possible state of health for the population, within the limited means."[11]

Efficiency in health administration can be achieved through proper policy formulation and its implementation. Health administration is the force which can help the health system in the formulation of sound health policy and its implementation. One of the best definitions of Health Administration is given by C.E.A.Winslow who defined it as "The science and art of preventing diseases; prolonging life, promoting health efficiency through organised community effort for the sanitation of the environment, the control of communicable diseases, the education of the individual in personal hygiene, the organisation of medical and nursing services for the early diagnosis and preventive treatment of disease, the development of social machinery to ensure to every citizen a standard of living adequate for the maintenance of health, so organising these benefits as to enable every citizen to realise his birth right of health and longevity."[12] Thus Public Health Administration is the application of administrative processes and methods which are used in carrying out the objectives of health in an organised community. The term community refers to the entire population of functionally defined geographics are that has developed common interests, activities and inter-relations.

According to Beaton :

"Public Health is the planning, carrying out and evaluation of health measures and systems services that both maintain and improve the health of a population group and prevent and control diseases within that population group."[13]

There has been an increase in the variety, number and complexity of functions that have to be performed by the health administration, because of scientific and technological advancement. The health administration has not been modernised correspondingly to make use of the new technology. A serious imbalance exists between aspirations and performances. There is a widespread belief prevalent among the experts in the field of Health Administration that there is an urgent need for better management of health services if higher standards of health and health care are to be achieved.

The following are typical of the symptoms that demonstrate the need for better management:

(a) Overlapping, conflicting and competing organisations within the health 'system'. Where the system is composed of unrelated parts, it is not possible to manage a coherent health programme because no administrative structure can execute it.

(b) Widely scattered funding mechanism with little control over costs. Many health services have little idea of the true cost of some of their facilities or services.

(c) Decisions on the mixture of facilities and services without reference to population needs and with no information about those who do not use the services. Medical management thus tends to be based on currently met demand, not a need.[14]

Good management provides the surplus investment which nourish the processes of industrialisation and modernisation of society. Good administration furnishes the infrastructure of services which secure the order, stability and security which are the prerequisites of economic and social development. Carefully recruited and periodically trained or re-trained personnel are needed for both spheres of operation.

We would, therefore, like to conclude with Charles Beard, who wrote at the end of his long career :

> "There is no subject more important that this subject of Public Administration. The future of civilised government, and even, I think of civilisation itself, rests upon our ability to develop science, philosophy and practice of administration competent to discharge the public functions of a civilised society."[15]

There is no doubt that medicine has accumulated a long list of triumps as regards the care containment, or amelioration of established somatic diseases. Yet, it knows almost nothign of social aspects of disease and its treatment. In the past not much attention has been paid by the medical an dother scientists to such causes of social disease as parental inadequacy, overcrowding, poverty, malnutrition, inadequate occupational and educational opportunities, the non-therapeutic uses of leisures, the misuse of mass media or the suppression of underprivileged section of the community. Medicine today with all its success or failures and the kind of demand it faces, is increasingly becoming a part of longer societal concern. The health administrators have to become aware of the fact that the obligatory relationship of social, mental and somatic disease requires looking afresh, at medicine's expanding role. They have to think in terms of planning and execution of comprehensive medical care programmes, including preservation of health and prevention as well as cure of disease. Already, continuity of home care has become a new slogan in the medical circle, particularly in the developing countries. While all these aims appear laudable, they are rarely achieved except for the `cure of disease part'. Obviously, as the successes of medical science pile up, the sub-division of medical labour increases with its attendant technical imcompetence, discontinuity of care and high cost. These consideratiosn coupled with the present defensive isolation of the medical world in the bastion of acute curative, specialised and technical medicine, the hospitals prevent the giving of comprehensive care and the development of the true "health centre" as a focal point for community health care. All this must be studied as the most crucial area of health administration.

In the developing countries in particular, the emphasis has changed from the physical environment to preventive medicine. A great deal of attention is now being paid to man's relationship with his total complex social environment. The occurrence and spread of disease is being looked at in relation to numerous interacting factors in man's physical, biological, socio-economic and cultural environment. Thus the discipline of health administration is faced with many new challenges and nothing much can be achieved by it without looking at health problems from a holistic point of view.

One fo the basic principles of public health administration relevant both to developed and developing countries should be that scarce sources, including that of medical manpower, should not be utilised only for the purpose of creating high power clinical establishments to treat rare diseases rather than using them for the successful functioning of public health services to combat common health problems, particularly of vulnerable groups, like pregnant women, lactating mothers and young children. Similarly, medical education can be reoriented and medical services reorganised with the involvement and cooperation of political and social scientists.

Objectives of Public Health Administration

There are numerous objectives of public health administration. The following deserve special attention :

(a) Increasing the average length of human life.

(b) Decreasing the mortality rate, particularly infant mortality rate, due to those diseases which can be easily prevented or remedied.

(c) Decreasing the morbidity rate.

(d) Increasing the physical, mental and social well-being of the individual.

(e) Increasing the pace of adjustment of individual to his environment.

(f) Providing total health care to enrich quality of life.

The important activities in the domain of Health which need the attention of health administration has been well-enumerated in the 'Charter of Health' adopted by the Regional Committee for South-East Asia. The objectives of the Charter include :

(a) The provision of primary health care services to the rural population and under-served groups in urban areas, aiming at full coverage.

(b) The development of health manpower which will maintain its sensitivity and relevance to the health service delivery system.

(c) The provision of safe water to rural and urban communities and improvement of the facilities for waste-water disposal and basic sanitation.

(d) The reduction of mortality and morbidity among infants, children and mothers; and the regulation of fertility so as to achieve a balance between population growth and economic development.

(e) The implementation of effective measures for the surveillance, prevention and control of the major communicable diseases, with prevention and control of malaria being given the highest priority and due importance being given to an integrated multi-immunisation programme.

(f) The promotion and formulation of national and regional food and nutrition policies and the development of common programmes jointly with the other economic and social sectors concerned.

The health Charter should serve as a spring board to renewed activities, for the health and happiness of humanity.[16] It is beautifully expressed in the Vedic benediction;

Hindi version

सर्वे भवन्तु सुखिनः सर्वे सन्तु निरामयाः ।

सर्वे भद्राणि पश्यन्तु मा कश्चित् दुःख भागभवेत ॥

May all humanity be happy
May all be without disease
May all witness auspicious sights
May none have to undergo suffering

In practice, it is difficult to achieve the ideals of public health as mentioned in the Constitution of World Health Organisation. Even the most advanced countries have not been able to meet this ideal. So, the Health Administrators in the developing countries must focus their attention on achieving a level of health which they can afford. They must proceed gradually in the pursuit of this ideal. Health Administration, whether in developed or developing countries, are faced with a number of managerial problems ranging from the provision of the most basic health and sanitary measures to the best use of finite resources in elaborate medical care system. All countries, however, have one basic problem in common — how can one best improve the health status of the population? This problem has become more passing owing to changes in the needs and expectations of communities to developments in health and other technologies, and to the urgent need to link health improvement with socio-economic development."[17]

The purpose of public health administration is to enrich the quality of life leading to ethical, artistic, material and spiritual development of man.

If the ideal of health administration is to provide better medical care to the people then we shall have to see that in a given situation we make the best possible use of our resources in terms of personnel and finance to achieve optimum results. For instance, in a developing country like India, the health administrator should normally be concerned with the following :

(a) that the patients are treated as close to their homes as possible in the smallest, cheapest and simply equipped unit such as a sub-centre which is capable of looking after them adequately;

(b) that the medical services should be organised and administered in such a way that the quality of medical care improves gradually;

(c) that medical care services should be organised from the bottom-up and not from the top-down.

(d) that the services planned should meet the needs of the people.

(e) that all members of the health and medical personnel function as a well-knit team;

(f) that new categories of health personnel such as multipurpose health workers and community health workers should be given suitable training to provide simple medical care and preventive services to large sections of the community.

In the case of virtual epidemic of behavioural disorders, modern health care must place a new emphasis on solving the human side of medicine. As stated by Maureen A. Backy, "The crucial link between the person providing health care and the persons receiving it, is often very weak indeed. Modern medicine tends to emphasise technical solution and to overlook the value of close personal contact and relationship."[17]

C. Nature and Scope of Health Administration

Health Administration as a Science and an Art

Health administration is becoming complex day-by-day. Man is acquiring undreamt of powers, for scientific progress makes him everyday more capable of shaping the world and his destiny. He has the potentiality to bring about socio-economic revolution for the harmonious and healthy development of the people. The world has the resources and know-how to achieve a significant improvement in health care. But improved health will not percolate to the majority of the people as a natural consequence of economic growth. It requires an efficient administrative and managerial system to translate the benefits of science and technology of the people. Unfortunately, developing countries have failed to produce the expected system. The weakness, ineptitude and general inefficiency of their governmental systems are massive obstacles not only in their development but even in their survival.[18] These deficiencies prevent the vast flood of money, talent and material from achieving their objective. It is accepted that inability to manage efficiently or utilise effectively the available and potential resources is the common ill of all the less-developed countries. It follows that successful development demands a sound programme for managerial improvement.[19] Thus, the administrative inadequacies in a national government have a retarding influence on socio-economic development. Charles F.Nicklas, Public Administration Advisor to the Philippines Government, remarked :

> "The success of management improvement efforts and indeed the quality of public administration depends to a very great and undeniable extent upon the concepts, philosophies, interests and characteristics of key officials at the top echelons of the government hierarchy. Without the proper attitude and impetus at these levels, the cause of improved management and operation in government faced constant frustration. It is, therefore, essential in the interest of progress that the individuals be endowed with the desire to see that the public service is administered in the most efficient, effective and economic manner possible and possess the knowledge and breadth of understanding necessary to fulfil that desire."[20]

Public health administration is an area of activity which calls for specialised knowledge and techniques which can help the people to achieve the health care. Until and unless, we understand all the implications of such an administration, we may not be able to reap the potential benefits of health organisations. This is a definite art which can be learnt and practised to produce pre-designed output. Health administration is an art as it can help to direct and guide the efforts of those involved in such an enterprise towards some specific ends or objectives efficiently. There is a great need to make this art perfect and professional. A professionally efficient and competent administration is able to serve the people better. Besides, the health personnel must be dedicated to their profession.

Dr. H. Mahler is very critical about the inability of health workers in contemporary society to influence those social and environmental factors which truly determine public health. He states :

> "There persist widespread negative attitudes among health professionals towards the health care of the poorest strata in the rural and urban populations in the

developing countries. Most of these attitudes imply — with a repetitiveness of an old gramophone record caught in a narrow, arrogant, condescending and indifferent groove — that these poor people are too apathetic, too superstitious, too illiterate to benefit from the health care potentially available to them... Health professionals and those who train them should be much more radical in accepting a social responsibility for the health needs of the people in these poor rural and urban communities so that they can act as agents for change."[21]

Thus, we can say that there is a need to train health administrators and workers in the new art of Public Health Administration so that they can take the benefits of the modern science to the common man and maintain the spirit of Geneva Declaration :[22]

"Now being admitted to the profession of Medicine, I solemnly pledge to concentrate my life to the service of humanity. I will give respect and gratitude to my deserving teacher. I will practice medicine with conscience and dignity. The health and life of my patients will be my first consideration. It will hold in confidence all that my patient confides in me. I will maintain the honour and noble traditions of the medical profession. My colleagues will be my brothers. I will not permit consideration of race, religion, nationality, party politics or social standing to intervene between my duty and my patient. I will maintain the utmost respect of human life. Even under threat I will not use my knowledge contrary to the laws of humanity. These promises I make freely and upon my honour."

The same feeling has been expressed in the Tokyo Declaration. To quote the preamble to the Declaration of Tokyo :

"It is the privilege of the medical doctor to practise medicine in the service of humanity, to preserve and restore bodily and mental health without distinction as to persons, to comfort and to ease the sufferings of his or her patients."[23]

Prof. J.S. Neki has rightly said in this connection that "to help, to heal, to reconstruct, to comfort -and all along the line to act with compassion — all these bear testimony to the moral consciousness of the doctor. Whatever the new strains imposed upon medical ethics, this structure will survive and continue to guide doctors in their professional conduct.. Legal and juridical obligations they have, of necessity, to fulfil. But these are not genuine ethics. Genuine ethics has to be ingrained into character and does not have to depend upon external controls."[24]

Now the question arises whether public health administration is a science or not. It is definitely not a science like the physical sciences as it cannot claim certainty. It is a science similar to other Social Sciences like Economics, Sociology, etc. We are applying scientific methods in health administration for careful planning, analysis and the design of the procedures. We can make the instruments of Health Care Administration more perfect through careful practice and research and thus reach definite universal principles. We should be clear here that the universal principles in human organisations would differ to a great extent depending upon the ecological differences prevalent in different areas. We can say that 'scientific societies, and the exchange of knowledge and hypotheses by natural scientists have advanced the exactness of knowledge in the domain of natural science, so we may expect administrative societies, and the exchanges among administrators to advance the exactness of knowledge in the domain of administration."

Thus public health administration is both a science and an art. In order to advance the cause of this budding discipline for the present and the future academic scholars and practitioners, we may concentrate on its principles, philosophy and practice. The developing world is faced with the problems of limited resources, infinite needs and competing demands in the domain of health. In order to provide the health services (preventive, promotive, curative and rehabilitative) to the total population—sick and the healthy, the developing world would have to provide an effective system of health administration. If these components are combined fruitfully, it is sure that the health administration can deliver the desired goods and services to its constituents.

Scope of Health Care Administration

In order to translate the aims and objectives of the public health organisations, the scope of health administration is expanding. Besides curative, preventive, promotive aspects, Health Administration studies social medicine which is concerned with the study of man as a total individual for the understanding of health and disease. The British Medical Association considers this concept from the angle :

> "That the health of the people depends primarily upon the social and environmental conditions under which they live and work, upon security against fear and want, upon nutritional standards, upon educational facilities and upon the facilities for exercise and leisure."

Social medicine includes social anatomy, social psychology, social pathology and social therapy.

There is also a new term, i.e., Medical Geography—linking medicine with geography. Medical Geography views disease as "maladjustment to the environment to which numerous factors contribute, disease, therefore, becomes an anthropological phenomenon with geographical distribution."

Thus, to understand the implications of health, it is necessary to have knowledge of the ecology of man. Such understanding would throw a flood of light on problems of diagnosis and treatment.

We can see the expanding and diversified field of medical science from the chart depicting the various stages of the development from 1850-2000. To quote W.L.Barton :

> "If this era is to have success there must be a move from the concept of health as being the total responsibility of a professionalised service to a new emphasis on self-reliant health care. . . The emerging science of the new era calls for a clear definition of objective, purpose and function, so as to identify the required competence. distinctive skills and body of knowledge in terms that can be clearly understood by the people and the politicians, as well as by the professional leadership involved. It demands daring leadership, not afraid to step forward from the basic professions from which they came, to face the challenges and difficulties of education in the new fields and to direct with courage, through competence in public health, the team of equals."[25]

Health administration is concerned with 'what' and 'how' of the health. 'What' is the subject matter, covering preventive, promotive, curative and rehabilitative services. It also covers professional training of the health and medical personnel and the role of the

International Health Administration and its impact on the national health administration. It is very difficult to classify the subject matter of health administration in watertight compartments. We have to focus on an integrated philosophy of health. The term medical care is defined by the WHO as :

> "a programme of services that should make available to the individual, and thereby to the community, all facilities of medical and allied sciences necessary to promote and maintain health of mind and body. This programme should take into account the physical, social and family environment, with a view to the prevention of disease, the restoration of health and the alleviation of disability. The extent of these services will vary according to local conditions."[26]

PROMOTION OF THE CONCEPT OF TOTAL HEALTH

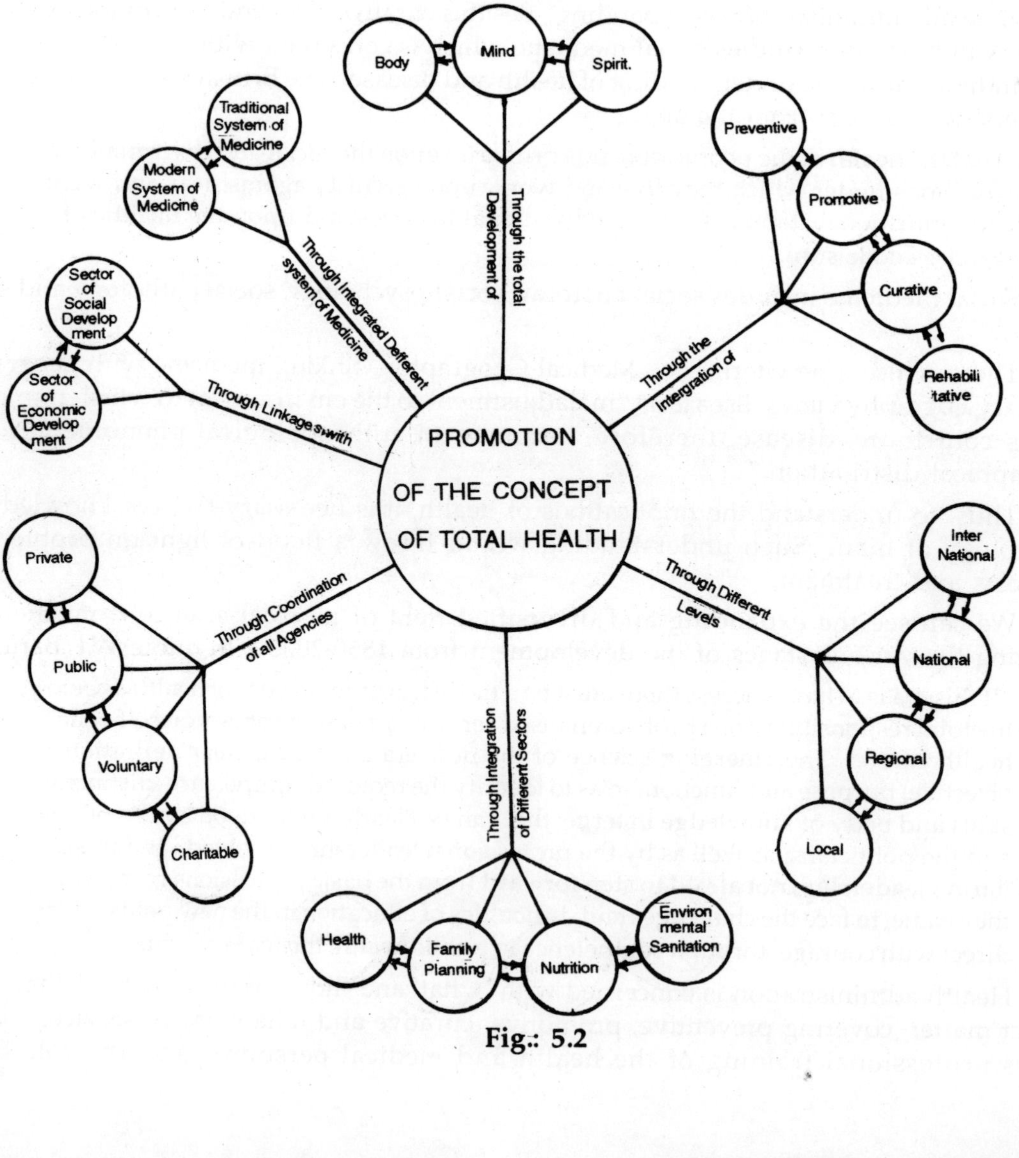

Fig.: 5.2

We have to view health administration from a broader viewpoint. It encompasses many other factors which influence health care administration. The broadening scope of health care administration can be seen from the chart given on previous page:

The various activities which can come under each sub-head can be seen from this chart entitled "promotion of the concept of total health."

As regards 'how', it is the technique of management i.e., the principles of management which can make the health administration successful and fruitful.

These principles have been classified by different management experts into a number of functions. Clough[27] gives only two—making decisions and providing leadership. R.C. Davis[28] gives three—planning, organising and controlling. Newman, Summer and Warren[29] list four—organising, planning, leading and controlling. Terry[30] notes planning, organising, actuating and controlling.

Koontz and O'Donell[31] list five functions : planning, organising, staff, direction and control. Hicks[32] covers six functions : creating, planning, organising, motivating, communicating and controlling. Dale[33] goes one step further, i.e., seven functions — planning, organising staffing, direction, control, innovation and representation.

Many experts on Administrative Management feel that management is a basic operative force in all complex, purposive organisations. It is the function of executive leadership anywhere. It means that management skills are transferable. But there are writers who argue that there are fundamental differences between managing one organisation and the other. Earnest Dale, for instance, says that the universality of management principles is contradicted by observed examples of the difficulties faced by managers who work in widely different type of organisation from the one in which they were successful. As such, we should be careful in applying the general principles of management to health organisations within the peculiar environment surrounding them.

We must understand the difference between administration and management, though, we have used the term interchangeably.

Orday Tead has made a distinction between these two terms in the following words : "Administration is the process and agency which is responsible for the determination of the aims for which an organisation and its management are to strive, which establishes the broad policies under which they are to operate, and which gives general oversight to the continuing effectiveness of the total operation in reaching the objectives sought." And he goes on to say that "management is the process and agency which directs and guides the operations of an organisation in the realising of established aims."

To quote Mcfarland : "In government agencies administration is preferred over managements, although in recent years the term management has become widely used in government agencies. Another possible distinction refers to the levels of organisation. In business, the term administration refers to the activities of the higher levels in the managerial ranks. Still another distinction related to organisational level is that administration refers to the determination of major aims and policies, while management to the carrying out of the operations designed to accomplish the aims and effectuate the policies. Here again, the distinction is not only widely followed but it exists."

Peter F. Drucker has rightly observed : "Our society has become, within an incredibly short fifty years, a society of institutions. It has become a pluralist society in which every major social task has been entrusted to large organisations from producing economic goods and services to health care, from social security and welfare to education, from the search for new knowledge to the protection of the natural environments."

Now let us discuss some of the definitions of management which can be understood and applied by Health Administrators and managers.

"Management may be defined as the art of securing maximum results with a minimum of effort so as to secure maximum prosperity and happiness for both employer and employee and give the public the best possible service."

Peter F. Drucker has rightly pointed out that, "Management is the crucial factor in economic and social development. It was obvious that the economists' traditional view of development as a function of savings and capital investment do not produce management and economic development. On the contrary, management produces economic and social development, and with it savings and capital investment. It becomes apparent that the developing countries are not underdeveloped, they are undermanaged."

Massie says that, "Management is defined as the process by which a cooperative group directs action towards common goals."

Terry has rightly said that, "management is a distinct process consisting of planning, organising, actuating, and controlling, performed to determine and accomplish the objectives by the use of people and resources."

According to A. Dasgupta, "Management is the creation and control of technological and human environment of an organisation in which human skill and capacities of individuals and groups find full scope for their effective use in order to accomplish the objectives for which an enterprise has been set up. It is involved in the relationship of the individual, group, the organisation and the environment."

To Stanely Vance, "Management is simply the process of decision- making and control over the action of human beings for the express purpose of attaining predetermined goals."

According to Lundy, "Management is principally the task of planning, coordinating, motivating and controlling the efforts of others towards a specific objective."

The health sector has wide and varied relationships with other sectors of the social system. Individual and community health depends on a multiplicity of factors, such as nutrition and other basic biological requirements, personal and psychological security, culturally supported behavioural patterns, legislation, education, opportunity for participation of the community in planning and implementation, protection against exposure to pathogens, and accessibility of treatment to reduce the impact of disease. Indeed, it is hard to think of a community activity that has no relationship to health. This view makes health the result of occurrences in many sectors of the social system; it implies that what occurs in those sectors may support, negate or offset the preventive and therapeutic interventions of the health sector. These considerations have enlarged the objectives of health administration from the mere provision of health services to the improvement of community health by all available means.

The health administration studies all aspects for the delivery of health care services. In this context health administration studies the role of public, private, and voluntary efforts in meeting health challenges. Health administration also studies the structure and functioning of international health administration, government administration at all levels, private administration and voluntary administration which help the people in improving their health status. A recent development in health administration has been the encouragement to the traditional medical systems to help the needy people. According to Dr. P.N.V. Kurup, Adviser to the Government of India for indigenous system of medicine,

> "In our anxiety to make an effective comprehensive health service available as soon as possible to the maximum number of people, the available material, financial and manpower resources that are rooted in traditional medical practices should not be overlooked. Against this background the traditional systems of medicine can play a vital role as an additional or alternative approach in a country's Health Delivery Programme."

China has used this system with definite results. Thus health administration studies the role of all the systems of medicine which help in the improvement of the health status of the people.

However, in order to make a really good contribution it has to adopt a multi-disciplinary approach. In the West, the health administrators are increasingly relying on the application of behavioural administrative sciences — anthropology, sociology, social psychology and public administration — in the identification and solution of administrative problems in the area of health. Thus this needs to be achieved with a much greater pace in a developing country like India. It cannot be delayed in view of the kind of problems we face today. In the present context, the health administrator has to acquire a broad outlook and a strong will and determination to grapple with the existing mind-boggling health problems.

Research and Monitoring in Health Administration

There is need for conducting systematic research on many aspects of health care administration. By using operational research methods and techniques one can assess the extent to which scientific knowledge is utilised for bringing about improvement in the health level of the bulk of the people at the lowest cost. Research in health administration is concerned with administrative, economic and organisational aspects of the delivery of health and medical services. Success of health care administration depends not only on research investigations in the medical field but also on the researches in other allied fields and particularly on the application of the procedures and practices as evolved in these fields. It may be stressed that operational research has special relevance to health administration in India because of inadequacy of organising health services as well as of several shortcomings of policy-making. However, nothing much can be achieved without providing the necessary training to personnel engaged in public health programmes and activities. The Central and the state ministries of health and family welfare have to play a special role in this regard. There is a definite need for studying the patterns of utilisation of health services both in the rural and urban areas. By identifying factors affecting delivery of health care services, they can possibly plan to overcome them. The Union Government has already done a good job in this direction by instituting an Institute of Family and Health Welfare Administration which is actively engaged in various types of researches relating to health and hospital administration. Some universities are also teaching an independent paper on health administration. It would be suggested that the universities must be encouraged to take up research projects in health and hospital administration as the dichotomy between the social scientists and medical personnel is fast fading.

Monitoring and Surveillance in Health Administration

Unplanned development in the area of health has led to many unforeseen problems, which are directly or indirectly related to certain deficiencies in the planning processes. Thus there is a great need to develop specific guidelines for monitoring the public health programmes and activities so as to yield maximum benefits to the largest number of people. The governments both at the Centre and the State levels need to be made aware of malfunctioning of health organisations in time so that remedial measures could be adopted. In all communities where a central organisation exists there are some devices to keep Government informed about the health of the people they govern. There is a need to examine these devices, so that these could be further modified to yield the desired results. By applying modified devices one could provide a sensitive indication of trends in health and development to the health planners for taking appropriate decisions regarding adoption of remedial measures.

Health surveillance is the comparison and interpretation of data generated through monitoring or from any other sources to determine the impact of health measures on the health status of populations :

> "Surveillance means the epidemiological study of disease as a dynamic process involving the ecology of the infectious agent, the host, the reservoirs, the vectors, and the environment as well as the complex mechanisms concerned in the spread of infection and the extent to which the spread occurs."

D. Indicators Measuring Impact of Health Care Administration

Health is generally referred to as a measurable quantity, but the concept is elusive and words cannot define it with precision. A WHO study indicated that among the problems of measurement of levels of living, that of the measurement of health levels occupies a central position. Health, a very broad concept, lends itself poorly to objective measurement; direct measurement of health status is often impossible and, in practice, indicators concern states that deviate from health but can be measured-indicators of the health status of individuals or groups; indicators of environmental conditions that may have an effect on health status; and the indicators of the activities of health services.[45] The distinction between 'health' and 'sickness' is not always well—defined. Most people would agree that it is desirable to prevent illness and premature death. However, the prevalent indices are :

Death Rate. All over the world death rates have been coming down and the average age at death has been moving up. During the thirty-year period between (1935-39 to 1980-81) it has been estimated that for the world as a whole life expectancy at birth has increased from 40 to 55 years—the developed countries averaging an increase from 56 to 72 years and the developing countries from 32 to 52 years.

Infant Mortality Rate. It means the number of infants who die under one year of age out of every 1,000 who are born alive. It has been going down. In England and Wales the infant mortality rate in 1941-45 was 148 while in 1981 it was 12. Several other highly developed countries have recently recorded still lower rates, e.g., Sweden with just under six in 1981. The same trend has been occurring recently in the developing countries, several of whom have records of infant mortality rate going back to at least half a century. For example, in Mexico the rate was 223 in 1922 and 23 in 1981; in Mauritius 156 in 1920 and 40 in 1981, and in Sri Lanka 171 in 1915 and 23 in 1981.

Incidence and Prevalence of Disease. In most countries of the world a system operates that enables both the local and the central health administration to know fairly and quickly about variations in the occurrence of the notifiable infectious diseases and about the outbreak of epidemics. The system has come in for heavy criticism because reporting is often patchy, incomplete and unreliable. But with all these limitations these statistics, looked at over the years do provide an enormously useful record of the long-term gradual decline of many infectious diseases as well as of sudden epidemics, their rise and fall, and their passage from one community to another or from one country to another. To give some random examples : in Japan in 1939 the number of cases of diphtheria reported was 39,801, but in 1980 the figure was only 300. In the United States in 1946 the number of reported cases of poliomyelitis was 25,698 while in 1980 it was 5.

Admission Rate of Patients to the Hospitals in the Area. Hospitalisation statistics are essential for administering a hospital service and for planning and evaluating the services. They cannot provide a full and undistorted picture of the health or ill-health, of the population served. However, with experience health statisticians and health administrators learn to interpret the statistics and can often determine what is going on in the community.

Surveys and Special Enquiries. Such health surveys or morbidity surveys can be of various kinds. They may involve medical examinations or special disease finding (surveys) tests or they may be performed through household visits and enquiries. National sickness surveys have been carried out in many countries including Canada, Denmark, Japan, India, UK, USA, for the past 20 years. However, although continuous health surveys have great value within a country, something less elaborate is needed for comparing levels of health in different places and for recognising important changes over the course of time. It would be good if we could devise a simple but general health index that would summarise the state of health of a population in one single figure that would be easy to monitor and interpret—something like the GNP in the economic field. But so far this has not been possible as health is not a readily quantifiable entity or attribute.

Proportional Mortality Ratio. It is defined as the number of deaths at the ages of 50 and over as the percentage of total deaths. If all persons survive up to 50 years of age, then the index would be 100, if no one reaches this age, the index would be zero.

Expectation of Life. The expectation of life at birth is generally considered to be the single indicator of the health status of a population.

It will be seen from the above mentioned indicators that there is no comprehensive measure of a nation's health.

Limitations of Health Administration

Health is concerned with qualitative improvement and it is not subject to exact measurement. Any health organisation can be successful if the following facts, peculiar to health management, are taken into consideration :

(a) The nature of the object being managed;

(b) Public attitudes to that object;

(c) The difficulty of placing a value on 'health';

(d) The multiplicity of aims and objectives and of the criteria applied to them;

(e) The long interval between decision and outcome and the associated uncertainty surrounding decision-making;

(f) Orientation to 'service' rather than 'production';

(g) The involvement of several professions in the management process;

(h) Political intervention;

(i) The scope for public involvement; and

(j) The need to coordinate many different agencies, official, private and voluntary.

All these factors must be taken into consideration while administering the health development. Health administrators should be sensitive to all these limitations and plan and administer health services most conducive to the satisfaction of the population. It is really difficult to have a single model to solve the health problems in a country or area. A single model has not been devised for the solution of health problems. However, we can design any workable model suitable to a given area.

The ideal index which combines the effect of a number of components measured independently, is yet to be developed, although it can be stated that such an index should satisfy the following requirements :

(a) *Availability.* It should be possible to obtain the data required without special and complex investigations.

(b) *Completeness to coverage.* The index should be derived from data covering the population of an entire country or that part of it to which the index is supposed to refer.

(c) *Quality*. The national data should not vary with time and place in such a way as to have any substantial effect on the index.

(d) *Universality*. The index should, as far as possible, be the expression of a group of factors that determine and affect the level of health.

(e) *Calculation*. The index should be calculated in as simple a manner as possible and the calculation should not be costly in terms of the resources required.

(f) *Acceptance*. The index should widely accepted and used and no doubts should exist in respect of the methods employed for developing the index or for interpreting it.

(g) *Specificity*. The index should reflect changes only in those phenomena of which it is the expression.

(h) *Reproducibility*. When the index is used by different specialists under different conditions at different times the results should be identical.

(i) *Sensitivity*. The index should be sensitive to changes in the phenomena concerned. Allowance should be made for the effect of inflation of the index.

(j) *Validity*. The index should be a true expression of the factors of which it is supposed to be a measure. Some form of independent external evidence of this should be provided.

Moreover, health cannot be measured in isolation. It is a part of much broader spectrum of inter-related and inter-dependent conditions, and no picture of health status can be complete without also taking account of the socio-economic and environmental circumstances—income, education, housing, environment, clothing, food, climate, pollution and still other facts that influence levels of health and disease at least as much as the activities of the health services themselves.

References

1. WHO, SEARO, S.E.A./RC/31/p.59.
2. Govt. of India, *First Five Year Plan*, p. 488.
3. WHO, *World Health*, May 1979, p. 23.
4. Seal, S.C. (1963), *Presidential Address*, 50th Science Congress, Delhi.
5. WHO, *Public Health Papers*, No. 49, 1973, p. 9.
6. Govt. of India, *First Five Year Plan*, p. 511.
7. WHO, *World Health*, December 1975, p. 3.
8. Simon H, *et al.*, *Public Administration*, p. 3.
9. Marx (ed), *Elements of Public Administration*, p. 3.
10. Pfiffner and Presthus, *Public Administration*, New York, p. 3.
11. WHO, *World Health*, May 1979, p. 14.
12. Hanlon, J.J. (1964), *Principles of Public Health Administration*, C.V. Mosby.
13. Beaton, G.H. (1974) *Canad J. Public Health*, 65, 463.

14. WHO, *Public Health Papers*, 55, Geneva, 1974, p. 8

15. Dimock and Dimock, *Public Administration*, p. 2

15a. Gunaratne, Therat V., *Challenges and Responses : Health in South-East Asia Region*,Tata McGraw Hill, New Delhi, 1977, pp. 44-46.

16. WHO, *Technical Report Series* (596), "Application of System Analysis to Health Management, Geneva, 1976, pp. 5-6.

17. WHO, *World Health*, December 1975, p. 6.

18. David Brown, S., "Improving the Administrative Capability of the Aid Receiving Countries," *Public Administration Review*, June 1964, p. 64.

19. Iboko, J.I., "Developing the Administration in a developing country," *International Review of Administrative Science*, Vol. XXXVIII, No. 2, 1972, p. 293.

20. Charles, Nicklas, E. in the book *Approaches to Development: Policies, Administration and Change*, Edited by Montgomery and Siffin, New York, 1966, p. 188.

21. Text of Address by Dr. H. Mahler, Director General, WHO, to thirtieth Session of WHO. Regional Committee for South - East Asia, 2-8 August, 1977, Bangkok, Thailand, published in South-East Asia, Region Office : *Final Report and Minutes of the Meeting of the Thirtieth Session*, New Delhi, September 1977, pp. 69-70.

22. Geneva Declaration.

23. "I Swear by Apollo" by Christians Viedma, *World Health*, the magazine of the WHO, July 1979, p. 28.

24. Medical ethics: "A viewpoint from the developing world," By J.S. Neki, *World Health*, July 1979.

25. "Alma-Ata : Signpost to a new health era", by W.L. Barton, *World Health*, July 1979, p. 14.

26. WHO, *Technical Report Series*, No. 176.

27. Clough, Donald J., Concepts in Management Science, Prentice-Hall, Englewood Cliffs, N.J., 1963, p. 2.

28. Davis, Ralph C. , Industrial Organisation and Management, Harper, New York,1956, p.54.

29. Newman, Sumner and Warren, *The Process of Management*, Prentice-Hall, Englewood Cliffs, N.J. 1967, p. 10.

30. Terry, Geroge R., *Principles of Management* (Homewood, III, Irwin 1965), p. 52

31. Koontz and O'Donnell, *Management—A Book of Readings*; McGraw-Hill Book Co., London, 1968, p. 1.

32. Hicks, Herbert G., *The Management of Organisations*, McGraw-Hill, New York, 1967, p. 156.

33. Dale, Earnest, *Management Theory and Practice*, McGraw-Hill, New York, 1967, pp. 57.

7

District Collector and Decentralised Health Planning

Seventh Five – Year Plan document of Government of India records: that the nation is committed to attain the goal of health for all by 2000 AD. To achieve this, primary health care has been accepted as main instrument of action. Again, the plan document states clearly that family welfare occupies an important position in the socio-economic development plans. Health and family welfare planning plays a crucial role in human resource development and in improving the quality of life of the people. Besides, maternal and child health (MCH) is intimately related to family welfare. So, the thrust of all developmental plans of the government for the betterment of people is an improvement in the quality of life of the people. This concern is reflected all through the various plans seeking better health care and population stabilisation in the country. However, this thrust had become more explicit in the current plan :

(i) to achieve the goal of health for all by 2000 AD and precisely for that hardly 11years are left to attain that target; and

(ii) to achieve the population stabilisation at the replacement level for India by 2000 AD.

In the area of population stabilisation, some success is there, but that is less than desired due mainly to :

(i) less than optimal use of available resources;

(ii) lack of infrastructure facilities, which hamper the quality of programmes;

(iii) high levels of maternal, infant and child mortality;

(iv) political, social, economic, cultural factors; and

(v) lack of desired effective administration, coordination, and integration of programme efforts.

Although, the demographic situation in India is a matter of grave concern and poses challenge for development, Government is confident on the basis of its national experience and also through the documentation of international experiences that the goals for demographic stabilisation, better MCH care and improved health can achieved.

Now, it has been very well understood that population stabilisation, improvement in MCH and general health care requires a multi-dimensional and multi-involvement approach. This is more relevant in the light of the recent focus on decentralised micro-planning. This, in fact, means revitalisation of planning process at district level and below. Though, the Planning Commission issued guidelines to the states for initiating district planning as far back as in 1969, yet it remained un-operational. This, at least, is more true for the health and family welfare sector.

IDEAL ADMINISTRATIVE AND ORGANISATIONAL LEVEL

In the context mentioned above, it is envisaged that the most ideal administrative and organisational level will be that of a district to make efforts for initiating the district level planning to solve the population and health problems. This could be achieved through multi-dimensional approach or multi-pronged strategy to be evolved at district level to resolve the problem. This is becoming more pertinent in the light of the considered thinking about decentralised planning, right from the grassroot level, for which district will be a suitable nodal and intermediate point for developmental efforts.

When it becomes an agreed preposition, then the functionary to be the 'kingpin' of such efforts is the District Collector or Deputy.

Commissioner as it is called in some states. Before indicating what role District Collector can play more effectively, it will be better to see what position and role the District Collector has which can be more effectively utilised for giving boost to family welfare, MCH, and health programmes in the district.

Position of District Collector in India

The First-Five Plan document points out that the structure of the administration developed during the past century was based on the district as principal unit with District Collector as the government's principal representative in touch with the people.

Besides, being in control of the administration of law and order and revenue in the district, the District Collector held a coordination responsibility for the activities of all departmental agencies within the district. In the hierarchy of administration, he enjoyed status and power which gave him considerable influence over the local population.

The district is still the most important single unit of administration and District Collector is the intermediatry between the State Government executives and people.

Changing Role of District Collector

Since independence (1947) and particularly from the advent of planning (1952), the primary emphasis in district administration is on the implementation of development programme in close cooperation and with the active support of people. This envisages integration of various development departments in the district and linking up in relation to all development work. This also requires coordination and supervision of district development programme by District Collector.

In this context, it is also recognised that it is at the district level that attention in implementation of programme is focused and it is at the district level again that the relationship of administration and citizen assumes significance. Not only district administration provides principal points of contact between the citizen and the process of government, but in it is also found a structure and organisation for influencing the policy decisions at the district as well as state levels. It is because the Collector is the principal representative of State Government in the districts in India. District Collector through its agencies in the field give him a position of prominence not only for informing himself and the government but also coordinating and integrating the developmental activities of government with the aspirations of the people.

As Coordinator and Facilitator

This is because of the fact that Collector in the district is the captain of the team of officers of all departments and is responsible for securing the necessary coordination and cooperation in the perpetuation and execution of the district plans in the community development. The position may vary from state to state but District Collector invariably is the Chairman of District Development Council/Zila Parishad, and in some States Collector is also the Chairman of the Standing Committee of Zila Parishad.

After having identified the position and authority of District Collector, let us try to illustrate :

(i) how his position of authority and importance is most suited for health and family welfare programmes; and

(ii) the backdrop of information, knowledge, and skills required by him for administering, gearing up, and coordinating the programmes related to population stabilisation and health care.

AUGMENTATION AND ENERGISING THE HEALTH INFRASTRUCTURE

Strategy document of Government of India (1986-1990) towards population stabilisation indicates, on the basis of documented studies, that the reach and utilisation of family welfare, MCH and health care services is low and not very much satisfactory quality-wise. This prevailing condition of low reach and utilisation of services by the people is one of the big bottlenecks in solving the problem of population stabilisation and better health care. Many factors are responsible for this. One of the most important factors is the 'inertia' of the functionaries delivering the health and family welfare services to rural areas and urban slums. Others relate to non-filling of the positions, uneven distribution of staff and the problems connected with logistics and supply of medicines, drugs, equipment and others items falling in the category of infrastructure.

MODEL ORGANISATIONAL SET-UP

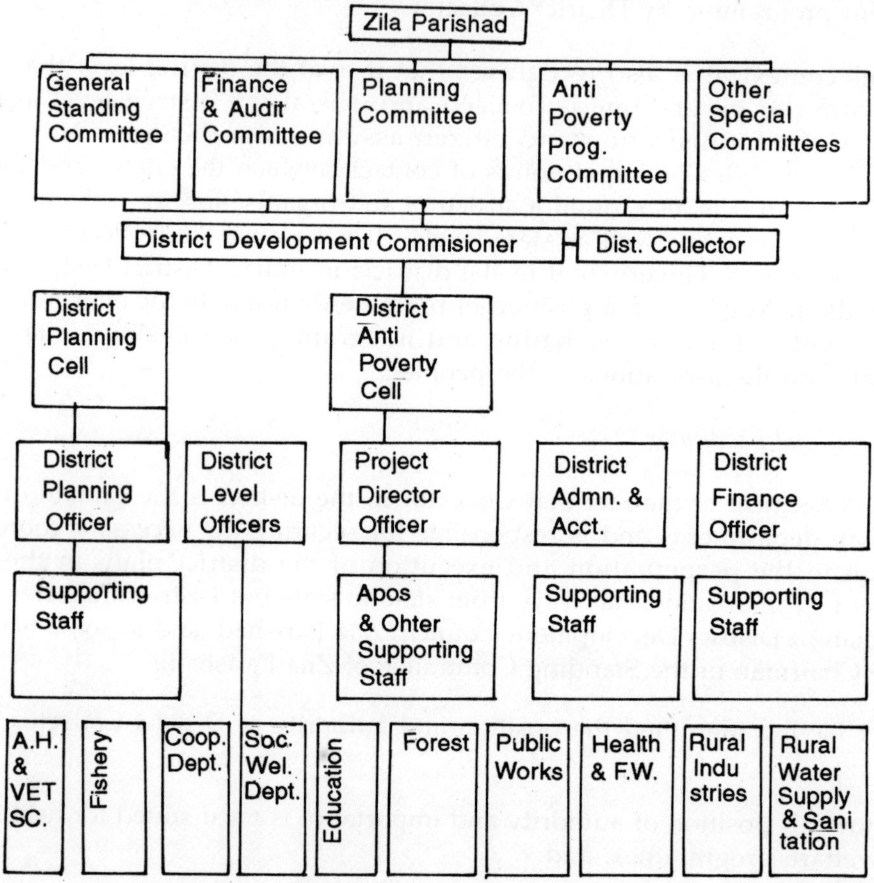

Source: *Report of the Committee to Review the Existing Administrative Arrangements for Rural Development and Poverty Alleviation Programmes*, Department of Rural Development, Ministry of Agriculture, December 1985.

What District Collector can do in the context of the district planning process for augmentation and energising of the infrastructure, particularly in rural areas, using his position and authority, has to be seen. District Collector can go systematically to find out all possible reasons prevailing precisely and mainly for the low reach of services and 'inertia' amongst the concerned staff. For example, on the part of health functionaries, the efforts may be lacking because of lack of basic facilities to them, like that of construction and allotment of residential accommodation, lack of transport, etc.

District Collector, first of all, may get a quick snap-shot observation-survey conducted to find out the precise and detailed reason for the low outreach of health and family welfare services in his district. For this District Collector can get prepared a map of the whole district, its blocks, villages and those pockets where outreach and utilisation of family welfare and health services remained : (i) low althrough, (ii) low only currently, and (iii) have never reached. This will give him the idea of his whole district for and with reference to health and family welfare planning. Thereafter, District Collector can call for or seek from the workers, their supervisors and also with the help of district intelligence machinery, the reasons for non-achievement of family welfare and MCH targets and low utilisation of health and family welfare services in the various pockets of the district. Getting this systematic exercise done will facilitate sorting out the problems in minute details, whether these are related to augmentation and energising existing infrastructure for 'inertia' or otherwise due to some other considerations.

When the quick analysis reveals that low performance is due to dormancy of the health and family welfare staff or inadequacy of personnel to man the positions, he can further probe, with district authorities, reasons for this sort of position and the efforts done by district level health authorities to overcome the prevailing situation. Here, he can play direct and indirect roles or he can provide direct and indirect support to the system to energise the infrastructure. District Collector can write a special note and report to the State Health Authorities to help improve the situation, particularly with reference to filling the positions, and improving the logistics so that health functionaries may be able to work more effectively. The direct role which he can play, exercising the position of his authority and leadership is as follows :

(i) Getting clearly delineated the job responsibility of all categories of employees;

(ii) Providing residential accommodation to all health functionaries right from periphery level (village level) to district level;

(iii) Sanctioning advances for purchase of transport to all health functionaries;

(iv) Getting the existing and available infrastructure facilities evenly distributed all the regions of a district;

(v) Developing a special constant monitoring mechanism in the collector's office; and

(vi) Making a cell to redress grievances of the health and family welfare functionaries.

Augmentation and Energising Other Departments

It is now well recognised that family welfare, MCH and health care is not the exclusive or sole responsibility of the functionaries belonging to health and family welfare departments. This is more true in the context of quick promotion and implementation of these programmes at the district level. Here, merely reducing or mitigating the inertia amongst health and family welfare staff may not pay full dividends. But the full and quick process of the programmes are related to moderation of fertility, reducing the mortality and improvement in the utilisation of health care services. This can happen when all other developmental departments join hands and work in a composite manner to the success of these programmes. In this context, District Collector can play a major role being captain at the district level. He can bring all the departments at one platform to contribute towards the goal of reaching health for all and population stabilisation levels in the district in due course. His directions in this regard are prone to show desired results. He can show how these programmes of health and family welfare will be helpful to their respective departments and their activities and how in turn these departments can extend help for health and family welfare activities while doing their own work. The real effort of a District Collector lies in the intersectoral coordination. For example, a District Collector may use his position to further energise and involve the department of education (the teachers) for improving school health programmes. He can get created a chain of school health clubs in all village schools for spreading education about immunisation, nutrition, health care and informing them about advantages of a small family norms. District Collector can make use of his being head of District Development Committee in his district and utilise departments of agriculture, forests, and social welfare in the efforts for improving the nutritional aspects of the programmes. Projects like that of 'Poshak Ahar' can vigorously be run with District Collector as a leader and monitor of such efforts in which even community financing can also be generated by him besides energising other departments. District Collector can use the mechanism of meetings with the staff of other departments and picking and choosing enthusiastic workers to assigning tasks and rewarding their efforts. Main role on the part of District Collector can be to convince other departments at District level about the importance of their contribution in social programmes like family welfare, MCH and health care.

Formation and Activising of Committees

Unless some formal official structure is not developed at : (a) the District, (b) Municipal/Corporation levels, (c) Block and Panchayat levels, and (d) Village level from amongst the functionaries of other departments operative at district level, the real, continuous and full involvement of various departments at these levels will not be possible. Without devising an organisational structure for the project, multi-sectoral involvement and action towards small family norm, increasing programme performance for health, family welfare and MCH will not be a workable preposition. After due orientation and sensitising various developmental departments about their prospective role and importance for contributing towards health and family welfare work, it will be in the fitness of the working that District Collector gives direction about formation of District/Block/Village level committees which would have in these committees functionaries from all developmental departments at these levels. These committees will have representatives from Department of Health and Family Welfare also and suitable action plans can be got drawn for implementation in the specified area in the specified time limit. Technical support can come from Department of Health and Family Welfare and these Committees would function under overall control and direction of District Collector as head of apex committee at the district level. Through these committees, small activities can be got initiated which will have integrated bearing on the improvement of health and family welfare programmes.

Orientation and Sensitisation

District Collector can take a special administrative responsibility in the orientation and sensitisation of the district level and block level officers belonging to various departments regarding the importance and gravity of problem of family planning and MCH and health care. District Collector can also have dialogue and informal meeting with District Officers to elicit what role they can play in augmenting the programmes for health and family welfare. This orientation and sensitising may be possible by holding : (i) initial contact meeting and (ii) arranging symposia inviting population scientists from State or the Centre. During orientation, the district officers from various departments can be briefed about the demographic, health and socio-economic profile of the district *vis-a-vis*, the State and the country as also that about possible solutions available or sought elsewhere. An outcome of these meetings, seminars, workshops, conferences could be that interaction will generate in other departments and may lead to develop a concrete thinking and action plans, to contribute towards health and family planning efforts at the district level through their respective machinery.

Coordination with Voluntary Organisations

Strategy paper towards population stabilisation (1986-90) indicates that voluntary organisation will be associated more closely and actively with the programme in order to fully exploit their potential for innovation and dedication to the cause, proximity to and credibility with the people. In this context, District Collector's role can be vital as he is the Government's representative in the district, directly in touch with people as well as people's organisation involved in welfare activities. District collector's role becomes more crucial in the light of the suggestions made in the Action Plan strategy of Government of India towards the priority programme of population stabilisation in the country. In the coming years, efforts should be made so that every district will have at least three voluntary organisations working for the health and family welfare programme. One of them may be designated as the lead voluntary organisation.

The efforts can be initiated at the district level by the District Collector for identifying suitable voluntary agencies operating in the district or adjoining area. District Collector's role is not limited only to identifying and recommending suitable voluntary organisation but also nominating a support committee for voluntary efforts in health and family planning. In this committee, people can be drawn from different walks of life including those from various voluntary organisations. This broad based committee, with District Collector as its chairperson, can guide, direct, consolidate the efforts being done by voluntary and other agencies in the area of family welfare and health care. This committee at the district level can have committees at block level for monitoring the efforts. District Collector can make financial assistance available through district funds as well as by approaching state authorities and foundations/enterprises operating in the district.

Generating Community Participation

The basis of primary health care depends on the effective role of the community. The community can play its role more effectively when it is induced for involvement, interaction, initiation and planning for participation towards health and family welfare efforts for their betterment. To start with, this is difficult. Hence, patience and perseverence are needed for generation of community participation, as a support mechanism to boost up programme component of primary health care, *viz.*, family welfare, MCH, etc. In this effort, role of District Collector as a chief catalytic agent at the district level is the most important. Through his position and authority, District Collector can induce and facilitate the efforts of mobilising the community. More than this, through his available administrative apparatus and set-up which functionally penetrates up to grassroots community level, District Collector can act as a manager of whole administrative set up to steer towards participatory efforts. He has multiple developmental activities to cater to the community, directly and indirectly and through these activities. District Collector can generate, manage and monitor participatory processes in the community. His position can enable him to combat the hindrances which come in the way of community participation. His administrative contacts and the administrative network of intelligence at his disposal makes his position unique to understand and control such factors.

Formation of Popular Committees

As a main instrument of generating positive and continuous community response from the community groups to promote family welfare, MCH and health care programme, official or departmental/governmental committees may not be able to do full justice to solve the demographic and health situations or problems at district level and below. Full implementation of policies and programme strategies devised at the official level is possible through formation and active participation of popular committees at different levels and developing their corresponding links with each other at all levels. The structure of such popular committees at all levels, *i.e.*, District/block/village, should, be such that it should have members from all sections of the society at large and those specifically of different communities. For example, District Collector can work-out a plan for formation of these committees to help the F.W.-MCH-Health programme efforts consisting of :

1. Elected representatives of people—MP/MLA/MLC/Member of Zila Parishad.
2. Members of different political parties;
3. People belonging to professional groups, like lawyer, doctors, engineers and teachers;
4. Members from cultural groups;
5. Religious leaders;
6. Media related people;
7. Members of voluntary organisations in the area;
8. Members from weaker sections, S.C./S.T.s; and
9. People belonging to artisans groups.

Involvement of Special Groups

For generation and management of community participation as an adjunct to the official efforts to push the family welfare, MCH and Health Care Programmes at the peripheri levels, involvement of special groups by District Collector is necessary. Such special population or community groups may be too many to enumerate. However, few important ones will be women's groups or Mothers Health Clubs, Student Groups or School Health Clubs, Youth Clubs, Farmers Group, etc. Not necessary that such groups would be already existing in the villages. Wherever these are not there in existence, these are required to be got created by District Collector utilising his district extension functionaries of health and other department. The village extension, block extension and district extension staff may be given the special task of inducing the participation of such groups and this work should be started with the formation or creation of groups like village womens health clubs, village school health clubs, etc. However, wherever such groups are already formed in whatever scanty and semi-organised manner, District Collector should direct, through meetings and circulars, his extension force in the district departments to further strengthen and activise such existing groups. This is possible through making these women, children and youth groups more broad—based and multi-functional. These Mother's Health and F.W. Clubs and young groups scan simultaneously be oriented through inputs like : (a) small training and demonstration courses, and (b) financial help for many diverse but interrelated activities of applied nutrition programmes, child care immunisation, family welfare and environmental sanitation.

Special involvement of students community is possible when District Collector takes it up with education department. This involvement can be started with his direction in initiating formation of school health clubs where students and teachers can participate at all levels, i.e., village, block and district. Through his direction, such special group of school health clubs can be utilised by him to augment various programmes at all levels, viz., school health programmes, etc. He can utilise the force of student community through his district extension machinery to activise immunisation and other programmes as school children are the potential health educators and change agents and women (mothers) are considered first and best provider of health care.

Involvement of Private Medical Practitioners

Intersectoral coordination for promotion of health and family welfare work envisages three types of coordination : (i) within the official health system, (ii) within the overall health system, including non-official health resources (manpower, etc.), and (iii) outside the health system. The District Collector is in position to take advantage of all the three tiers of intersectoral coordination. But his most potential resource will be the involvement of private medical practitioners for the promotion of health and family welfare efforts in his district. The specific reason for this resource being most important is that private medical practitioners penetrate deep in the community life up to the grassroots level. Not only these practitioners — whether Ayurvedic, Allopathic, or indigenous traditional health healers—are available at the doorsteps or in village corridor to the people but they have also earned faith and reputation of the people over the period of time. Such a medical manpower, howsoever inadequately qualified it may appear in terms of qualified medical standards, is definitely a force to reckon with.

District Collector can mobilise this potential medical manpower arranging orientation and sensitising camps for them. Private medical officers can be involved through calling them in workshops, meetings and informal dialogues initiated by District Collector from time to time at various levels and on various occasions, both formal and informal. He can generate feeling through his 'managerial leadership', so that the private medical practitioners, particularly in rural areas may start feeling concerned about national programmes for the people. A blueprint of action plans for private medical practitioners can be got developed at district level and District Collector can act as a 'monitor' of such action plans which may have some reward and appreciation mechanism for sustaining private medical practitioner's interest in the programme.

SOME THRUST AREAS

For contributing towards solutions of problems related to population stabilisation and MCH care, etc., District Collector has lot of scope, authority, and managerial and administrative opportunities. He can energise and electrify the whole situation directly through the programmes within the purview of health services as well as via special developmental measures which are beyond family planning. Many thrust areas for District Collector's direct and immediate concern can be identified and listed. Few thrust areas are discussed here which may have some bearing and relevance to the programme efforts and in which he can play a major and important role :

1. Child survival and immunisation;
2. Increasing age of marriage; and
3. Implementing differential strategy.

A stage has come in India's demographic scene where it's future fertility goals will be difficult to achieve unless these goals are intimately and deliberately linked with some developmental variables. Developmental variables are to be taken in broader sense. For realising and sustaining one such goal of development is the reduction in infant and child mortality. Universally low infant mortality has been found to be linked with decline in fertility. Keeping this contention in view, District Collector may start special drives with the help of district health authorities and also utilising infrastructural support from Agriculture, Veterinary, Tribal and Social Welfare and other allied departments and developing 'institutional linkages' for nutrition-cum-immunisation and child care programme. District Collector's working in this perspective, particularly for weaker sections not only would bring forth more chances of tackling various developmental problems but he will also be able to provide and develop a 'motivational base' for pushing and programmes for family welfare, MCH and health care in his district.

Actions Plans for Special Thrust Area Programmes

District Collector can have specific role in bringing the concerned department and agencies, particularly for two special programme drives : (i) successful implementation of universal immunisation at District/Block/Village level; and (ii) Oral Rehydration Therapy programmes. District Collector may use his good offices in getting detailed action plans developed for these important strategies of child survival and through his specially appointed committees, in which Village Health Guide and Trained Dai should be a member at village level. At block level, District Collector can get organised special *Bal Swasthya Melas* where demonstration for ORS and child nutrition benefits of immunisation, etc., should be demonstrated to people. Initiation of such efforts by District Collector will give boost to family welfare and MCH efforts at the district and lower levels.

Raising Mean Age of Marriage

In our country, although legal age of marriage is 18 years for girls yet in practice seven per cent females get married in the age group of 10-14 years and about 44 per cent married females are between 15-19 years of ages. Nearly three million estimated marriages (of 4 million total) annually take place in the age group of 15-19 years. This situation is worst in some states. Similarly, there are many districts in India where this situation further gets aggravated.

This dimension of low female age of marriage results in many complex problems of ill health, too early pregnancy and mortality of children and high fertility. What District Collector as an administrator can do in this regard depends on his innovative approaches and thinking. With his efforts, he may counteract this problem which is mainly confined to villages and more so in particular classes and communities.

Mere administrative authority of sending circulars/letters/wireless messages may not be sufficient for implementation of this social legislation regarding restraining the child marriages. More than its legality or legal consequences, the health, social and economic benefits to the individual and family, particularly belonging to weaker sections, are required to be highlighted through extension efforts organised at his level. District Collector can constitute a committee, which can be called Social Consciousness Committee, drawing people from all departments and all walks of life who have been social activists to promote social change programmes like that of shifting the attitude of the people towards increase in age at marriage. His efforts as monitor-manager and coordinator of social change for increasing age of marriage will rest not much in negative manner of emphasising deterrent punishment for breach of law relating to minimum age at marriage. Rather, as the highest administrative representative for managing social change, District Collector would be able to do a lot in this direction as discussed below :

(i) Forming 'Social Consciousness Committees' at village / block / district level for: (a) creating awareness about the legal age at marriage, and (b) transmitting benefits, particularly health and social benefits, to family.

(ii) Involving voluntary organisations to create social climate for raising marriageable age for females.

(iii) Promoting female education facilities through incentives to those families of weaker sections who educate and marry of their daughters beyond prescribed legal age of marriage. Since this measure requires multisectoral support, District Collector through his control and authority may make use of district education set up for augmenting female education.

(iv) District Collector may get generated funds and resources from the public and other private establishments to arrange mass simple and dowry less marriages for the daughters of weaker sections, who participate in programmes of upholding legal age of marriage and having small family.

(v) District Collector, as manager of the social affairs in the district, can workout various schemes of giving incentives through IDRP funds, and funds from wasteland development schemes to the newly married women who not only confirmed to the minimum legal age at marriage but also properly spaced their children after marrying above the legal age of marriage, and got their child immunised.

(vi) As a multisectoral departmental move, District Collector may involve women welfare agencies, human resource department functionaries, students, teachers and media infrastructure at the district level for propagation, in village and urban slums, efforts for raising marriageable age of females and its positive benefits to family, women and children in particular.

Throughout the district, all the time and over the years, same uniformed and identical strategy of functioning, coordinating and integrating of family welfare, MCH and health care may not be viable and very effective. Wide differences exist not only in Blocks and Tehsils in a district but also within Blocks area and cluster of villages where the performance and acceptance of family welfare, MCH and health care services are either very low or very high. District Collector can take special cognisance of such situations prevailing in the area. District Collector may evolve, with the help of his associates at the district, different and corresponding strategies workable in different blocks/pockets and regions within the district. His approach in solving such problems may generate out of his 'fact finding' and analytical style to go into the details about the minute reasons of prevailing situation. In some pockets of the district, the reason for lesser success may be unapproachable all whether road, non deployment of staff or political resistance. At some other places, the better success in certain blocks and pockets may be due to commitment of functionaries working in the area, active interest of voluntary organisations better logistics, etc. District Collector can derive suitable insights from factors associated with low or high performance, *i.e.*, factors which either push or block the programmes. His managerial skills and authority can help mitigating or lessening the blocking factors and further pushing the positive ones. So, his strategy will be a blending of many aspects of efforts, including involvement of few social scientists from the district institutions in the social council and that of some social workers to work for the programmes, in order to help correct the inhibiting factors.

Revitalising The Mass Media

For meeting or reaching and contacting more people, a multipronged strategy of revamping the media activities and the whole communication programme is required. In this context, the special role of District Collector will be with reference to energise the media efforts already going on and also developing more interest in the development of the folk media in the district. High technology based medium for propagations of messages about health and family welfare, MCH, etc., may have higher reach in terms of their respective wave length, etc., or physical recording. However, the reality now is that the impact of traditional and folk art is greater and deeper in this regard.

The special campaigns, utilising appropriate technology and local talents, particularly in the rural areas, for popularising the preventive and promotive aspects of health care along with the importance of small family norm, advantages of well spaced children, maternal-child health care, etc., are required to be got developed using Collector's good office and powers at the district level. Special efforts in this campaign could be on immunisation and de-emphasising the preference for male children. In this social venture, District Collector's meeting with the Village Groups and Village Associations will be of great advantage. These meetings can both be formal and informal and such meetings could also be tagged with other developmental meetings.

Informal Meetings With Village People

District Collector as communicator or in the role of a communicator can make an effective dent on the thinking of people with the informal dialogue mechanism than merely issuing the leaflets, circulars, appeals or orders, etc. Mere his presence in the meetings, particularly with rural folk, may build a strong bridge between family welfare, MCH and health programmes and people than through any formal and sophisticated communication mechanism. By virtue of his being a strong link between people and Government, District Collector knows the language of the people. His authority and power enables District Collector to get the programme efforts translated in reality more quickly through his day-to-day involvement in developmental efforts. Much, however, depends on his style of functioning.

Role of OTC and Small Newspapers

Two more mechanisms that the District Collector can find more useful as operational strategies for revamping the whole communication programmes are : (1) strengthening and streamlining of orientation training camps (OTCs), and (2) involvement of small newspapers for creating a positive atmosphere for implementing programmes related to health and family welfare and MCH. These two strategies can form a strong base for convincing the people. District Collector can encourage these organs through his liberal financial support and other mechanisms, *viz.,* inviting the editors and writers in these small newspapers at the district level to the official meetings for discussions on health and family welfare programmes. Some financial allocation can be made for feature writing for propagation of health and family welfare themes in the press.

Decentralisation and Financial Process

ICSSR and ICMR document on *Health For All : An Alternate Strategy* indicates that the allocated budget should reach the most peripheral body that controls the health activity (*e.g.*, the Gram Panchayat for the village and sub-centre, the Panchayat Samiti for the Community Health Centre and Zila Parishad for the District Health Centres). In this respect, the District Collector's role can be very crucial in seeing whether such delegation of administrative and financial responsibility to the local authorities—and ultimately to local communities — is taking place or not. District Collector can work for and towards decentralisation of such efforts which may contribute towards promotion of health and family welfare programmes. His efforts will be most beneficial through strengthening the whole procedure of sanctioning and simplifying the procedures for disbursement of money.

Monitoring and Review of Progress

Monitoring and evaluation of District Action Plans to boost up family welfare, MCH and health care programmes are not isolatory exercises to be operationalised in vacuum. Instead monitoring and evaluation can be linked through the intervention of District

SUGGESTED STAGES AND MECHANISM FOR PLANNING , IMPLEMENTATION, MONITORING AND EVALUATION OF DISTRICT ACTION PLAN FOR HEALTH, FAMILY WELFARE AND MCH

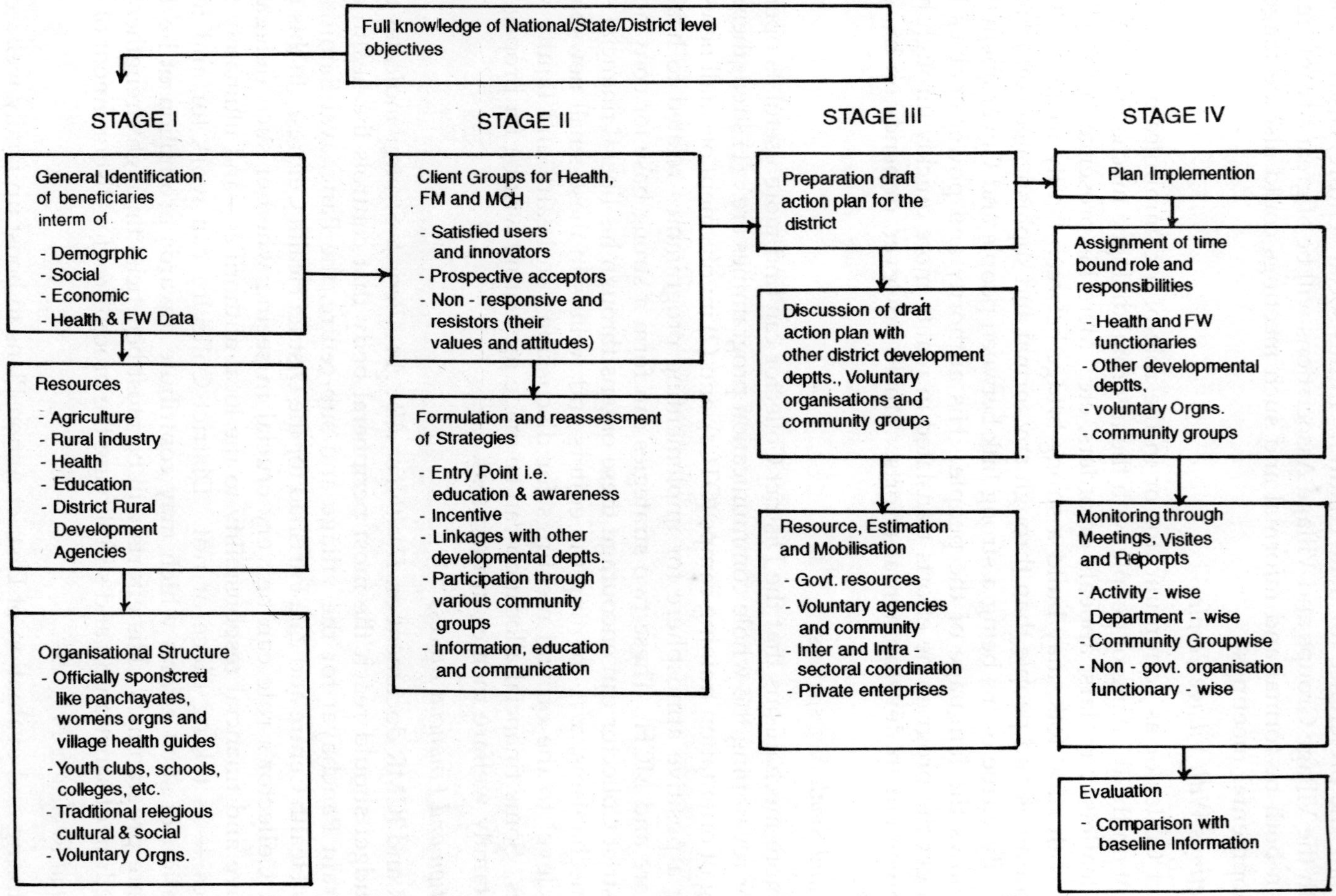

Collector with various stages and mechanisms for planning and plan implementation. No doubt, without a good monitoring system, whether it is a sophisticated Management Information System (MIS) or a simple lay reporting, the programme cannot succeed. A successful monitoring system has to pass through various stages. Few of these suggested stages/steps and mechanism for planning, implementing along with monitoring and evaluation, to be directed and administered by District Collector, are given in the chart on page-164. These are not exhaustive but tentative. District Collector may get an exercise done to redo and reshape these steps and stages that are more relevant to his district situation. This exercise should form part of the Action Research Plan at District/Block/ Village Level.

The suggested first step—which would help overall planning, implementation, monitoring and evaluation—is having full knowledge of national objectives/goals, *viz.*, National Health Policy, National Population Policy, National Nutrition Policy and National Education Policy. Besides this, District Collector's detail knowledge about state level objectives/goals will help him formulate District level goals/objectives, etc. This would give him thematic idea of arriving at practicals solutions about his own district while remaining in conformity with state/national goals and objectives. Thereafter stage one will include : (i) identification of prospective beneficiaries in terms of demographic, social, economic health and family welfare, (ii) identification or listing of resources under health and family welfare, agriculture, rural industry, education, district rural development agency, (iii) identification of available organisational structures—official as well as non-sponsored ones like women's organisation, youth clubs, traditional, religious, cultural and social organisations, voluntary organisations, private medical practitioners, village health guides, village trained dais; and (iv) identification of documentation of special schemes like that of rural employment, etc.

After having identified the prospective beneficiaries and client groups, knowing their values and attitudes, the strategies so developed will be monitored from time to time. The plan objectives or goals set for the district has to be monitored and evaluated with a time frame or time-scale, with a quality recording scale and 'change scales' developed with the assistance of District Statistical unit and other health programme machinery at his disposal. The suggested 'entry points' can be education, incentives, communication of information, participatory efforts through groups, etc. For plan formulation monitoring, knowledge and identification of entry points will be necessary.

Assignment of time-bound roles and responsibilities to individuals and groups of various departments, besides health resource estimation, mobilisation and allocation for the activities and their monitoring would have to be done through meetings at all levels, developing quick reporting system and getting prepared PERT charts, etc., for scheduling and Gantt charts, etc. Preparation of Gantt charts for activity monitoring would help District Collector to make needed 'mid-course adjustment' at the interval of three to six months for solving the problems and making the programme delivery of family welfare, MCH and health care more effective.

References

1. Government of India, *Report of the Working Group on District Planning*. Vol. I, New Delhi, Planning Commission, 1984, p. 167.

2. Government of India, *Report of the Working Group on District Planning*, Vol. II, New Delhi, Planning Commission, 1988, p. 220.

3. Government of India, *Seventh Five Year Plan* - 1985-90, Vol. II, New Delhi, Planning Commission, 1985, p. 421.

4. Government of India, *Revised Strategy for National Family Welfare Programme : A Summary*, New Delhi, Ministry of Health and Family Welfare, 1985, p. 32.

5. J.P. Gupta and B.B.L. Sharma, "*District and Block Level Planning for Health* ", Paper presented at the *Thirteenth Annual Conference of Indian Association for the Study of Population*, 1988, p. 19.

8

Aging, Aged and Age Care

Aging is considered a very serious problem. While children pass out of the stage of dependency with an alarming speed, the aged become increasingly dependent on others. It is generally believed that old people are helpless, isolated, ignored, physically weak, disengaged from active work and economically dependent. Serious concern has also been shown for the gradually rising proportion of such people in the total population According to UNESCO estimates, the number of old people in the world, above 60, is likely to go up from 350 million in 1975 to 590 million in 2005 and 1120 million in 2025 A.D. About half of them live in developing countries. In India, there were about 70 million old persons in 1981.

It is in this context that the World Health Organisation has made an appeal to discard the stereotype idea of the old as helpless and useless. While increasing concern is being expressed everywhere for the welfare of the old, the view held by the aged themselves about their later years has not been seriously studied, nor taken seriously. The aged certainly hold a better and more optimistic view of the state of their life. A limited study has revealed very fascinating results.

India's large population base accounts for a sizeable number of people 60+ even though the proportion continues to be small when compared to the developed countries. However, due to increase in the life expectancy rated and gradual decline in the birth rates, the proportion of elderly persons above 60 in the population reflects an increasing trend from 5 per cent in 1901 to 5.97 per cent in 1971 and 6.91 per cent projected for 1996. The census figures indicate that number of elderly persons in the age 60+ in 1901 was 12 million which rose to 20 million 1951 and 43 million in 1961 and it is expected to increase 67 million by 2000 A.D. The another significant dimensions of the elderly population is the higher rate of increase as compared to the increase in the general population. It is evident from the fact that as against 21.51 per cent increase in total population, people of 60+ age group increased at the rate of 22.40 per cent during 1951-61; during 1967-71 their increase was of the order of 32.32 as against general population growth of 24.80 per cent; during the 1971-81 their number increased at the rate of 31.60 per cent as against general population increase of 24.75 per cent. In all likelihood, this trend is expected to continue in the coming decades also. One of the major reasons for such a trend is the increase in the life expectancy from mere 23.63 years for males and 23.96 years for females in 1901 to 60.1 years for male and 59.8 years for females projected for 1991-96.

AGED IN TRADITIONAL SET UP

The most positive aspects of our aging population is that most of them continue to remain active earners in the family. It is mainly because these people are engaged in such sectors of economy in which there does not exist any specific age of retirement. Data rather show that the percentage of persons above 60 classified as workers are higher than those of the percentage of workers in all age groups in the total population. Likewise, the percentage of elderly persons in the working population worked out to be higher than their percentage in the total population.

India is a land where the elderly have been traditionally enjoying a place of honour, respect and power as prescribed by religious texts and social values and norms. The sons are expected to look after the parents. The failure to do so earns people social stigma.

The important role played by elderly persons is not confined only to ceremonial occasions; they actively participate in familial and community life too. Their power and status in the family are reinforced by their rights over the ownership of the means of production and property. As they grow older they tend to withdraw from their day to day affairs depending upon their state of health and the availability/willingness of other members in the family to discharge their responsibilities. The transition from active work participation to the roleless status has so far been voluntary and smooth.

EFFECTS OF RECENT CHANGES

However, the recent changes in society particularly those resulting from rapid industrialisation, urbanisation, western education and migration have caused stress and strain on the aged in varying degrees which have tended to increase the vulnerability of the aged.

The traditional Kinship and family organisation is being replaced by nuclear family norms. The people are increasingly becoming more materialistic and individualistic in their orientations. They are no longer able to maintain the same relationship with elderly numbers as they did in the past because of several social and economic circumstances. The shortages of housing accommodation in the cities, high rentals, limited earning and host of other factors compel young members of the family to leave the parents in villages without any care. The increasing employment of women in cities in offices and factories led them to spend much less time on the care of elderly members. The high cost involved in the upbringing of children and education, and need to maintain a reasonable level of leaving offer disincentives to look after the aged properly.

AGED IN THE WELFARE STATE

Under these circumstances, the problems of the care of the growing aging population is a matter of great concern and calls for special treatment. It is particularly so in view of their declining income, growing age and deteriorating health conditions. These people cannot be ignored in a society which claims to be democratic and welfare-oriented.

Our Constitutional provisions, Directive Principles of State Policy and legislative measures provide recognition to the need to receive adequate attention in matters of care, work and security. Article 41 clearly states : "the State shall within the limits of economic capacity and development, make effective provision for securing the right to work, to education, and to public assistance in cases of unemployment, old age, sickness and disablement and in other cases of undesired want." This is an important provision of the Directive Principles of State Policy. The Article 37 stipulates that, "it shall be the duty of the state to apply these principles in making laws." Section 125 of the Criminal Procedure Code 1973 expects every person having sufficient means to maintain his father or mother who are unable ot maintain themselves. The Section 20 (3) of the Hindu Adaptation and Maintenance Act 1956 also considered it obligatory for a person to maintain his or her aged or infirm parents.

Several committees and governments have initiated steps to combat the problems being experienced by the aging population. The Study Group on Income and Wages (1978) recognises the need for providing security to the old persons covered by pension and other retirement benefits. It suggested some norm to be adopted by different states to grant old age pension to the old destitutes. The Seventh Finance Commission (1978) also expressed the need to have uniformity among different states with regard to old age pension. The Sixth Five Year Plan recognised the vulnerability of certain categories of population including the aged and the need for development programmes to meet their requirement.

The analysis of various provisions available for the welfare of the aging population in India indicates that the persons working in government, semi-government, public undertakings and in many corporate sector enterprises are given the benefit of some measure to maintain incomes after retirement. These persons are eligible for pension, gratuity, leave encashment and provident fund. In government and organised sector these provisions are being gradually liberalised including payment of pension to the family in the event of the death of the employees during service. Two other measures are of great significance for the welfare of the aged which have been introduced by the central government of its employees. One is an Insurance Scheme which assures payments on retirement or death and the other is general Provident Fund. Another measure was permitting the government servant to undertake employment after retirement that ensures regularity of income and work in the old age.

In the organised sectors of industries also several retirement benefits are available for the benefit of aged. Under Employees Provident Fund Miscellaneous and Provisions Act 1952, three schemes were introduced: (i) Employees' Provident Fund Scheme, (ii) Employees' Family Pension Scheme, and (iii) Employees' Deposit Linked Insurance Scheme. Under the first scheme the establishments employing about 20 or more persons are made to provide matching contribution in the Provident Fund. On attaining the age of 55, the employees are entitled to full refund of contribution by him together with that of employer plus interest. Under the second scheme, the benefits are given only to the deceased member. Under the third scheme the person is given his provident fund amount plus assurance benefit in the event of his death. The provision of gratuity is also available under payment of gratuity act 1972. This is applicable to factories, mines and plantation covering employees earning less than a specified amount.

MEASURES BY STATE GOVERNMENTS

Different state governments have introduced old age pension schemes in the nature of public assistance. However, the eligibility criteria varies from state to state. While most of the states have kept 65 years as the minimum age for eligibility, a few others have kept it as 60. In some states, a lower age limit has been prescribed for females, widows, and for the physically and mentally handicapped. The requirement of continuous residence in that state for a period varying from 3 to 10 years have been made essential in almost all the states. The old age pensions are given to persons with little or no source of income with no one to support them. The period of entitlement also varies from state to state; in some states it is for a limited period while in others it is on a continuous basis.

It is heartening to note that the government of Haryana has also initiated an old age pension scheme for persons in the age group of 60+. Since the scheme was launched only during 1987-88, its impact on the welfare of the aged can be assessed only after sometime. The step is, however, bold in the sense that benefit is offered to all the aged who are 60 and above irrespective of their socio-economic conditions to bring about a favourable change in the attitude and behaviour of other family members towards the elders in receipt of old age pension. The delay in the payment of subsequent person, however, is causing some resentment among the people. The State government also appears to be critical of this fact and is planning to devise ways and means to avert this kind of situation.

HEALTH CARE OF THE AGED

Much of the problems experienced by the elderly persons have their roots in their poor health and declining physical capacity. Aging is often found to be associated with respiratory and digestive problems, deficiencies and functional disorders. Failing eyesight and hearing capacity, slow and faltering steps, declining work capacity, blindness and forgetfulness also plague the old. The situation becomes most serious in the case of women and persons having no income and no family support.

There does not exist a separate health care system for the aged; it is rather integrated with the overall health system, In rural areas where most of the population resides, medical services are offered to them through Primary Health Centres and Sub-Centres. India is committed to achieve "Health for All by the Year 2000" through a provision of minimum package of health care services to all including the aged. In the organised sector the employees continue to receive benefits of health care on nominal payments even after retirement.

In a large establishments like the post and telegraph, railways and defence services specific medical services are made available to the retired employees. Most state governments also provide some health facilities to the retired employees and their families. However, this constitute only a negligible part of the whole problem as the most aged particularly from poverty groups have little or no access to any of the health care services. If some kind of service is available locally, it is not easily accessible. A long way has, therefore, to be traversed in order to provide health care services to the aging population on a priority basis. The provision of medical camps, mobile medical care facilities and after care services need to be arranged. The use of the services of retired medical staff may be suggested as a possible steps for providing adequate health care for the aged. Special outdoors facilities in the hospitals may help the aged greatly.

The scheme of common residence for the aged which is often advocated as a solution does not seem to be practical in view of the emotional and social ties that the elders have for their families. The shortage of housing accommodation in the cities and the high rentals make their sons who migrate unwilling to carry elders with them. Moreover, there does not exist any separate housing schemes for elderly. However, in the recent years the state sponsored housing schemes earmark certain percentage of houses for the retired employees of the government and organised sectors. The housing loans provided by the employers provide some security after retirement as far as housing is concerned

ROLE OF VOLUNTARY ORGANISATIONS

A significant role has to be played by voluntary organisations in providing security to the aged. This can be done by providing them recreation, work opportunities, health care and by increasing their access to development programmes. The most significant step is to create a feeling among them that they can contribute effectively in the community activities. The stereotype idea that they are helpless and weak needs to be changed. Opportunities should be provided to increase their participation in community activities. The experiences of the elders could be used for solving our day to day problems. The more we can make the aged engaged in some kind of constructive work better it is for them.

9

Health Needs and Health Care of the Aged

Aging is an inevitable process involving a change in the state of mind. Today, we are witnessing the beginning of revolutionary change in that state of mind. In the yester years, old age meant enforced retirement, loss of physical functions and mental capacity involving all too often an isolation from normal activities of society. The aged person was considered as suffering from an irreversible form of illness and was treated like a sick child.

The recognition of aging as a social problem is recent and recognition of aging as a social and scientific problem is more recent. Accordingly, the image of the aged person as one who is tottering towards the grave, battered by illness and afflicted by disease, beyond the capacity for loving and incapable of taking care of himself much less rendering service to others, is false. Recent studies of healthy individuals show that, even at seventy years of age, they can do far more than take care of themselves. They can do a good day's work, use their minds creatively, carry on loving relationship and play an active role in the community.

Apart from the aforesaid nature of aging, the number of older people aged 65 years and above has increased world over the 63 per cent over the last 20 years. It is expected that the percentage of the aged would increase at a higher rate in more developed countries as compared to the lesser developed countries. A study of the United Nations shows that by 2000 AD, the aged (65 and above) would constitute 11.4 per cent of population of the more developed countries and 4.6 per cent of the less developed countries with a world average of 6.1 per cent. At present, over 50 per cent of aged (over 60) live in developing countries and it is anticipated that this proportion will reach to 72 per cent by 2025 A.D.

India is a developing country and the number of aged persons is bound to increase with better health and medical facilities, control of communicable diseases, reduction in death rate and decrease in birth rate. Inspite of all these developments the population growth in India is not expected to decrease much in case of substantial decrease in growth the proportion of aged to total population would increase.

Aging people require a wide range of preventive, curative and rehabilitative care. They have special needs in nutrition, in hygiene, in exercise and in immunisation. Housing, transport and personal security should be adapted to their particular needs. Research in all these areas and into the whole social and biological process of aging should receive new impetus. Keeping this in view, an attempt is made to assess their health status in the present context in order to recommend the health services needed for the aged.

Only a few studies on health problems of aged have been carried out in India. Choudhuri et al. surveyed the inmates of the home for aged women in Calcutta for geriatric in 1965. Raj and Parsad (1970) attempted to assess the health status of the rural aged in India. A similar work has been initiated by Raja, in the year 1971 by attempting a medico-social study of the aged in certain villages. Purohit made an appraisal of the socio-medical problems of aged in 1973. Purohit et al. (1976) completed a study on general health status of the aged, 60 and above, in a rural health training centre area. Sen Gupta and Chakraborty (1982) added to the above series by conducting a research study on assessing the health status of males aged 55 years and above, in a slum area of Calcutta.

MATERIAL AND METHOD

The present study was conducted in Hisar district of Haryana state. A cluster of four villages was purposively selected where a household survey by the state ICDS programme was being conducted, to estimate the total number of children and women who need the programme services. The sample of 25 subjects aged 55 years and above were selected randomly from each village making a sample of 100 respondents. Besides the above mentioned samples of the aged, all the aged who happened to visit Medical College, Rohtak for treatment, were also interviewed over the period of two weeks simultaneously. The total respondents counted as 13, thus making total sample size 113 respondents. These respondents were personally interviewed with the help of structured interview schedule.

Respondents schedules were edited and responses were tabulated. Simple percentages were calculated for both the type of respondents.

RESULTS AND DISCUSSION

Field Results

The selected field sample comprised of more females and less males, 54 per cent and 46 per cent respectively, which strengthens the fact if women can survive the hazards of child bearing potential they live longer than males.

Out of total 100 field subjects, the majority that is 88 per cent belonged to joint families and a minority (12 per cent) represented the nuclear families. This observation adds to the information that the concept of joint families still dominates the rural sector.

As far as the marital status of field subjects is concerned, it had been observed that a majority, that is, 65 per cent were married and the remaining, that is, 35 per cent were either widow/widower or unmarried. The substantial section in this category at this age indicates the probability of creating feeling of isolation amongst these citizens.

With regard to educational status, it was revealed that as many as 86 per cent were literate, whereas 4 per cent were found to be educated to the level of matric. The low educational status indicates slow improvement in all other aspects of life including health.

Analysis of occupational status of the respondents revealed the fact as many as 30 per cent were unable to do any work. In other words, they were dependent upon other family members for their livelihood. Again, quite a large number, that is, 35 per cent were found engaging themselves in only household work. This category of respondents, (women) though quite helpful indirectly in production, can be termed as partially dependent for their livelihood thus making the category of dependent quite a large that is, 65 per cent. The remaining 35 per cent (23 per cent engaged in agriculture and 12 per cent engaged in household as well as in agriculture) were those who actively participated in productive work or they were not dependent upon their family members. A significant percentage of the selected group's dependency on family members for their livelihood is partly the product of the biological phenomena and partly the cultural heritage of being free from productive engagements the moment their sons become productive members.

An income analysis of the selected group of subjects revealed that 27 per cent of farm families were having total annual income less than Rs. 10,000 on rough estimates. These can be treated below poverty-line (low income group) and 31 per cent of families having annual income more than Rs. 20,000 (High income group) and majority that is 42 per cent were having income more than 10,000 but less than Rs. 20,000 annually (middle income group).

Clinic Results

A majority that is 84.8 per cent of the aged who came for treatment to hospital were males and only 15.2 per cent were females. This observation highlights the male-dominated society which gives men preferential treatment.

As far as their educational level is concerned, a sufficiently large portion that is, 69.2 per cent were illiterate whereas 23.1 per cent were middle school level passed and only 7.7. per cent were found to be graduate.

STATE OF HEALTH AT THE TIME OF SURVEY

Field Results

Old persons were classified into three groups : healthy, sick and chronically ill. The groupings revealed that 76 per cent of the total chosen subjects were sick at the time of survey. Sen Gupta and Chakraborty (1982) observed that 75.6 per cent were sick at the time of the survey whereas Raj and Parsad (1970) and Purohit (1973) found 59.6 and 62.8 per cent ill respectively in their studies. The morbidity rate as found in the present study is higher than that of last two studies and in line with the first one.

Variation in morbidity prevalence rate with the last two studies may be due to two major causes, environmental variability at the places at the time of data collection and different parameters in collection of research information, because of the objectives specifications.

A majority of the sick subjects that is, 92.1 per cent were found suffering from chronic illnesses.

This observation of chronic ailments amongst aged exceeds the observations (69.1 per cent chronic morbidity) made by other scientists, namely, Sen Gupta and Chakraborty, Raj and Parsad and Purohit.

Clinic Results

All the persons who happened to visit the clinics at Medical College hospital were sick and they all were chronically ill. (Table 9.1).

Table 9.1 :

State of Health at the Time of Interview

Field Results

Sr. No.	*Category*	*Number*	*Percentage*
1.	Health	24	24%
2.	Sick	76	76%
	Total	100	100%

Number of sick persons = 76

Number of chronic patients = 70 (92.1%)

Clinic Results

Sr. No.	*Category of Health*	*Number*	*Percentage*
1.	Healthy	-	-
2.	Sick	13	100%
	Total	13	100%

Number of sick persons = 13
Number of chronic persons = 13 (100%)

MORBIDITY PATTERN OF THE GROUP STUDIES

Field Results

The highest prevalence that is, 46 per cent was claimed by muscle-skeleton connective diseases followed by ill-defined ones and others 18.5 per cent (Table 9.2). Circulatory respiratory diseases also affected a sufficiently large number of the selected field respondents that is, 15.8 per cent, followed by infective parasitic and mental, nervous system and sense organs that is 5.3 and 5.3 per cent respectively. Other diseases listed in the Table 9.2 had just a minimal prevalence rate.

Though it was not possible to compare the complete morbidity pattern mainly because of different strata selected for the study, yet the comparison lead to some other clues needed for better health planning. The findings revealed dominance of muscle-skeleton connective disease in rural areas and circulatory, respiratory in slum areas of the same region. This necessitates the assessment of health needs of various broadly defined stratas separately and this variability can be delineated to the different socio-physical environment of the communities.

In this regard, it would be worth-nothing that only 6.6 per cent subjects were found suffering from multiple ailments (Table 9.2).

Table 9.2 :
Distribution of Illness (Morbidity-Pattern)

Field Results

Sr. No.	*Disease*	*Prevalence*	*Percentage*
1.	Infective parasitic	4	5.3
2.	Mental, nervous system	4	5.3
3.	Circulatory, respiratory	12	15.8
4	Digestive	1	1.3
5.	Muscule, skeleton connective	35	46.0
6.	Accidents, poisoning, violence	1	1.3
7.	Ill defined, others	14	18.5
8.	Infective, parasitic muscule skeleton, accidents, poisoning, violence	1	1.3
9.	Infective parasitic ill-defined, others	1	1.3
10.	Digestive, genitourinary	1	1.3
11.	Infective, parasitic, digestive	2	2.6
	Total	76	100.0

Clinic Results

Sr. No.	*Disease*	*Prevalence number*	*Percentage*
1.	Circulatory, Respiratory	3	22.7
2.	Genitourinary	3	22.7
3.	Muscule-skeleton connective	1	7.8
4.	Circulatory, respiratory muscule, skeleton general weakness	1	7.8
5.	Infective parasitic circulatory, respiratory	1	7.8
6.	Circulatory, respiratory, digestive, genitourinary muscule, skeleton	1	7.8
7.	Circulatory, respiratory, muscule-skeleton	1	7.8
8.	Infective, parasitic, muscule, skeleton	1	7.8
9.	Infective parasitic muscule skeleton Genitourinal	1	7.8
	Total	13	100

Clinical Results

The maximum percentage, that is, 45.4 per cent who visited the Medical College Hospital, Rohtak for treatment were suffering from circulatory, respiratory and genitourinary diseases. It was interesting to note that remaining percentage, that is, 54.6 per cent represented varied and multiple symptoms of multiple diseases. This finding suggested that people come to the hospital or come for specialists's services, when they fall sick seriously (Table 9.2).

STATE OF HEALTH OF THE AGED

Field Results

A large percentage of subjects, that is, 80.5 per cent were found to be sick, the proportion increased to 88.9 per cent in the next age group. The fact can be due partly to physiological and partly due the socio-economic change. In the next age group, a relative decrease in morbidity rate had been reported, that is, 78.9 per cent, followed by a sufficient decrease in morbidity prevalence rate in the following two age categories which could be explained by the fact that once they become accustomed to the socio-economic changes, the morbidity also got affected. But in the last category, that is, 80 years and above the tremendous increase in morbidity rate, that is, from 50 per cent to 71.4 per cent was found which revealed the fact that the more advanced the age period, the more vulunerable its membes are (Table 3).

Clinic Results

A majority of sick persons who visited the Medical College Hospital for treatment were in the Ist age group ranging between 55-59 years which supported the aforesaid fact that the onset of old-age is vulnerable period in this regard (Table 9.3).

Table 9.3 :

Distribution of Population by Age and State of Health

Field Results

Age Group (In yrs)	*Number*	*State of Health* (III)	*Per cent*
55-59	36	29	80.5
60-64	26	21	88.9
65-69	14	11	78.9
70-74	6	3	50.3
75-79	4	2	50.0
80+	14	10	71.4
Total	100	76	76.0

Clinic Results

Age Group (In yrs)	*Number*	*State of Health (III)*	*Per cent*
55-59	9	9	100%
60-64	1	1	100%
65-69	-	-	-
70-74	2	2	100%
75-79	-	-	-
80+	1	1	100%
Total	13	13	100%

PHYSICAL DISABILITIES

Field Results

A majority, that is, 61 per cent of the aged who become the subject of study were free from any disability.

Of the remaining, 36 per cent of respondents were partially blind. Only one per cent were totally blind where as 2 per cent of the selected subjects were found having disabilities of eyes and ears. The prevalence of disability of vision could be attributed to environment.

Clinic Results

A majority that is, 76.6 per cent of aged who come for treatment to the Medical College Hospital were free from physical disabilities; 23.4 per cent of the aged however suffered from physical disabilities and had multiple disabilities (Table 9.4).

Table 9.4:

DISTRIBUTION OF DISABILITIES

Field Results

Nature of Disability	*Prevalence Rate (Number)*	*Percent to Total*
Nil	61	61%
Partially blind	36	36%
Completely blind	1	1%
Partially blind & deaf	2	2%
Total	100	100%

Clinic Results

Name of Disability	*Prevalence Rate (Number)*	*Percent to Total*
Nil	10	76.6%
Partially deaf	1	7.8%
Partially blind + kyphosis	1	7.8%
Parkinsonism + kyphosis	1	7.8%
Total	13	100%

HEALTH SERVICES

To ensure better health care for the elderly, India has recommended that certain specific facilities for old people should be set up, including special geriatric departments in hospitals and out-patients clinics with facilities for elderly patients. It has also recommended mobile medical units exclusively for the aged population. The study of geriatrics should not only introduced as a separate subject in medical schools but nurses caring for elderly patients should be given special training to enable them to understand and fulfil their job better. A simple manual on self care in the health field based on the World Health Organisation recommendations should be produced for the elderly and widely distributed and they should be entitled to free or subsidised medicine.

Apart from general recommendations made at national level, a few specific services needed for the aged are laid below which are the outcome of the findings of this research study :

1. In order to improve the health status of the aged, the first and the foremost necessity is to improve their economic level, which could be improved on the following lines:
   (i) to educate them to participate as long as they can, in production work; this would necessitate them not to follow traditional heritage of being free the moment they find their sons and daughters capable of looking after the productive work.
   (ii) sufficient loaning facilities should be made available to poor and skilled aged.
   (iii) pension should be made available to all the aged irrespective of their caste and creed.
2. Special provision for the treatment of the aged may be made at the hospitals and dispensaries such as O.P.D. counter exclusively for them, issuing of identification or health cards which entitle them preferential treatment in terms of reduced charges and waiting hours.

3. Some sort of education and welfare programmes need to be initiated for the aged on the lines of I.C.D.S.
4. Occasional rural medical camps especially the eye camps and mobile medical care facilities maybe initiated so that aged need not cover a long distance for seeking treatment for minor ailments.
5. Simple literature need to be produced which may provide help and guidance to the elderly person for solving elementary health and
6. Post treatment/after care service may be initiated to check the reversal of diseases.
7. Wherever possible, health clubs for the elder persons may be initiated which can be used for keeping the aged physically active.
8. Suitable and balanced diets should be worked out for the aged and the efforts need to be made to make the same popular.
9. The services of retired doctors, nurses, compounders and para medical staff may utilised in health services for the aged.
10. Planners and architects should be requested to look into suitable housing designs for the aged and Central Building Research Institute at Roorkee may be involved in this task.

References

1. Choudhary, R.N., Chhetri, M.K., Saha, T.K., and Basu, S.P. "A Geriatric Survey of the Inmates of a Home for Aged Women in Calcutta". *J. Indian Med. Assoc.* 44,401,1965.
2. Purohit, C.K. "Appraisal of Medico-Social Problems of Rural Aged." *Indian Med. Gaz.* 13, 44, 1973.
3. Purohit C.K. and Sharma, R. 1976, "A study of general health status of persons aged 60 years and above in rural health training centres area". Naila, Indian, J. Med. Res., 64, 202.
4. Raj. B, "A Medico-Social Study of Aged Persons in Certain Villages." *Indian Med. Gaz.* 19, 25, 1971.
5. Rab, B. and Prasad, B.G., "Health Status of the Aged in India—A study in Three Villages", *Geriatrics*, 25, 142, 1970.
6. Statistical Abstract of Haryana, Economic and Statistical Organisation, Planning Department, Govt. of Haryana, 1981-2.
7. Sen Gupta, D.K. and Chakraborty, A.K., "Health Status of Males Aged 55 years and Above in a Slum Area of Calcutta", *Indian J. Pub. Health.*, 27, 112, 1982.

10

Population Policy and Family Planning Administration

A. Population Trends and Implications of Population Explosion

Population Trends

We are witnessing a trend of accelerating growth of world population which began some 200 years ago. This phenomenon coincides with the birth of industrial revolution in Europe. It took more than 1,000 years to double the population before the industrial revolution. The growth has been explosive during the last two centuries. It gathered momentum during the first half of the twentieth century (50 per cent increase between (1900-1950). At the present rate, numbers can double in 37 years (See Table 10.1 and 10. 2).

Table: 10.1

GROWTH OF WORLD POPULATION

Estimated Population

(*Millions*)

Year	*World total*	*More developed regions*	*Less developed regions*
1750	719	201	590
1800	978	248	730
1850	1,262	347	915
1900	1,650	573	1,077
1950	2,506	857	1,649
1960	2,995	976	2,019
1970	3,621	1,084	2,537
1980	4,401	1,183	3,218
1990	5,346	1,282	4,064
2000	6,407	1,368	5,039

Table 10.2

Period	*Annual Increase (millions)*			*Annual rate of growth (millions)*		
	World total	*More developed regions*	*Less developed regions*	*World total*	*More developed regions*	*Less developed regions*
1750-1800	3.7	0.9	2.8	0.4	0.4	0.4
1800-1850	5.7	2.0	3.7	0.5	0.7	0.5
1850-1900	7.8	4.5	3.2	0.5	1.0	0.3
1900-1950	17.1	5.7	11.4	0.8	0.8	0.9
1950-2000	78.0	10.2	67.8	1.9	0.9	2.2
1950-1960	48.9	11.9	37.0	1.8	1.3	2.0
1960-1970	62.2	10.8	51.8	1.9	1.0	2.3
1970-1980	78.0	9.9	68.1	2:0	0.9	2.4
1980-1990	94.5	9.9	84.6	1.9	0.8	2.3
1990-2000	106.1	8.6	97.5	1.8	0.6	2.2

Source : UN Statistical Year Book, 1975, p. 8.

An interesting feature of this table is the uneven distribution of population increase among the regions of the world. Most of the increase has registered in those regions where socio-economic standards are poor. The rate of growth in less developed regions was more than two times.

In contrast with the low-growth potential regions, *i.e.*, Europe (.6) and North America (1.0), are the countries of Africa and Asia which can be classified into high-growth potential regions.

The age distribution of the population in developing countries is not on average altering significantly in this quinquennium. In 1980, children and youth under 15 years represented 40 per cent of the population as compared to 27 per cent in developed countries. Let us now discuss in depth the demographic situation existing in India.

India with a population of 685.0 million (1981) is the second most populous country in the world (next to China) and seventh in land area. The rural population is 79.4 per cent of the total population, 40.1 per cent of the population is below 15 years. One sixth of population of the world is living in an area of 2.4 per cent of the world's land area. This trend in the growth of India's population can be seen from the following table 10.3.

Table 10.3
GROWTH OF POPULATION IN INDIA
(1901-1978)

Census year	*Population in crores*	*Decimial increase or decrease (in crores)*	*Percentage increase or decrease during the decade*
1901	23.6	—	—
1911	25.2	+1.6	+5.7
1921	25.1	–0.1	–0.3
1931	27.9	+2.8	+11.0
1941	31.9	+4.0	+14.2
1951	36.1	+4.2	+13.3
1961	43.9	+7.8	+21.5
1971	54.8	+10.9	+24.8
1981	68.5	+13.7	+25.0

The table clearly reveals that growth in population in the recent years is due to high birth-rates and declining death rates. There is a need to control birth-rate to check population growth. The Census Commissioner has rightly mentioned that :

> "The growth-rate of population of 25 per cent in just one decade of 1961-71, is no doubt very high. It is to be hoped that with the mortality rate brought down to the minimum level possible, the control of fertility will start yielding fruitful results on the overall growth rates of populations."

Rate of growth of population is a function of birth and death rate. Birth rate minus death rate is known as annual growth rate. The birth and death rate for India are given in table no 10.4.

Implication of Population Explosion

The growth rate in population absorbs the national income and lowers the standard of living. The world population conference indicated in the population plan of action that population growth and population policy must be viewed not in isolation, but in the context of development. It was mentioned by the Secretary-General that "Current and potential world-wide population trends evidently cannot continue for as long as even one century without causing serious dislocations and crisis in many areas."

Currently, India's population is more than the total population of USA, USSR and Japan put together. It is estimated that over 55,000 babies are added to the population every day. After deducting the 8 million deaths, there is an addition of 13 million people every year to the population (population of Australia). The population is increasing at an alarming rate.

Table 10.4
AVERAGE ANNUAL BIRTH AND DEATH RATES IN INDIA

Decade	*Birth per 1,000*	*Death per 1,000*	*Annual growth rate %*
1901-11	48.1	42.6	—
1911-21	49.2	48.6	
1921-31	46.4	36.3	
1931-41	45.2	31.2	
1941-51	39.9	27.4	1.33
1951-61	41.7	22.8	2.13
1961-65	41.0	17.2	2.38
1966-70	37.0	15.9	2.11
1970-75	35.2	15.9	1.93
1975-80	33.3	12.5	2.08

Source : Census of India, 1981

The 1981 census placed the country's population at a level higher than expected. However, it also revealed certain redeeming features. For the first time in over four decades the population growth rate stabilised at a more or less constant level. Compared to the preceding decade (1961-71) as against 8 states and union territories (with 13 per cent of the population) which had shown a declining growth rate, 15 states and union territories comprising 47 per cent of the population which had shown a declining growth rate, 15 states and union territories (comprising 47 per cent of the population) showed such decreasing trends during 1971-81. Birth rate which was around 40 in 1951 came down to 33 in 1981 but this birth rate is still very high.

Myrdal in his book *Asian Drama* gave a stern warning to the world in regard to population explosion when he said, "Demographers are of the view that if fertility does not decrease, a time will come when mortality will lose its relative independence of levels of living and begin to rise again."

Thus there is a great need of stabilising population. According to Frank W. Notestein:

> "The ultimate goal of the worlds population policy must be to achieve an equilibrium based on low birth and death rates that can be sustained throughout a distant future for the world and its several parts."

As long as the birth rate is not restricted in these countries, it would not be possible to bring about improvements in the living standards of the people.

In a 'capital poor' and technologically backward country, growth of population diminishes the rate of capital accumulation, increases the amount of disguised unemployment and lowers the standards of living of the people *i.e.*, resources go to the formation to population, not capital. According to Prof. A.W. Singir, population growth has a negative effect on the rate of economic development.

According to him :

$$D=SP-r$$

Where, *D*=rate of economic development

S=rate of net savings

P=productivity of new investment

r=rate of increase of population

In the above equations. r appears as a negative factor with a minus sign.

Let us examine the impact of population growth on the socio-economic development.

(1) *Need of More Investments to Sustain Population Growth.*

The population growth requires more investment while at the same time reduces the capacity of the people to save. This creates a serious gap between investment requirements and the availability of investible funds resulting in the low rate of growth of an economy.

According to Coale and Hoover, " The significance feature of population as such is that a higher rate of population growth implies a higher level of needed investment to achieve a given per-capita output, while there is nothing about faster growth that generates a a great supply of investable resources."

(2) *Reducing in the Rate of Capital Formation*

The composition of the people in underdeveloped countries (40-50% of the population in unproductive age-group) is such that it reduces the capacity of the people to save which affects the rate of capital formation. According to Prof. Meier, "This high dependency requires the economy to divert a considerable part of its resources, that might otherwise go into capital formation, to the maintenance of high percentage of dependence who may never become producers or, if so, only for relatively short working life."[6]

Recognising this, the Third Plan States :

> "In an underdeveloped economy with very little capital per person, a high rate of population growth makes it even more difficult to step up the rate of savings which, in turn, largely determines the possibility of achieving higher productivity and incomes. Moreover, for a given investment, a larger proportion will need to be devoted to the production of essential consumer goods at the expense of investment goods industries thereby still further slowing down the potential rate of growth."

(3) *Food Problem*

The demand of food is rising faster than the production of food. In a study carried out by Food and Agricultural Organisation, it was found that the failure of food production to keep up with population growth was especially pronounced in the case of the developing countries. Out of the total of 106 countries studied, 72 were classified as developing; but in 24 of these (or one-third) food production lagged behind the growth of population. In the more recent period, it was mentioned, the situation was even less favourable.

(4) *Unemployment and Underemployment*

The result of more population would affect the employment situation as there is already a back-log of unemployment and underemployment in these countries. The growing unemployment of these countries is not only an economic but it is also a social evil.

(5) *Poor Health Standards*

Family planning and health are intimately related. Family planning can promote women's health through the prevention of unwanted pregnancies, limiting number of births, and proper spacing, timing of births and foetal health. Family planning also promotes the health of the child through the reduction of child mortality, and promotion of the child development. Maryellen Fullam stresses the importance of family planning as instrument for the promotion of health. He says :

> "Uncontrolled fertility directly threatens the health of mothers and infants and may undermine the health of other family members. Today, no health programme can be considered complete unless it offers ready access to the appropriate family planning measures for all potential parents."

(6) *Social and Psychological Tension*

Rapid population growth leads to social and psychological tensions, and breakdown of a distribution system. Civil amenities such as water and power supply, housing, transport and social utilities like schooling, educational, health and medical services fall much short of demand in spite of their constant expansion. Besides, it leads to political and social corruption and accentuates economic disparities.

Thus, we can say that the problem of growing population has reached such menacing proportions that it has become a real threat to the socio-economic stability of the country. The excessive growth in population does not affect the stability of the national economy alone, it disturbs the stability of the entire body politic. It poses a colossal threat to our social structure. In our fight against poverty, disease, hunger, malnutrition and unemployment, checking the rapid growth of population is as important as raising production in the farms and factories and provision of social services. Population control is one of the chief issues which the country has to resolve and accord top priority in its march towards social and economic development. The programme of family planning is of vital importance of our country. It is a positive and constructive approach to the betterment of the quality of life of the community. Thus, it is evident that the key to India's economic future based on social justice lies in the immediate and effective implementation of a nationwide population programme.

Recent Developments

Realising the magnitude of the population problem, the United Nations declared the year, 1974, as World Population Year to focus international attention on various aspects of the population dynamics. The World Population Conference held at Bucharest, Romania, from 19 to 30 August, 1974, was the third in a series of population conferences convened under the auspices of the United Nations. The first two conferences, which took place in Rome in 1954 and in Belgrade in 1965, were purely professional in nature. The Bucharest Conference convened under Economic and Social Council Resolution 1484 (XLVIII) of April, 1970, reflected the increasing concern with populations in the world today and was a global conference of governments which devoted its attention to the national and international populations policies and action programmes needed to promote human welfare and development.

Four United Nations symposia on population issues were held prior to the conference, in which experts addressed themselves to the substantive aspects of the complex inter-relationships between population and the multiplicity of socio-economic and other factors which affect it and are in turn affected by it. These were : the Symposium on Population and Development (Cairo, 4-14 June 1973); the Symposium on Population and the Family (Honolulu, 6-15 August, 1973); the Symposium on Population Resources and the Environment (Stockholm, 26 September–3 October 1973); and the Symposium on Population on Human Rights (Amsterdam, 21-29 January 1974).

Besides, the two conferences – Stockholm Conference (September 1974) and the World Conference of the International Women's Year in 1975 also discussed the population problem. All these conferences highlighted the fact that the growth of population had outstripped the natural resources in many countries and needed careful planning for remedial measures.

B. Meaning and Scope of Family Planning Programme

Meaning

Family planning programme makes a planned and scientific approach to the issues and problems of family life and attempts to solve them to make the family life happier, harmonious and fruitful. Family planning was thought of as a public heath problem. It was stated in the First Five-Year Plan :

> It is apparent that population at a level consistent with the requirement of national economy should be established. This can be secured only by the realisation of the need for family limitation on a wide scale by the people. The main appeal for planning is based on considerations of health and welfare of the family. Family limitation or spacing of the children is necessary and desirable in order to secure better health of the mothers, and better care and upbringing of children. The measures described to this end should, therefore, form part of the public health programme.

A distinction must be made between population control and family planning. Population control is influenced and determined by a government policy motivated by socio-economic considerations. Family planning, on the other hand is a responsibility of the family. WHO has given various definitions of family planning.

An Expert Committee (1971) of the WHO defined family planning as : "a way of thinking and living that is adopted voluntarily upon the basis of knowledge, attitudes and responsible decisions by individuals and couples, in order to promote the health and welfare of the family group and thus contribute effectively to the social development of a country."

Another Expert Committee (1971) defined and described family planning as follows : "Family Planning refers to practices that help individuals or couples to attain certain objectives :

(a) to avoid unwanted births;
(b) to bring about wanted births;
(c) to regulate the intervals between pregnancies;
(d) to control the time at which births occur in relation to the age of the parents; and
(e) to determine the number of children in the family."

Scope of Family Planning Services

Family planning is not synonymous with birth control. It encompasses more than mere birth control.

As the term 'Family Planning' had a narrow connotation, it was replaced by the term 'Family Welfare' in India, a much larger concept consistent with the philosophy of integrated welfare, on which the family constitutes the basic unit. In a broader sense, family planning is concerned with the quality of life. In the context of family health, it is a way of helping families to be healthier and happier. With family planning, pregnancies can be spaced so that a women can regain all her strength and take good care of a new child. Many different methods of family planning are available today which enable couples to determine when and how many children they wish to have.

Families can play an important role in this direction as the young couples may be motivated by their families to limit the number of children for the welfare of the family. In this context, families are playing a negative role in India. Old ladies want their sons to have many children and especially males. Therefore, the education of the elder members of the family is also important to generate the proper atmosphere for population education.

To quote John D. Rockefeller : "My final conclusion is that the ultimate objective of our work in family planning is not the restriction of human life but rather its enrichment. To me, it is disturbing that so many people think of the population problem only as number of people versus available food. This seems to equate man with animal and food with fodder."

A WHO Expert Committee (1970) has stated that family planning includes in its purview (1) the proper spacing and limitation of births, (2) advice on sterility, (3) education for parenthood including pre-natal and post-natal care, (4) sex education, (5) screening for pathological conditions related to the reproductive system (e.g., cervical cancer), (6) genetic counselling, (7) pre-marital consultation and examination, (8) carrying out pregnancy tests, (9) marriage counselling, (10) the preparation of couples for the arrival of their first child, (11) providing services for unmarried mothers, (12) teaching home economics and nutrition, and (13) providing adoption services. These activities vary from country to country according to national objectives and policies with regard to family planning. This is the modern concept of family planning.

Policy-making and Planning for Family Welfare

Family planning as an official programme was adopted in India in 1952. Before this, the Family Planning Association of India was formed in 1949 in Bombay. On April 1951 the Advisory Panel on Health Programmes appointed a sub-committee on Family Planning. The sub-committee strongly recommended that family planning should be recognised as an official programme to protect the health and welfare of mothers and children and to aid the national economy by reducing the birth rate concurrently with the death rate in order to stabilise the population. During the first two Five Year Plans (1951-61) the programme was taken up in a modest way with a clinical approach. During the Second Plan period, 549 urban and 1,100 rural clinics were set up.

The programme was reorganised in the Third Plan after the publication of the 1961 census result which showed a higher growth rate than anticipated. It was towards the middle of the Third Plan that the emphasis was shifted from the clinical approach to the more vigorous extension educational approach for motivating the people for acceptance of the small family norm and for provision of services. The major activities envisaged during this Plan were :

(a) education and motivation for family planning;

(b) use of voluntary organisations for diffusion of family planning message and practice;

(c) provision of services integrated with rural health services including facilities for sterilisation;

(d) supplies; and

(e) research.

A full-fledged Department of Family Planning was created in the Ministry of Health. During the three annual plans (1966-69), The programme which was described as the 'kingpin' of the plan was made time-bound and target-oriented with vastly increased funds. In the Fourth Plan, the programme was accorded the highest priority. More emphasis was given to training, research, publicity, organisation, supplies and evaluation. Medical Termination of Pregnancy Act, 1971, was passed which came into force from 1 April, 1972. With this Act, State Governments were empowered to constitute relevant boards to certify the registered doctors who were willing to perform the operations causing termination of pregnancy. Though the MTP Act is mainly a health measure, it also supplements the family welfare programme because a large percentage of women undergoing medical termination of pregnancy readily accept family planning measures to avoid future conceptions.

During the Fourth Plan, the approach had been to integrate family planning services with those for health, maternal and child health and nutrition.

On the eve of the Fourth Plan, five central training institutions and 43 regional family planning training centres were functioning and were preparing to train 10,000 medical and 1,50,000 para-medical personnel required to implement the programme vigorously. There were 4326 rural family welfare planning centres. 22,826 rural sub-centres and 4,797 urban family welfare planning centres in operation. The Fourth Plan stated :"Family planning will remain a centrally sponsored programme for the next ten years and the entire expenditure will be met by the Central Government. It will be ensured that performance does not lag behind the expenditure. The effort will be to achieve enduring results through appropriate education and motivation. Central health services will be fully involved in the programme."

The Fourth Five Year Plan outline referred to family planning as 'kingpin of the Plan' and 'limitation of family' as an essential and inescapable ingredient of development. The high priority given to family planning was reflected in the formation of a Cabinet Committee with the Prime Minister, Shrimati Indira Gandhi, as the Chairman. Similarly, committees have been established in most States. A Department of Family Planning was formed within the Ministry of Health and Family Planning. A Cabinet Minister is in overall charge, with a Minister of State guiding the programme, and a Secretary to the Government of India exercising administrative control.

The Fifth Five Year Plan had two basic objectives–to be economically self-reliant and removal of poverty. As regards population growth the approach is to tackle it more effectively : "The high rate of growth of population constitutes an important constraint on progress towards removal of poverty. It has an adverse effect on domestic saving which is detrimental to the growth of the economy. There is, in addition, an adverse impact on the pattern of growth, for the needs of sheer subsistence have to be given a greater weight. The higher the rate of growth of population, the lower is the rate of growth of *per capita* income, corresponding to a particular rate of growth of national income. For all these reasons, the objective of removal of poverty calls for more effective restraints on the growth of population. The family planning programmes need to be evaluated carefully with a view to evolving a package of practices that holds better promise. The large provision of Rs. 560 crores for family planning in the Fifth Plan should provide the means to put through a more effective programme."

The Fifth Plan aimed at reducing the birth rate further to about 30 per thousand by the end of the Plan period and to 25 per thousand by the end of 1983-84. Operational targets were laid to achieve the required reduction in the birth rate. The operational targets involved a little over 18 million IUD insertions and about 9 million Conventional Contraceptive Users (CC users) by 1978-79.

The Government of India, in the year 1976-77 announced a National Population Policy. The policy covered a broad range of individual policies including such vital matters as raising the age of marriage, freezing representation of Members in Parliament, linking the distributing of federal resources to the performance in family planning, promoting female literacy, increasing the monetary compensation for sterilization operation. The policy statement emphasised the urgent need for a direct attack on the population problem as a national commitment. It suggested a series of measures which, it was hoped, would reduce the birth rate to 25 per thousand of population by the end of the Sixth Plan.

Some of the Important Measures of This Policy Were

1. Age of marriage to be raised to 21 for boys and 18 for girls. Offences under the new law have been made cognisable.
2. Representation in the Lok Sabha and State legislatures to be frozen till the year 2001 A.D. at the level determined after 1971 Census.
3. Eight per cent of Central assistance to State Plans to be specifically earmarked against performance in family planning.
4. Monetary compensation for both male and female sterilisation to be raised so as to provide a motivation to couples to have lesser number of children.
5. No Central legislation is proposed for the time being on the question of compulsory sterilisation. States were left free to introduce compulsory sterilisation if they were well-equipped to meet its demands.
6. Group incentives to be introduced for panchayats, teachers and the labour.
7. Scheme for aiding voluntary organisations to be expanded to make family planning a mass movement.
8. Special measures to be undertaken to raise the level of female education.

9. High priority to be introduced in the educational system to sensitise younger generations.
10. Change to be made in the Service and Conduct Rules of Central Government employees to ensure that they adopt small family norm.

In the wake of this population policy, the Prime Minister, Smt. Gandhi asked the Chief Ministers to accord a very high priority to family planning. The top leadership of the ruling party, both in the government and outside, extended its full support to the new population policy as well as to the new specific programmes set forth for the year 1976-77 in the light of this policy. In the then prevailing state of Emergency in the country this was generally taken as a mandate by the states. Coercion of various kinds and even outright compulsion thus became rampant in the campaign for mobilising people for sterilisation. This created resentment among the people. The evidence of this was that the people resorted to violent defiance of authority, resulting in firings, lathi charge and arrests. On January 10, 1976, Dr. Karan Singh told the consultative committee of MPs attached to the Ministry of Health and Family Welfare that it is necessary to introduce some sort of compulsion in the implementation of the programme. A few days later, Mrs. Indira Gandhi told a Conference, "We must now act decisively. We should not hesitate to take steps which might be described as drastic."

The quantitative performance as a result of the implementation of this policy had been quite impressive. The performance under the different methods in relation to the targets for the year 1976-77 with comparative figures for 1975-76 is given in Table 10.5.

Table 10.5 reveals that the number of sterilisation went up steeply to 8.26 million as against 2.67 million in 1975-76 and 1.35 million in 1974-75. There has been similar increase in other methods as well. There was, however, a decline in the number of conventional contraceptive users under the free distribution scheme from 2.39 million in 1975-76 to 2.27 million in 1976-77.

On qualitative examination, one is shocked to learn that the people were compelled to adopt family planning measures during the emergency. The programme was administered with negligence and carelessness resulting in many deaths and side effects. Many people having no children were sterilised. The programme was implemented indiscriminately. Compulsory sterilisation was done to large numbers of males and females including sometimes the very old and the very young. Dr. Karan Singh in his interview to the *People* said that, "it must, however, be admitted that an extra-constitutional centre of power and authority was operating at that time, and it was this phenomenon that was responsible for the unfortunate manner in which the programme was implemented in some states causing revolution and anger in the public mind."

All this created a fear and revulsion about the family planning programme resulting in permanent damage to the programme.

The Family Planning Programme became a major political issue and the Opposition coalition or Janata Party used it in the election campaigns against the ruling party. This gathered momentum and the Congress lost the election at the hands of the Janata Party. The new party changed the name of the Family Planning Programme to the Family Welfare Programme. The Janata announced the revised policy on the Family Welfare Programme on 29 June 1977.

Table: 10.3

COMPARATIVE ACHIEVEMENTS OF 1976-77 VIS-A-VIS 1975-76

Method	*Target*		*Achievement*		*Percent Increase (+) Decrease (-) in performance*	*Per cent achievement of target*	
	1976-77	*1975-76*	*1976-77*	*1975-76*		*1976-77*	*1975-76*
	*(Figure in millions)**						
1	2	3	4	5	6	7	8
Sterilisation (a+b)	4.30	2.49	8.26	2.67	(+) 209.3	192.1	107.1
(a) Vasectomy		—	6.20	1.44	(+) 330.6	—	—
(b) Tubectomy	—	—	2.06	1.23	(+) 67.5	—	—
T.U.D	1.14	0.91	0.58	0.61	(-) 5.0	51.1	66.6
Other methods	4.69	4.36	3.69	3.53	(+) 3.6	78.7	80.9
Eq Users (a+b)							
(a) C.C. Users							
(i + ii)	—	—	3.63	3.50	(+) 2.9	—	—
(i) Free	—	—	2.27	2.39	(-) 6.3	—	—
(ii) Commercial	1.50	1.50	1.36	1.10	(+) 23.6	90.7	73.4
(b) Oral pills users	—	—	0.056	0.032	(+) 75.3	—	—
Total acceptors	10.13	7.76	12.53	6.81	(+) 85.5	123.3	87.8

*Based on actual (unrounded) figures.

1.5 In relation to the target, the performance in 1976-77 was 192% in the case of sterilisation 51% in the case of IUD and 76% in the case of other methods (C.C.and O.P) as compared to 107% in sterilisation, 67% in IUD and 81% in the case of other methods in 1975-76. All the States and Union Territories except Jammu and Kashmir, Kerala, Arunachal Pradesh, Goa, Diu and Daman, Lakshadweep and Mizoram over-reached their, targets in terms of total acceptors.

2.1 Sterilisation during the year under review, all the states and territories has exceeded their sterilisation performance of 1975-76. Andhra Pradesh, Bihar, Haryana, Himachal Pradesh, Karnataka, Madhya Pradesh, Manipur, Meghalaya, Rajasthan, Uttar Pradesh, West Bengal, A&N islands, Delhi.

The new approach towards family planning by the Janata Party Government is known as the 'Cafetaria Approach'. Under this approach, the people can choose any method suitable to them. There is no undue emphasis on sterilisation. It is available only to those who desire it. The main features of this policy are :

(a) Ruling out compulsion or coercion of any sort in the field of family welfare for all times to come; while all methods of contraception will be promoted with equal emphasis, it will be left to each family to make its own choice of the method for maintaining the small family norm.

(b) Assigning a vital role to maternal and child health care by providing maternity services to all those who may need them and expanding the immunisation programme further.

(c) Raising the age of marriage for girls and boys. Although the statement envisaged raising the minimum age of the marriage for girls to 16 years, it was decided subsequently that the minimum age for girls would be raised to 18 years for the time being while that for boys would remain 21 years.

(d) Giving higher priority to the improvement of women's educational level through formal and non-formal channels.

(e) Using the population figures of 1971 as a base till the year 2001 in all cases where population is a factor as the allocation of Central assistance to State plans, devolution of taxes and duties and grants-in-aid.

(f) Linking of 80 per cent of Central assistance to the State Plans with their performance and success in the Family Welfare Programme.

(g) Giving population education the attention it deserves, specially in the courses for schools and colleges aimed at influencing that segment of population which would soon be entering reproductive age and marital life.

(h) Emphasising a multimedia motivational approach in which all media units of the various departments in the Centre and the State would be fully associated.

(i) Involving actively all voluntary bodies and the organised sector as agents of change.

(j) Allowing full rebates in the income tax assessment for amounts given as donations for the family welfare purposes.

(k) Paying special attention to the necessary research inputs in the field of reproductive biology and contraception.

(l) Soliciting active cooperation and involvement of all ministries and departments of the Government of India as well as the States in the programme.

(m) Monitoring of the programme intensively and carefully. Annual review of the situation in depth is to be made by the Union Cabinet.

(n) All restrictions aimed at limiting the size of the family in the case of government employees through conduct rules and the disincentives introduced by the Ministry of Finance in respect of those who violated the small family norm have been withdrawn.

One of the important decisions taken by the Government during the year in the light of the new policy was to set up a Grievance Cell to deal with numerous complaints received in the ministry and to ensure redressal of grievances. At the same time, the state governments were requested to ensure prompt payment of the *exgratia* relief of Rs. 5,000 to the dependents of those who died as a result of sterilisation.

It is very difficult to assess the impact of this policy. However, the quantitative performance has been poor. There has been steep fall in the performance. While the ideals of the new policy were no doubt noble it was in the field of implementation of the programme that there was a perceptible fall. The year 1977-78 was bad for the programme as the number of sterilisations fell to as low a level as 0.9 million as against 8.2 million in 1976-77. There was a sharp decline in the IUD insertions (60 per cent) and users of conventional contraceptives (18 per cent) compared to the corresponding period of the earlier two years. To quote Dr. Karan Singh,

> The national population policy was directed towards achieving a target of reducing the birth rate from 35 per thousand in 1974 to 25 per thousand in 1984, thus reducing the growth rate to 1.4 per cent. It is now clear that not only will this target not be achieved but it is even possible that the growth rate might increase with all the disastrous consequences that will entail for the future of our nation in the 21st century.

There is still a belief that the cooperation of the people can be secured through persuasion and that lasting success can be obtained through this approach. The real purpose of family planning is not the prevention of the baby boom temporarily but the creation of a spirit of planned and responsible parenthood by instilling in every citizen a sense of social awareness and obligation.

Coming to the existing political scene in India, which has emerged with the Congress (I) back in power under the leadership of Mrs. Indira Gandhi, it is hoped that a strong political will and determination would be created to make the programme a success. The Fifth Plan objective of reducing the birth rate from 35 per thousand population at the beginning of the Plan to 30 per thousand population by 1978-79 could not be achieved. In fact, the level of effective family planning couple protection has come down from 23.6 per cent in 1976-77 to 22.21 per cent in March 1980. However, in 1982 and 1983, the position became good. Till March 1983, 25.9 per cent of the total eligible couples were effectively protected. Of these 22 per cent were protected by sterilisation alone. Details of couples protected from 1971 to 1983 can be seen from the graph appended. This trend needs to be maintained.

The non-attainment of the birth rate targets adopted in the Plans is largely on account of our inability to carry forward the programme throughout the country with the active involvement of the people. Public enthusiasm and community participation in the programme which is necessary for its success has not been generated in adequate measure. This programme is still viewed by public as a routine government act. Some voluntary organisations have no doubt done creditable act in the field of family planning, but their out-reach is mostly conferred to the urban areas. There is need for projecting the programme as a people's programme backed by support from governmental and non-governmental agencies. Inadequacy in infrastructure available for implementation of the programme have also been partly responsible for the slow progress of the programme. In some cases, even the infrastructure available had not been put to effective use or properly maintained. There were shortages of trained manpower under the schemes of appointment of multi-purpose workers and maternal and child health which are so important to the programme. The performance of the family planning staff in motivational work on the basis of well-maintained and updated eligible couple registers, left much to be desired.

Table: 10.6

OUTLAY AND EXPENDITURE ON FAMILY PLANNING PROGRAMME OVER DIFFERENT PLAN PERIODS IN INDIA

(in lakhs of rupees)

Periods	*Outlay*		*Expenditure*	
First Plan				
1951-56	65.00		14.50	
Second Plan				
1956-57			8.70	
1957-58			26.00	
1958-59	497.00		31.50	215.60
1959-60			51.00	
1960-61			98.40	
Third Plan				
1961-62			139.30	
1962-63			277.20	
1963-64	2,697.60		217.20	2,486.00
1964-65			652.30	
1965-66			1200.00	
Annual Plan *(Inter Plan Period)*				
1966-67	1,493.00		1,342.60	
1967-68	3,100.00	8,293.00	2,652.30	7,046.4
1968-69	3,700.00		3,051.50	
Fourth Plan *(Plan Outlay 33,000.00)*				
1969-70	4,200.00		3,618.42	
1970-71	5,200.00		4,890.43	
1971-72	6,060.50	28,576.20	6,175.56	28,443.30
1972-73	7,630.70		7,974.80	
1973-74	5,485.00		5,784.59	
Fifth Plan *(Plan Outlay 49,735.73)*				
1974-78				
1974-75	5,413.60		6,204.80	
1975-76	6,319.50		8,061.37	
1976-77	14,910.74		17,298.21	
1977-78	9,817.67		9,330.70	
1978-79	11,093.39		10,418.13	
1979-80	11,519.23	47,554.10	11,851.13	51,313.2
1980-81	13,949.75		14,191.91	
1981-82	15,477.56		18,389.89	
1982-83	24,470.50		28,831.96	
1983-84	32,973.42		—	

Table 10.7

FAMILY PLANNING PERFORMANCE IN THE DIFFERENT FIVE YEAR PLANS

Period	*Sterilisation through Vasectomy and Tubectomy*	*IUD*	*Conventional Contraceptive Users*	*Percentage of couples protected (currently) by all methods*
1	2	3	4	5
Second Plan (Jan.1956 to Dec.1960)	1,52,677			0.2
Third Plan (Jan. 1961 to March 1966)	13,73,166	8,12,713	5,82,141	3.0
Inter Plan Period (1966-67 to 1968-69)	43,91,996	20,57,436	9,60,896	8.7
Fourth Plan (1969-74)	90,03,626	21,49,160	30,09,995	16.5
Fifth Plan (1974-79)	14,710,000	25,00,000	1,65,90,000	22.8
(1979-80)	17,40,000	6,20,000	29,90,000	22.5
(1980-85)	22,00,000	79,00,000	11,00,000	36.56 (Targets)

Apart from the constraints on the supply side, the generation necessary acceptance in favour of the small family norm proved to be a far more elusive problem. Quite a large segment of the population is steeped in poverty, bound by traditional value systems. Certain sections have no doubt adopted the small family norm, but their number is small. A large majority of the population has not been adequately motivated and made aware of the benefits of a small family. The communication channels, both formal and informal including the educational system, have by and large not succeeded entirely in imparting the knowledge and information which the community needs.

The prevalent high rates of mortality in general and very high infant mortality in particular is inhibiting acceptance of family planning and creating a psychological barrier against the programme. The estimates of infant mortality for 1976 available from the Sample Registration Scheme (SRS) of the Registrar General of India shows that this rate is still as high as 139 in rural areas, 80 in urban areas and 129 for the country as a whole. The pre-school death rate among 0-4 age group is also around 51 per thousand population.

COUPLES EFFECTIVELY PROTECTED UNDER FAMILY PLANNING PROGRAMME (1971 TO 1983)

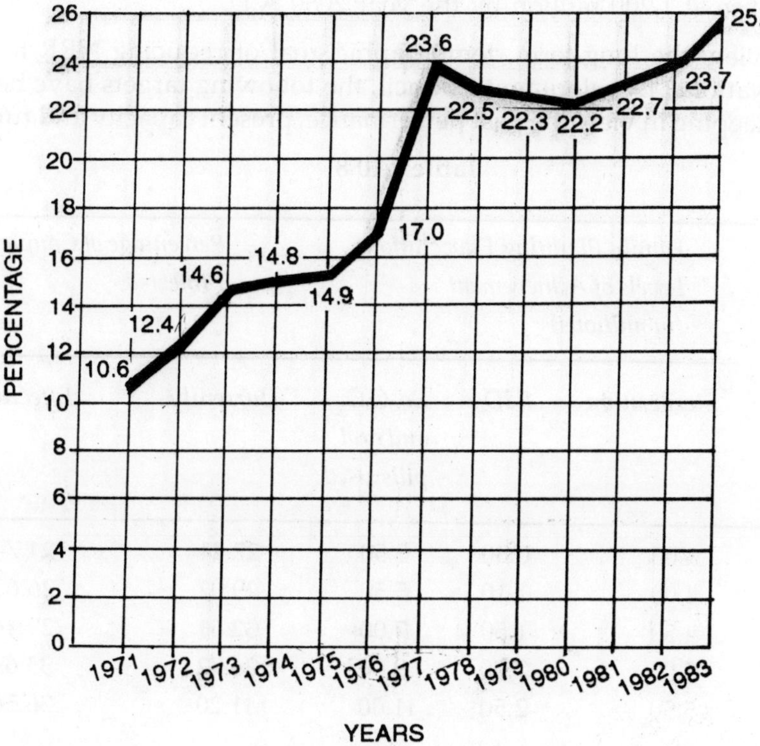

*** As on 31st March of the Year**

***Source*: Annual Report, Government of India, Ministry of Health, 1983-84**

Objectives of the Sixth Plan

The Working Group on Population Policy set up by the Planning Commission has recommended the adoption of the long-term demographic goal of reducing the Net Reproduction Rate (NRR) to one by 1996 for the country as a whole and by 2001 in all States from the present level of 1.67. The implications of this are as follows :

(i) The average size of the family would be reduced from 4.2 children to 2.5 children.

(ii) The birth rate per thousand population would be reduced from the level of 33 in 1978 to 21.

(iii) As against 22 per cent of the eligible couples protected with family planning at present, 60 per cent would be protected.

(iv) The death rate per thousand population would be reduced from about 14 in 1978 to 9 and the infant mortality rate would be reduced from 129 to 60 or less.

(v) The population of India will be around 900 million by the turn of the century and will stabilise at 1,200 million by the year 2050 A.D.

Keeping in view the long-term demographic goal of reducing NRR to 1 by 1995 as approved by the National Development Council, the following targets have been envisaged for the Sixth Plan keeping in view the past performance, present capacity and future potential:

Table : 10.8

	Family Planning Expectation/ Levels of Achievement (in millions)			*Percentage of Couple Protected*	
Year	*Sterilisation*	*IUD*	*Eq. C.C. and oral pills used*	*Currently*	*Effectively*
1980-81	3.00	0.80	5.50	27.21	24.74
1981-82	4.00	1.10	5.50	29.07	26.63
1982-83	4.50	1.50	7.00	32.51	29.46
1983-84	5.00	2.00	9.00	36.72	33.69
1984-85	5.50	2.50	11.00	41.20	36.56
Total for Sixth Plan	22.00	7.90			

The number of sterilisations which were around 1.74 million in the base year (1979-80) will go up to 5.50 millions in the terminal year of the Plan. The number of IUD insertions will go up from 0.62 million in 1979-80 to 2.50 million in 1985. The percentage of effective couple protection envisaged by 1985 is 36.56 against the present 22.5. This calls for a tremendous motivational effort backed by adequate infrastructural facilities which have to be taken care of in the Plan. It needs mention, that a total of 15.5 million sterilisations will be required during the Plan period 1980-85 for maintaining the birth rate at the existing level, assuming present levels of IUD and CC Users. This is because the proportion of women in the reproductive age will be rising. Even if age-specific fertility rates are held constant, the birth rates will rise unless matched by vigorous family planning promotional efforts. We have not been able to meet the targets as planned.

Table : 10.9
TARGETS FOR 1982-83 AND COMPARATIVE PERFORMANCE DURING 1982-83 AND 1981-82

(Figures in millions)

Sl. No.	*Method*	*Targets 1982-83*	*Achievements 1982-83**	*1981-82*	*% change $$ in performance in 1982-83 over 1981-82*	*%Achievement $$ of annual target for 1982-83*
1.	Sterilisation	4.52	3.98	2.79	(+) 42.5	88.0
	(a)Vasectomy	—	0.58	0.57	(+) 1.9	—
	(b)Tubectomy	—	3.40	2.22	(+) 53.0	—
2.	I.U.D	1.51	1.09	0.75	(+) 45.6	72.2
3	Other methods					
	(Eq. Users)	7.00	5.95	4.56	(+) 6.6@	84.9
	(a) C.C. Users	6.50	5.77	4.44	(+) 5.4@	88.7
	i) Free Dist.					
	Scheme	3.50	2.42	2.13	(+) 13.5	69.1
	ii) Commercial					
	Scheme	3.00	3.358	2.31	(–) 2.2@	111.7
	(b) Oral Pill	0.50	0.18	0.12	(+) 49.1	35.5
	Users					
	Total Acceptors	11.02	8.10			

* Figures Provisional

@ Worked out after excluding the figures of full cost commercial sales of condoms.

$ Includes 1.09 million C.C. Users under full cost commercial sales of condoms directly from manufacturers.

$$ Worked out on the basis of absolute figures.

Source: Annual Report, Government of India, Ministry of Health and Family Welfare, 1983-84, p. 214.

If we compare the targets set for the Sixth Plan and the current working of 1981-82, 1982-83, and targets for 1982-83 (Refer table 10.9); we find that we have not been able to achieve as planned. For example, the targets for 1982-83 for sterilisation were 4.50 million while achievement is 3.98 million. For IUD, the target was 1.50 million while achievement is 1.09. For other methods the target was 7 million while the achievement is 5.95 million. Similarly we provided to ensure the couple protection to 29.46 per cent but we could achieve only upto 25.9 per cent.

The Family Welfare Programme was included in the New 20-Point Programme of the Prime Minister announced in January 1982. It envisages promotion of family planning on a voluntary basis as people's movement.

A well-defined long-term strategy has been evolved to ensure that the adoption of the 'small family norm' is done entirely on a voluntary basis. The salient features of this strategy consist of intensified efforts to spread awareness and information through imaginative use of multimedia and interpersonal communication strategies, providing services and supplies as close to the doorsteps of the acceptors as possible, developing facilities for rapid increase in female literacy, extending population education to youth in schools and colleges as well as those out of schools, assisting and supporting the association of elected representatives of the people at all levels with the programme, developing linkages with other concerned ministries and departments, ensuring effective observance of the law relating to minimum age for marriage of girls and boys and ensuring close monitoring and follow-up of the programme at all levels.

A critical examination of the existing and past population policies indicate that the family planning programme has become more political rather than technical. Well-designed and articulated public policy can keep the structural components and their elements integrated. We should not change the population policy so often. There are not two different opinions regarding the need for control of population and reducing the growth rate to zero. The views differ regarding the methodology and strategy. We must try to evolve the strategy in cooperation with the people.

> Although many dedicated and wise people have been working on the Indian population problem for several years, there are few ideas, and less agreement, about what needs to be done to recruit significantly large numbers of acceptors.

A national population/family planning policy should clearly prescribe guidelines for administrative action, but should be sufficiently adaptable to permit a high degree of programme innovation at different stages of programme development. Increased concern is being given to the "necessity of formulating population policies and programmes as integral parts of the social and economic processes."

Performance Appraisal

On examining Table 10.6 relating to outlay and expenditure on Family Planning Programme over different plan periods in India, we find that the expenditure has been increasing substantially. It has increased from 14.50 lakhs in the First Plan to 10,100 lakhs in the Sixth Plan (1980-85), As compared to the Fifth Plan, the increase, till Sixth Plan would be doubled.

Let us now review the performance in terms of the achievement of the targets set for the programme.(Table 10.7) "Family Planning Performance in the Different Five Year Plans" reveals that the performance has been unsatisfactory. The performance in respect of sterilisation (vasectomy and tubectomy), IUD, conventional contraceptive and percentage of couples protected by all methods has been unsatisfactory as compared to the resources devoted for this challenging task (see Tables 10.7 and 10.8). There is a need to re-examine the population policy so that the fruits of investments can yield better results. There is a need to devise radical and innovative policy which can motivate the people to adopt family planning in the interest of family health and the development of the country.

Suggestions to Formulate Reliable and Realistic Population Policy

We have already mentioned the various policy measures adopted from time to time to encourage the adoption of family planning measures. There is a need of a population policy which should be clear and acceptable to all sections of the people. This would be possible only if the policy is formulated after considering the views and suggestions of the people, intellectual elite, health experts, political elite, etc. The following suggestions are given, which may be considered while formulating a new policy or revising the earlier population policies.

(a) The framework for the implementation of the policy must be designed afresh. We have been attending so far to the objectives, goals and targets of the family planning programme. We have paid very little attention to the framework which needs a change to secure cooperation and success. It is suggested that the policy-makers may design a suitable structure to ensure autonomy and flexibility at all levels.

(b) The developing countries cannot afford massive expenditure being incurred for the Family Planning Programme. The policy measures must ensure the tapping of voluntary resources of men and women, particularly women lying idle and untapped, to do this challenging task. It can be done by giving legal recognition and status to the organisations providing such services. Such recognition at public functions can go a long way in the success of the programme.

(c) The policy measures should adopt and spell out clearly the disincentives if the Family Planning Programme is not adopted by the family having two or more children especially among the government employees. The government is the model employer and the government employees can act as the standard setters for the rest of the population.

(d) A policy decision must be taken to wind up all the organisations which have not been serving any useful purpose. There are many voluntary agencies which are wasting the grants obtained for this purpose. We must develop a well knit set up to avoid wastage of efforts and resources.

(e) All the compensation for this work should be withdrawn and the money saved on this account may be used to provide effective and efficient services. One cannot believe that a family can take a decision to limit its members for meagre monetary considerations.

(f) No new institution or organisation may be set up. The policy to streamline the existing organisations may be devised so that the emphasis may be on achieving the results rather than building massive and costly structures.

(g) Population education should be an integral part of population policy and it may be imparted through the existing educational institutions or the machinery of adult education. The population education should also include sex education. If sex education is imparted by dedicated personnel through careful planning and methodology, it can sublimate the energy of youth which can be utilised for national reconstruction and socio-economic development like the water of Bhakra Dam which was causing floods and havoc earlier but is being used now to generate electricity, and irrigate the barren lands.

C. Existing Administrative Set-up of Family Planning Programme in India

The success of the well organised family planning programme depends to a great extent upon administrative skill and competence. We shall discuss in brief the structure and administration of the programme at various levels.

1. Organisation at Union Level

The apex body at the centre is a cabinet committee which is presided over by the Union Minister of Health and Family Welfare. It includes Ministers of State for Finance, Social Welfare, Home Affairs. It also includes a member from the Department of Electronics and Scientific and Industrial Research. This body has the overall responsibility for the formulation of national policies on family planning and for reviewing the progress in their implementation.

The Central Family Planning Council is an advisory body for policy making. It includes Health Ministers from all the States and is presided over the Union Minister of Health and Family Welfare. Other members are from the Planning Commission, representatives of major voluntary organisations, labour organisations and selected members of Parliament. It has representatives from a wider section of interests in family planning, including those that are directly charged with the implementation of the programme.

The Department of Family Welfare (earlier Family Planning) within the ministry is responsible for the implementation of policies. The Secretary to the Government of India in the Ministry of Health and Family Planning is overall incharge of the Department of Family Welfare. An Additional Secretary assists the Secretary and provides overall direction to programme implementation. He is known as Additional Secretary and Commissioner for Family Welfare. There is a Joint-Secretary who supervises the working of the Technical Wing of the Department which provides technical guidance to the various programme activities i.e., Sterilisation, IUD, Post Partum, M.C.H., Training, Mass Education, besides Evaluation and Research. The Additional Secretary's duties include policy formulation, programme planning, supervising the programme implementation and coordination of activities of the department with other related ministries and departments of the government of India.

There are two wings of the department (A) Administrative Wing (the Secretariat) and (B) Technical Wing with many divisions.

On the secretariat side, there is a Policy Division, Aided Programme Division, an organised sector and Voluntary Organisations Division and a Plan Budget Division.

(i) The Policy Division looks after formulation of policies concerning family welfare.

(ii) The Aided Programme Division looks after the activities of organisations which receive extra government assistance and aims at improving upon the scope and quantum of medical and health care services.

(iii) The Organised Sector Division coordinates Departmental Policies and Measures affecting the family planning activities of public bodies and private organisations which are collectively called institutions in the Organised Sector.

(iv) The Voluntary Organisations Division assigns programmes to voluntary agencies and aims at assessing the efficiency and effectiveness of these agencies.

On the technical side, the following divisions are functioning. The functions are clear from the names of the divisions.

(i) Programme Appraisal, Coordination and Training and Sterilisation (including Research) Division.

(ii) Technical Operations Division.

(iii) Maternal and Child Health Division

(iv) Evaluation and Intelligence Division.

(v) Mass Education and Media (including population education) Division.

(vi) Nirodh Marketing Division.

(vii) Transport Division, and

(viii) Projects Division (Area Projects).

Advisory Bodies

A number of committees advise the Ministry on various aspects of the programme. A committee on Socio-Economic Studies on Family Planning advises on the coordination and development of research on various dimensions of family planning and population matters. The committee ceased operations in 1974 and consideration was given at that time to the creation of the Indian Council on Population Research to replace it.

A Family Planning Communication Board has been set up, with the Minister of Health and Family Welfare as Chairman, the Minister of Information and Broadcasting as Vice-Chairman, and Secretaries of various concerned ministries and co-opted experts as members. The Board advises on improving the mass communication programme of the department with a view to closing the gap between awareness and actual practice in family planning.

An Inter-Ministerial Coordination group advises the ways and means of involving Panchayats in the programme, and a Tripartite National Committee on Family Planning seeks to secure the cooperation of workers, labour leaders and employers in government projects in family planning. A Steering Group on Population Education composed of representatives from the Ministry of Health and Family Welfare and Ministry of Education and Social Welfare, advises on the development of educational materials on population matters for use in the public school curricula and in reaching out to school youth and other groups.

ORGANISATION CHART : DEPARTMENT OF FAMILY PLANNING

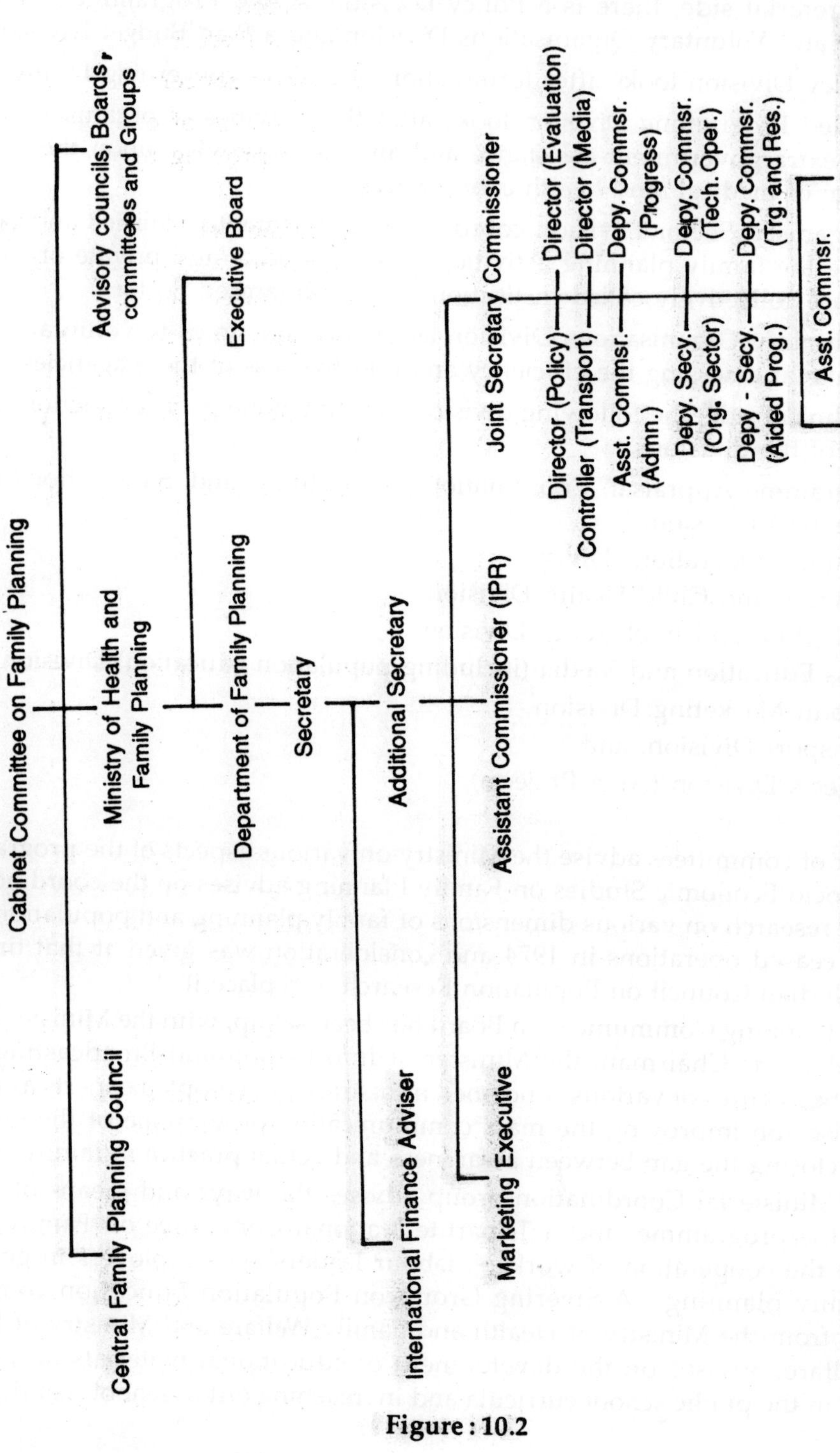

Source : Adopted from the Ministry of Health and Family Planning, Report : 1974-1975 (New Delhi Government of India Press, no date), p. 123

Figure : 10.2

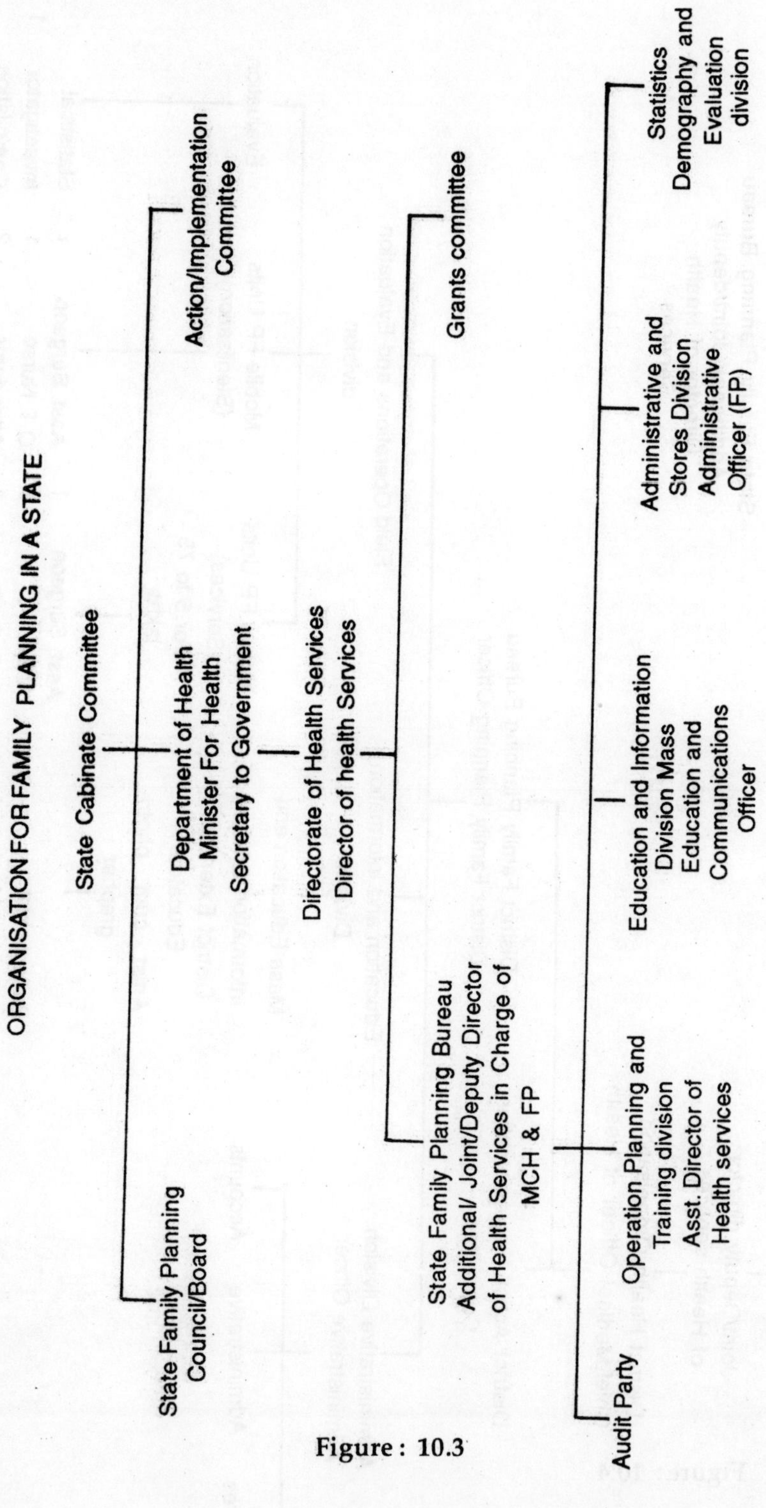
ORGANISATION FOR FAMILY PLANNING IN A STATE
State Cabinate Committee
State Family Planning Council/Board
Action/Implementation Committee
Department of Health Minister For Health Secretary to Government
Directorate of Health Services Director of health Services
Grants committee
State Family Planning Bureau Additional/ Joint/Deputy Director of Health Services in Charge of MCH & FP
Audit Party
Operation Planning and Training division Asst. Director of Health services
Education and Information Division Mass Education and Communications Officer
Administrative and Stores Division Administrative Officer (FP)
Statistics Demography and Evaluation division

Figure : 10.3

ORGANISATION FOR FAMILY PLANNING IN A DISTRICT

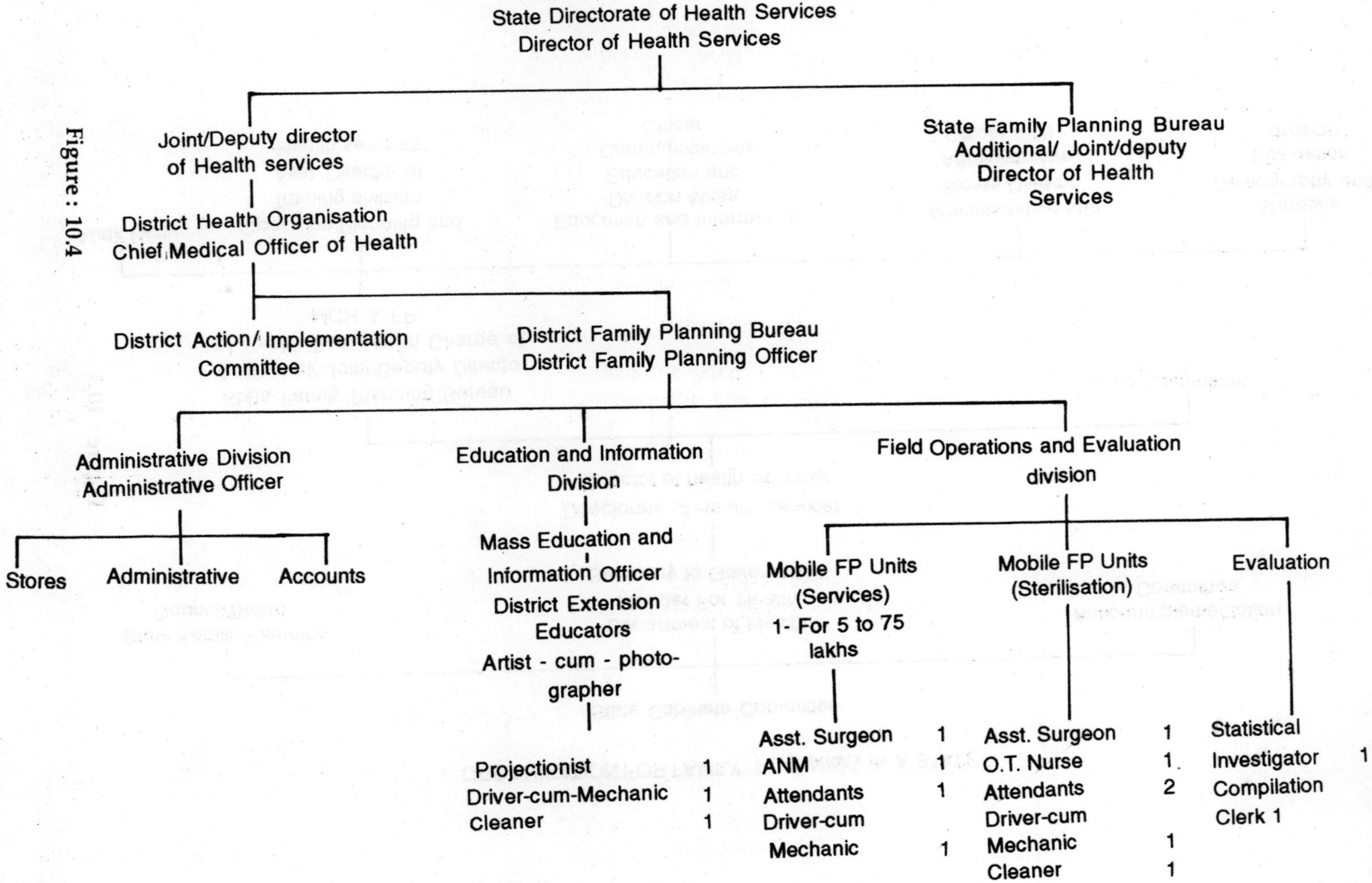

Figure : 10.4

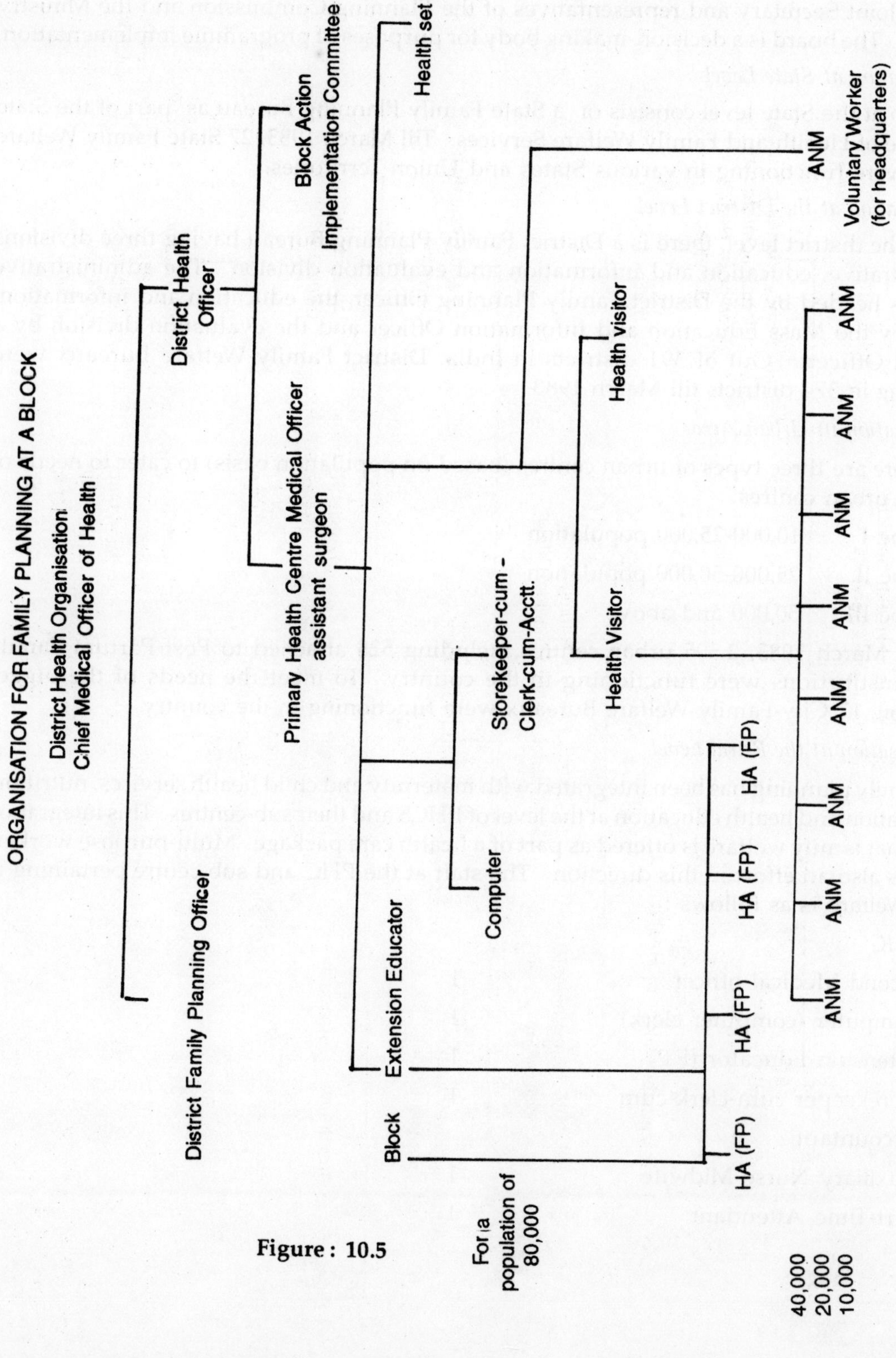
ORGANISATION FOR FAMILY PLANNING AT A BLOCK
District Health Organisation
Chief Medical Officer of Health
District Health Officer
District Family Planning Officer
Block Action Implementation Committee
Health set Up
Primary Health Centre Medical Officer assistant surgeon
Block
Extension Educator
Computer
Storekeeper-cum-Clerk-cum-Acctt.
Health Visitor
Health Visitor
ANM
Voluntary Worker (for headquarters)
HA (FP)
HA (FP)
HA (FP)
HA (FP)
ANM
ANM
ANM
ANM
ANM
ANM
ANM
ANM
For a population of 80,000
40,000
20,000
10,000

Figure : 10.5

The Department of Family Welfare has an Executive Board composed of the Additional Secretary, Joint Secretary and representatives of the Planning Commission and the Ministry of Finance. The board is a decision-making body for purposes of programme implementation

2. Organisation at State Level

The set-up at the State level consists of a State Family Planning Bureau as part of the State Directorate of Health and Family Welfare Services. Till March 1983, 27 State Family Welfare Bureaux were functioning in various States and Union Territories.

3. Organisation at the District Level

At the district level, there is a District Family Planning Bureau having three divisions : administrative, education and information and evaluation division. The administrative division is headed by the District Family Planning Officer, the education and information, division by the Mass Education and Information Officer and the evaluation division by a Statistical Officer. Out of 391 districts in India, District Family Welfare Bureaux were functioning in 374 districts till March 1983.

4. Organisation in Urban Areas

There are three types of urban centres (based on population basis) to cater to needs of people in urban centres.

Type I	10,000-25,000 population
Type II	25,000-50,000 population
Type III	50,000 and above

Till March 1983, 2,505 urban centres including 528 attached to Post-Partum Family Welfare institutions were functioning in the country. To meet the needs of the bigger population, 17 City-Family Welfare Bureaux were functioning in the country.

5. Organisation at the Rural Level

Family planning has been integrated with maternity and child health services, nutrition, immunisation and health education at the level of PHCS and their sub-centres. This integration implies that family welfare is offered as part of a health care package. Multi-purpose workers scheme is also an effort in this direction. The staff at the PHC and sub-centre pertaining to Family Welfare is as follows :

At the PHC

Second Medical officer	1
Computer (computer clerk)	1
Extension Educator (F.P)	1
Storekeeper cum-clerk-cum Accountant	1
Auxiliary Nurse Midwife	1
Part-Time Attendant	1

At the Sub-centre (for 10,000 population)

Auxiliary Nurse Midwife	1	
Voluntary Worker (to act as female attendant)	1	
Male FP Field Worker	1	(For 2 sub-centres)
Lady Health Visitor or Public Health Nurse	1	(for 40,000 population)

Till March 1983, 5,959 Rural Family Welfare centres (an integral part of the PHC) had been established. Besides, the State governments have set up 158 Rural Family Welfare Centres at such PHCs which do not have one at present. There are 65,643 sub-centres under PHCs.

Coordination Between the Union and the State Governments

To coordinate the family welfare activities between the State governments and the Centre, there is one family welfare cell to give adequate support to the State Health and Family Welfare Departments. There are 16 Regional Health Offices to liaise with the respective State Government/Union Territories for speedier implementation of the programme. There is a proposal to integrate all the unipurpose regional offices set up for supervising the implementation of national health programmes.

Aspects of the Programme

Let us now discuss some of the important aspects of the Family Welfare Programme.

1. *Facilities*

(a) *Post-Partum Programme*. Post-Partum Programme is maternity-centred hospital based approach to family welfare. This is a programme for motivating women to adopt the small family norm, through education and motivation during ante-natal and post-natal period when they are by and large most receptive to the idea of limited family and voluntarily accept the method of contraception.

The programme began with 59 medical institutions in 1969 and by the end of March 1983, it covered 604 institutions, which include 110 medical colleges and 400 district and other big maternity hospitals.

(b) *Medical Termination of Pregnancy Programme*. Since the coming into force of Medical Termination of Pregnancy Act 1971, abortion in India has been liberalised. Abortion is now considered as essentially a health measure, particularly for the welfare of women. Till March 1983, there were 2,813 MTP centres which provided services to a total 28 lakh cases.

(c) *Promotion of Conventional Contraceptives*. Nirodh which is one of the conventional contraceptives occupies a pivotal position claiming about 90 per cent of the total contraceptive users. However, as a part of a cafetaria approach, other contraceptives like jellies, foam, tablets, diaphragms and oral pills are also promoted and the choice of selecting a method is left entirely to the eligible couples.

(d) *Sterilisation*. Sterilisation may be effected by vasectomy in the male and tubectomy in the Female.The camps are organised in the areas where the normal facilities for male and female sterilisations are inadequate and where it is possible to provide the facilities by pooling the manpower and equipment for the duration of the camp.

(e) *Intra-Uterine Devices (IUD)* This is effected by introducing a foreign body into the uterus.

(f) *Compensation Money*. The Central assistance to States/Union Territory and other agencies for sterilisation is Rs. 108 per case of vasectomy and Rs. 200 per case of tubectomy. A similar amount of Rs. 8 is provided as compensation money for each case of IUD insertion. If any acceptor of sterilisation operation/IUD insertion unfortunately dies, an amount of Rs. 5,000 shall be paid to the legal heirs.

2. *Training*

The need of efficiently trained workers in a programme for social change cannot be over-emphasised. NIHFW imparts training to health administrators holding key positions. The International Institute for Population Studies, Bombay formerly known as Demographic Training and Research Centre, set up in July 1956, serves as an institution for training and research in population studies for the countries of the ESCAP region. In the last 22 years, the institute has trained 624 students from twenty countries in the ESCAP region and two countries in Africa. The Family Welfare Training and Research Centre, Bombay, imparts training to various categories of workers under the MPW Scheme and CHW Scheme. There are many other institutes which impart such training.

3. *Education and Motivation*

The aim of education and motivational efforts in support of the family welfare programme, is to inform the people about various aspects of the family welfare programme and to promote increased acceptance of the small family norm by the people voluntarily. All available media are utilised for this purpose. The message of family planning is also carried through mobile publicity units of the Directorate of Field Publicity, Song and Drama. The other media units of the Union Ministry of Information and Broadcasting are also actively engaged in mass motivation of the people in favour of family planning.

4. *Evaluation and Research*

Research is carried out on Reproductive Biology through a number of institutions. Recently, a coordination committee for Bio-Medical Research was reconstituted under the Chairmanship of the Secretary, Ministry of Health and Family Welfare, with the following objectives :

(a) To coordinate and review the progress in the entire field of bio-medical research including health care delivery system and operational research at national level;

(b) To fix up national priorities for research in different areas.

(c) To consider availability and utilisation of grants and assistance available from foreign agencies and international organisations for research work;

(d) To provide additional grants for such projects as are considered important and for which funds were not adequate;

(e) To evaluate the progress of research in different fields;

(f) Besides the Central Council of Research in Indian Medicines and Homoeopathy has been engaged in screening a number of plants considered to possess contraceptive potentiality with a view to bringing out an acceptable non-steroid contraceptive agent.

Besides the Biomedical Research, the research in demographic and communication aspects are also undertaken through Population Research Centres. The Research studies undertaken by these centres included fertility and family planning surveys, covering cross-sections of population and special groups of population such as scheduled castes and industrial workers, studies on fertility differentials, characteristics of family planning acceptors, evaluation of family welfare programme, differentials in family planning practices, role of voluntary organisations in the family welfare programme, developing of an action methodology programme among the resistant group, integrated child development programme and family planning, follow-up studies of oral pill acceptors etc.

Role of Voluntary Organisations

The efforts of the government are supplemented by the voluntary organisations. At present voluntary organisations are running nearly three hundred Urban Family Welfare Planning Centres, and a large number of ANM Training Schools with assistance from the department. These organisations also undertake educational and motivational activities for which funds are provided.

To further involve these bodies, a Conference of Voluntary Organisations was held in New Delhi on 1 and 2 May, 1978, in which a large number of voluntary organisations participated. Among other things, it was resolved in the conference, that the voluntary organisations should undertake the provision of clinical and non-clinical services as also educational and motivational work in closer cooperation with the government. It was also recommended to delegate financial powers. As a result of it, the State governments have been delegated powers to sanction grants-in-aid upto a limit of Rs. 2.5 lakhs in each case annually to voluntary organisations for all on-going approved schemes.

National Institute of Health and Family Welfare

History and Need

The National Institute of Health and Family Welfare came into being with effect from 9 March, 1977, by the amalgamation of the erstwhile institutes, namely the National Institute of Family Planning and the National Institute of Health Administration and Education. It has been established as an autonomous body (registered under the Societies Registration Act, 1860) and its object is to act as an apex technical institute for promoting the Health and Family Welfare Planning Programme in the country through education, training, services, research and evaluation. The overall objective of the Institute has been to play a leading role in orienting training and research in health administration and education to the newer concepts of administration and education and thereby strengthen and accelerate India's health and family welfare programmes.

Organisation

The Institute is governed by a General Executive Council with the Union Minister for Health and Family Welfare as the President/Chairman. The day-to-day activities are administered by the Director. The Institute is supported in its activities by International Agencies such as WHO/ SEARO and UNICEF. Closer contact and collaboration exist between the Institute and numerous other organisations in the country. The finances for the functioning of the Institute are provided by the Government of India through grants-in-aid.

Structure

As health administration is based on the concept of 'multi-disciplinary' approach, the Institute has departments embracing various disciplines. These are the departments of Public Health Administration, Hospital Administration, Family Welfare, Maternal and Child Health Programme Planning, Evaluation, Social Sciences, Epidemiology, Health Education, Public Administration, Bio-statistics, Education and Training, Field Training, Public Health Nursing and Field Services. A field practice area in the Rohtak district of Haryana State exists for experimentation and field training exercises of the participants of the institute. Research in the field of Health Administration is reckoned to be a key factor for the development of the activities of the Institute and is therefore, an integral part of the functioning of all departments of the Institute. The new Institute has been renamed as the National Institute of Health and Family Welfare.

Activities

The main activities of the Institute are :

(a) Education and Training

(b) Research

(c) Evaluation of Health Programmes

(d) Consultation Services

(e) Clearing House Functions

(f) Publications and Documents.

(a) (i) *Education and Training*. NIHFW is concentrating on the education and training of health personnel engaged on administrative jobs. The main objective of the Institute is to develop a corps of able and competent health personnel to occupy positions in health administration in the country. The education and training facilities at the Institute are aimed at imparting a better appreciation of the concepts of integrated health care through the improvement in the discipline of health care administration. Education and training is sought to be provided through doctoral level education programme, staff college courses, seminars, conferences and other short courses and workshops etc. The staff college and hospital administration seminars, by and large, continue to be the main instruments of training. These two courses have been attracting participants from neighbouring countries and the Institute is, in fact, engaged at present in framing condensed staff college courses for participants from Asian and African countries, who have shown an interest in attending such courses of short duration.

(ii) *M.D.(Community Health).* This is a two year duration course run by the Institute under affiliation with the University of Delhi. It is designed to give a broad base of education to prepare doctors for leadership in senior posts for the administration of the integrated health administration. A comprehensive curriculum has been drawn up, keeping in view the needs of an integrated health service. Apart from research methodology in health administration for purposes of meeting the thesis requirement, practical field experience in a variety of situations from the hospital to the rural health centre, the administrative headquarters of the health services, the health organisation at the district, municipality, the public health laboratory etc., forms part of the intensive training. Special emphasis is given to the teaching of social science epidemiology, statistics and principles of public administration.

(iii) *Staff College Course.* In addition to the above, it has been found necessary to run shorter courses for bringing together experienced and busy executive officers (both medical and non-medical) working in the field of health, to give them an opportunity of examining different administrative practices in their special fields in order to equip them to discharge their present assignments efficiently and also prepare them for higher responsibilities in the future. It is found useful for those entrusted or likely to be entrusted with the position of top management in the health field, to be given the opportunity for discussing their problems with others having different but comparable experience and training with a view to improving themselves. By this interchange of ideas and experiences it is hoped to enrich their personalities leading to greater administrative efficiency in individual performance.

For this purpose, the Institute has been organising staff college courses for senior categories of health administrators. This course is of 8-10 weeks duration and presently is being held once in a year regularly, for the inception of the Institute. The teaching methods employed for this course are :

(a) Syndicate-discussion groups on specific problems;

(b) Prepared case studies;

(c) Lecture-seminar discussion on different aspects connected with family welfare and health administration; as also panel discussions; and

(d) Observational field visits to the institutions in and around Delhi.

It may be pertinent to mention here that the Central Council of Health in its 14th meeting held in New Delhi in October 1967, had suggested that attendance of the Staff College Course be treated as one of the requirements for appointment or promotion to posts entailing administrative responsibility.

(iv) *Country Course Health Planning.* The Institute has also started holding courses on health planning for health administrators who are primarily connected with planning in the states.

(v) *Hospital Administration and Other Seminars.* Besides the Staff College Course, the Institute is also holding seminars on different aspects of administration of health and family welfare. One of these is the seminar on Hospital Administration to focus attention of the administrators on different facets of hospital activity. These seminars are of two-week duration and are repeated twice every year. These are meant for senior administrators of hospitals and medical care programmes as well as senior nursing personnel. The main objectives of this course are to discuss the role of the hospital in comprehensive community health programmes, hospital care aspects of health service and the importance of planning and proper management of hospitals to improve patient care and better utilisation of resources; discussion on the methodology of evaluation of medical care and on the planning of hospital and other medical care facilities. The contents of the seminar include lecture discussions on different aspects of organisation and management of hospitals, panel discussions, case studies, group and syndicate discussions and field visits to hospitals. The Institute has received requests for holding hospital administration seminars in other parts of the country.

Other seminars of short duration have been on health planning and evaluation, integration of health services, civil defence and orientation of new entrants to health services, health education planning, nursing administration, social sciences, teaching of bio-statistics in medical college and teaching methods and management development.

(vi) *Workshops.* Another method of education and training utilised by the NIHFW is the 'Workshop' on specific problems. These are usually of a short duration of 3-6 days and are essentially for a group of already well-informed people to work out recommendations for solution of a particular problem.

(b) *Research.* In addition to education and training programmes, research in Health Administration and Family Welfare is another activity of the Institute. Some of the research studies undertaken by the Institute are as follows :

1. Study of evening out-patient department in hospitals of Delhi.
2. Study of the job satisfaction of scheduled caste and scheduled tribe employees in a large hospital in Delhi.
3. Study of factors associated with adoption of practices related to health aspects of family planning by hospital patients and relatives (WHO project).
4. Action project on Mothers Club in a locality in South Delhi.

The Institute has completed a number of research projects in the field of health administration. Some of these are :

1. Multi-purpose Workers Health Project.
2. Appraisal of MCH & FP services rendered through an Urban MCH & FP centre and Urban Maternity Home (M.D.)
3. Study to evolve staffing pattern for MCH & FP centres of Municipal Corporation of Delhi.
4. A study of trends of administrative research in health by preventive and social medicine departments of medical colleges in India.
5. Pilot study of "Feasibility of Involving School Teachers in Providing Health Care to Rural Communities."

6. A comparative study of emergency services to three large Delhi hospitals.
7. Norms of management of environmental cleanliness in the hospital.
8. Profile of Rural Field Practice Areas attached to medical colleges in India.
9. Health and education status in a teaching hospital.
10. Case studies in hospital administration.
11. Utilisation and pattern of demand for the CGHS Ayurvedic dispensaries in Delhi.
12. Study of utilisation of hospital beds (ICMR - sponsored).
13. Study of collection of charges in Delhi hospitals.
14. Study of the laboratory services of Willingdon Hospital, New Delhi.

(c) *Evaluation of Health Programmes*

The Institute also provides assistance or consultation in the evaluation of health programmes in their various aspects viz., technical, administrative and training. In this connection the Institute assisted the Programme Evaluation Organisation (PEO) of the Planning Commission in their evaluation study of national family planning programme in 1968-69. Similarly, at the request of the Christian Medical Association of India, a Consultation Committee was appointed by the Institute to study their family planning project in 1969. The Committee submitted its report containing recommendations for streamlining and making the activities of the family planning project more productive.

(d) *Consultation Services*

Consultation services is yet another important area of activity being developed in the Institute. It maintains close contact with the Union Ministry of Health and Family Welfare, and State Health Department. The Director, NIHFW attends most of the conferences organised on health and family welfare matters as well as the meetings of the Central Council of Health. The Institute provides advice and guidance to the State governments on development of health services and allied issues. It also takes up the study of problems in the field of Health Administration and Training on request by the Central and State Departments of Health. It offers guidance to voluntary health agencies in conducting studies for solution of problems of health and related subjects.

The faculty of the Institute collaborates with other sister organisations in their training programmes. In the course of visits to States, faculty members meet participants and render advice and guidance on problems that come up during discussions with them.

(e) *Clearing House Functions*

The Institute prepares background papers on various subjects as well as extracts from current literature, committee reports and review and provides these to the various course participants. Publications relating to various conferences and seminars organised by the Institute are brought out and supplied. The Institute through its own journal published every quarter, keeps participants and health administrators in touch with the activities of the Institute and developments in the field of health administration. The Institute has a modest but rich library with about 20,000 mimeographed papers, 60,000 books and bout 150 journals both Indian and foreign which are received regularly. Upon request, preparation of bibliography on various subjects is undertaken and supplied to indenting parties. Important articles appearing in various journals on different disciplines are regularly being indexed.

(f) *Publications and Documents*

The Institute publishes a quarterly journal *Health and Population: Perspectives and Issues*. Though just six years old the journal has established a place of its own in the current literature on problems of health administration planning. In addition to this journal, reports and recommendations of various seminars and conferences and research studies are published from time to time as Technical Reports and Research Reports.

CRITICAL APPRAISAL

1. *Improper utilisation of trained personnel*. It has been found that most of the persons who are sponsored for the training programme at the Institute are not utilised for the assignment for which they have been trained. This results in a lot of wastage. Training can be effective only if the knowledge and skills acquired by the trainees are used for performance improvement and career development. Further training cannot be considered in isolation from other aspects of personnel administration or from other aspects of performance improvement. In fact, training *per se* can become a wasteful effort if it is not harmonised with a programme of administrative improvements and reforms.

2. *Absence of researches suiting Indian conditions*. The research conducted by the Institute has mostly been based on the models of the Health Administration in the advanced countries.

   The Institute can do a great service if the models of the Health Administration are designed to suit the needs of this country.

3. *More emphasis on theoretical aspects*. During the training courses more emphasis is laid on theoretical aspects rather than on its practical application. When the trainees go back to their jobs they find it difficult to implement the theoretical ideas into concrete practice. While imparting training, emphasis should be given on such ideas which are practical in the given situation of the country.

4. *Poor Coverage*. At present the training is being imparted to the senior and middle executive of the health administration. There is also a need to train the para-medical and clerical staff working in the Health Department and hospitals.

5. *Absence of links with States*. The Institute may set up its branches in the various States, to encourage the research in health administration like the Indian Institute of Public Administration which has its regional branches in most of the States.

6. *Absence of active liaison with medical colleges*. The Institute should have active liaison with the medical colleges and post-graduate institutes. The Institute in collaboration with the Ministry of Health and Family Welfare, Medical Council of India, Indian Council of Medical Research, etc., can frame certain syllabus in health care administration which can be incorporated in under graduate and post-graduate

medical education. In this way the future experts of health in various disciplines would have some idea of training and research in health care administration.

7. *No practical training to the trainers.* The success of training programmes to a large extent depends much on the trainers : "Investment in a trainer is a gain to the hundreds who he trains in turn".

But most of the trainers have bookish knowledge. They are not fully alive to the problems of health care administration. Lack of duly qualified trainers is one of the serious handicaps in making the training programmes effective. In the words of Laidlaw, "You could not teach surgery to medical students out of a textbook; only a surgeon with a long experience can teach others to be a surgeon"

D. Critical Appraisal of the Administrative Adequacy and Performance

The performance of the family planning programme has been very poor as compared to the resources put in the programme till the Fifth Five Year Plan except the Emergency period. The actual achievement has always fallen short of the targets laid for each year. However, since 1981 to 1983 the performance is satisfactory as compared to previous years. For example, the total number of acceptors of different family planning methods during the year 1982-83 reached a figure of 11.02 million against 8.10 million enrolled during 1981-82; 5.4 million enrolled during 1979-80. The progress has been satisfactory method-wise as well.

However still, it is not so encouraging as we see in other developing and developed countries of the world. We must strengthen our efforts till family planning is accepted as a way of life by the people.

Even the Government of India has itself admitted that the non-attainment of the stipulated reduction in the birth rate may largely be due to the highly ambitious targets set earlier, coupled with insufficiency of efforts to project the programme, throughout the country as a mass movement and rather slow build up of the infrastructure in some of the populous regions for extension efforts and provision of services. A comparison of India was made recently with other developing countries of the region, and it was found that the achievements of India's family planning programme are the lowest. It was stated that by 1974, family planning programme in India covered only 15.1 per cent of all married women between 15 and 44 years while the percentage was 60.1 in Singapore, 55 in Hong Kong and Taiwan, 31 in Colombia, 30.5 in South Korea, 24.8 in Thailand and 20.5 in Egypt. The figures stated by the Population Council of New York in *A Fact Book on Population and Family Planning Programme*, have revealed that in 1972 India's birth rate of 37.39 per one thousand was higher than 17 other countries. Even the 25 per thousand rate we are trying to achieve by 1986 was already achieved by Mauritius, Hong Kong, Singapore, Taiwan, Barbados and Puerto Rico. On the other hand it is quite strange that India's per capita family planning expenditure of 13 US cents in 1973 was higher than that of 11 nations. Besides, as a per cent of the total national budget, India's budget on family planning was the highest. Thus, the people at large in India have not yet adopted family planning as their way of life.

From the above observations and facts, it is quite obvious that there is something wrong in the organisation and administration of the programme. This has been ultimately responsible for the unsatisfactory performance of the programme.

> It is accepted that inability to manage efficiently or utilise effectively the available and potential resources is the common ill of all the less-developed countries. It follows that successful development demands a sound programme for managerial improvement.

It was also reported by the UN that "a principal obstacle everywhere to the development of successful official family planning programme lies in the area of organisation and administration. The challenge for Planners and Administrators is to work out effective means for delivery of this technology and service to the public."

Now, let us analyse the organisational and administrative factors in the context of family planning programme. On the basis of facts presented, we shall draw conclusions and make suggestions for a more effective programme.

Organisational Problems

Mr. Gaus defines organisation as : "Organisation is the arrangement of personnel for facilitating the accomplishment of some agreed purpose through the allocation of functions and responsibilities. It is the relating of efforts and capacities of individual and groups engaged upon a common task in such a way as to secure the desired objective with the least friction and the most satisfaction to those for whom the task is done and those engaged in the enterprise."

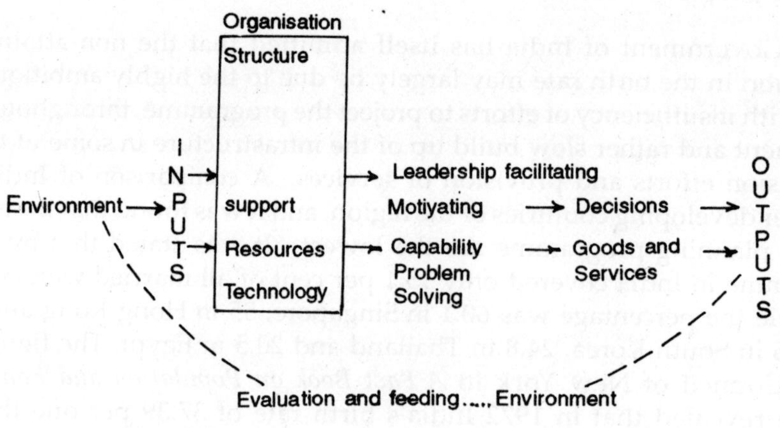

Figure : 10.6

Nowadays, organisation are defined, in terms of the systems approach (input and output). We can represent it diagrammatically.

Organisations are not simply structures but an action system and the success and failure of the organisations are to be measured in terms of this action system. Action system is a structured device in which resources are mobilised and transformed by use of certain skills and technology to produce pre-designed output, all taking place by influence of leadership within an environmental context. Let us now discuss the organisational problems and the improvements at various levels.

AT THE UNION LEVEL

The family planning programme in India is based on a flexible approach but the total programme seriously lacks the benefits of decentralisation and autonomy in the matter of implementation.

(a) While the entire programme is centrally sponsored its implementation is the responsibility of the State governments. The programme sets a uniform pattern right from Central to the district administration depriving completely the implementing agency from attempting any experimentation with alternative methods. Family planning programmes are very much influenced by changes in their operating environments and their programme usefulness depends upon quick response to differing situations and new social needs and demands. This would be possible only if the authority to adjust according to the prevailing environment is decentralised from the Union to the State Governments.

(b) The highly centralised nature of the programme ensures uniformity of staffing pattern but it lacks the inbuilt flexibility to change as and when necessary to entire efficient and effective programme implementation. There is a need to decentralise the development of personnel policy for this programme.

AT THE DISTRICT LEVEL

The most serious administrative problems in family planning efforts are found in the personnel area. Finding capable, technical and managerial personnel and training, motivating and keeping them in the programme are quite difficult tasks. Let us illustrate the point with the help of the organisation of the Family Planning Programme at the district level. In the administration of family planning programme, the District Family Planning Bureau is the most important link as the district is an important and strategic unit of administration. The District Family Planning Bureau is headed by a District Family Planning officer. He is a senior person with medical qualifications. He is to work under the overall supervision and direction of the Chief Medical Officer. He has been entrusted the responsibility without authority as he has no real administrative control over the staff working under him. There is hardly any difference in terms of status and qualifications between the CMO and DFPO(Chief Medical Officer and District Family Planning Officer) except that of seniority. This has given rise to many disputes between these two functionaries thus damaging the delivery of the programme. This needs to be carefully examined. It can be corrected either by giving administrative powers to DFPOS and only reserving appellate powers with the CMO of replacing the former with persons of general qualifications as the family planning programme is more motivational and educational programme than a technical one.

AT THE VILLAGE LEVEL

The supervision and management of family planning in the villages through the Primary Health Centres complex need leadership qualities, interest and experience in family planning but medical officers who are appointed to these posts lack these qualifications. There is a need of training the PHC doctors in the art and science of family welfare.

Administrative Leadership

Administrative leadership or capability is an important means of converting or processing programme inputs into outputs such as goods and services. It has been mentioned by Gabriel that "what makes the leadership variable so crucial in the implementation process is its dynamic, not passive quality i.e., its capability to act and react on these critical inputs. It is this manipulative and transferring quality of leadership that could significantly determine the administrative capability of implementing organisations."

Such leadership is not available in the tip and middle level administrators working in the family planning programme. Most of the administrators are not committed to the programme as they have been forced to work on this programme. They should stimulate others to a high level of performance. They should be willing to experiment new innovations and approaches especially to adopt the programme to differing and changing circumstances. Family planning is given only peripheral attention in the curricula of medical schools. In practice, only a few doctors seem to find family planning work professionally challenging. Instead of accelerating the momentum of the programme, these administrators are always on the look out for their transfer to the medical side. Because of their lukewarm attitude, their contagious effects spread in the whole organisation. Thus the success of the programme can only be achieved if adequate number of motivated persons are made available for accelerating the tempo of this difficult and arduous task. *The Tribune* editorial has rightly commented that,

> If picking good men is the most important of them all, dumping the bad ones is the next most important.

Walter R. Sharp has also mentioned the importance of the personnel in the organisation. He says :

> Even poorly devised machinery may be made to work if it is manned with well-trained, intelligent, imaginative and devoted staffs. On the other hand the best planned organisation may produce unsatisfactory results if it is operated by mediocre or disgruntled people.

So we must find out the administrators to carry out this challenging task who should possess the following qualities.

> First, there are certain specialised knowledge and skills which are programme relevant such as substantive knowledge of engineering in infrastructure programme. Second, managerial expertise and skills are paramount in effective implementation, coordinating

and scheduling work, planning and allocating resources and so on. Third, modern administrative leaders need human relations ability to deal with a major resource in organisational life. Motivating people to perform beyond normal requirements to instill a strong sense of programme commitment and integrity and to incite programme personnel to unfetter the suffocating bonds of anachronistic administrative values, traditions and practices are additional requisite skills. Finally, there are certain 'political skills' required to sustain support and cooperation from the volatile public (legislators and ministers), mass media, clientele, local political notables etc.

Besides, they must have faith in the ideals of the family planning programmes, be willing to accept hardships and the prepared to work in the spirit of service. Their ambition and enthusiasm should not be dampened by local conditions which may not provide them with the necessary facilities.

> Unfortunately, the sense of dedication has been the rarest casualty of the prevailing atmosphere of cynicism bred by increasing propensity towards expediency.[30]

Action Programme

The policy of the Family Planning Programme Organisation in terms of targets are made only for the state or country as a whole. No attempt has been made so far to prepare action plans for each sub-centre/primary health centre or urban centre in terms of money, equipment, personnel, time, physical targets etc. Such action programme if designed would help in effective implementation and monitoring, Here, we can make use of the new techniques of management—PERT/CPM for proper programme planning and resource deployment.

Environmental Linkage

It is understood that the implication of family planning programme is a quite complex process in which medical, cultural, psychological, social, economic, administrative and even political factors are involved and intermingled. A good organisation must respond to and react to the changes in the environment and establish environmental linkages. Linkages are points of interactions with the environment. They can be classified into four categories—enabling, functional, diffused and normative linkages

Enabling linkage ensures and protects the organisational authority to operate its access to resource and its power to achieve results. One of the most important factors which impinges on the programmes from its formulation to execution is political and its impingement on both the programme and its executors occur at all levels (national, regional, provincial, district) and at the programme input levels (financial allocations, personnel, material resources). The impact of politics and the political processes on the programme is both positive and negative and this insight provides the directions and options available to ensure greater success programme implementations. Since political constraints are neither permanent nor inseparable there is urgency in adopting measures designed to optimise the positive contributions of political support as well as minimise and mitigate the harmful effects of partisan interferences.

For administrators to operate successfully in this political environment they must acquire not only the knowledge and skills required in running the programme but also a deeper insight of the 'political games' as well as the 'political skills' needed to serve and thrive in that environment. An important asset is the capacity of programme leaders to seek and maintain support from key political elites both at the national and local levels.

Functional linkage is to link the programme with the task environment university, research institute, hospital etc.

(i) *Collaboration with the universities* : In this connection it is suggested that there should be effective collaboration between the universities and the family planning programme as the universities can be a source of strength to the programme from the policy formulation to evaluation. At the moment there is a dichotomy between the social sciences and the medical specialists which must fade away as early as possible. In South Korea, one of the reasons ascribed for the success of the programme is the association of the university with the family planning programme.

(ii) *Collaborations with the hospitals* : The success of family planning programme depends to a great extent on the way the programme can be operated through the health services network in the country. The hospital provides a good platform from the educational and motivational point of view. About 200 million people approach the hospitals every year in the country and there the people are most amenable to advice upon any aspect of their personal behaviour including family planning. Maternity wards are special places for such work. Moreover, the hospital is the best place for family planning as it can provide all the services to deal with after effects. Conventional contraceptives are not being used by the people in India because it requires high motivation and good standard of living e.g., the sale of Nirodh has touched 50 million mark in India, while in USA with half the population, sale is about 600 million per year, in Japan with one-fifth of India's population, the sale is 250 million per year. Therefore, the country should rely on sterilisation, IUD etc. Both of these require supervision of a high order. Hence, we must streamline the administration of the hospitals so that the hospital staff can also take up Family Planning Programme, work with more earnestness and seriousness.

Diffused linkage : "Life enlighten movement" means to reach the clients through mass media. Organisational family planning programme requires a high level of user participation. Any successful family planning effort must be understood and accepted by the people and be based on public trust and confidence. It cannot be solely dictated or legislated. Family planning is such a multifaceted personal and intimate subject that its practice can only occur on an individual, voluntary basis.

The art of developing common understanding among people is vital to bring about change of attitudes and behaviour. Sociologists have classified the diffusion process which leads to a widespread acceptance of the programme into five stages :

Awareness (The individual's first introduction to a new idea or practice).

Interest (the stage at which he actually seeks further information and background data).

Evaluation (the stage of assessment on theoretical grounds).

Trial (a limited phase of experiment), and finally *acceptance* or *adoption*.

Naturally the duration of the process depends upon personality factors which differs with individuals. Mass-media helps in creating awareness, in providing stimulation and motivation and in giving ready access to information. But at the specific stage of evaluation, trial and adoption, inter-personal, face to face, communication counts for much more and the inability of the mass media to maintain a two-way dialogue with regular feedback restricts their utility. Therefore, no medium of communication is effective.

> The process of social and economic development is a process of human development for people are the targets as well as the essential variable in development. Communication being a two way process, provides for participation at whatever stage of enlightenment of the individuals composing a society find themselves. Change agents are key factors in both the communication development processes since they are instruments for getting facts to the people upon which decisions can be based.

This function is to be performed mostly by the field workers. At present, the field workers are not fully equipped to do this interpersonal communication resulting into much misinformed criticism of the programme. For example, on the personal discussion of the writer with a group of rickshaw-pullers, it was revealed that they were not undergoing family planning operations as they thought that they would not be able to ply their rickshaws afterwards. Similarly, in a discussion with educated people one finds that they think that the adoption of family planning programme would lead to many social and psychological maladjustments. It was found in a survey that assistant field workers felt a need for more training to develop skills and techniques to contact, communicate and persuade their clients in their own particular setting/identity of personality. Even the Haryana Government has admitted that training of the workers in the field needs reorientation and pre-service training of multipurpose workers is absolutely necessary.[34]

It is even suggested that the field workers may be selected from that area, where the workers are to be assigned so that there may not be any cultural lag. Besides, it may be made compulsory for these workers to stay in the area of operation. Other than this method, population education through formal education can also serve the purpose. In order to enlist the support of the people for the family welfare programme, there is a need to educate the people about the dynamics of population. Educational approach is a healthy method and will motivate people to accept family welfare voluntarily. Any other scheme without educational base will miserably fail as it will generate reaction. We must encourage population education through formal and informal education to imbibe the confidence of the people in the family welfare programme. Population education is an educational programme to develop in young men rational and responsible attitude and behaviour towards population problem. NCERT suggested the following curriculum at the higher secondary stage :

(1) The population growth.
(2) Economic development and population.
(3) Social development and population.
(4) Health, nutrition and population.
(5) Family life and population.

Wayland suggests six basic topics for study :

(1) Basic instructions in population dynamics.

(2) Development of basic understanding of the process of human reproduction.

(3) Understanding of health problems concerned with bringing up of children.

(4) Appreciation of relationship between quality of life and family size.

(5) Government policies regarding population growth and economic development.

(6) Familiarity with the family planning programme of one's own country.

Normative linkage : There has been little attempt to incorporate the family planning behaviour into the existing value system of the society. Social values act as a hindrance to ready adoption. For example, if people talk about birth control behaviour naturally related to sex, it is traditionally regarded as impolite. Besides, the demand for sons to carry on the family line has been predominant in the Indian society. Not only social values but also religious values often act as a hindrance. Therefore, the mass-media and communication officers and family planning workers must dispel all these false impressions and taboos after a careful survey and research in demography. Mass media and communication officers may intensify their efforts by organising public meetings of different groups—labourers, farmers, workers, union leaders and extensive use of various media like cinema, exhibition, radio, TV etc., may be made. At present, the full use of mass-media is not being made in the real sense in spite of the availability of the arrangements. More attention is to be paid to uneducated rural people and economically depressed classes. Family planning and fertility control behaviour of the client group especially eligible women have been affected by their socio-economic background. It is found that the higher educated women tend to have a small number of children and the use of contraceptives and induced abortion is more prevalent among them. The socio-economic status as well as the urban-rural diffusion of client groups are clearly pronounced in their family planning behaviour. The Government of India, Ministry of Health, has also admitted that "high fertility rates have been identified as more a function of poverty than of anything else." Therefore, more attention must be paid to groups living under conditions of poverty.

Coordination with Voluntary Agencies

Voluntary agencies can play an effective role in mobilising the public opinion in support of the programme. The Family Planning Association of India and its branches in the States are rendering useful services. In this connection, it may be suggested that to revolutionise the programme, FPAI may take initiative in setting up the 'Women's Club' in every village as in South Korea. At present, the 'Mother's Club' having a membership of 20-40 women in each of 19,000 villages has become a multipurpose basic organ for the nation-wide. 'New community movement' since 1971, in Korea. It is significant to note that the family planning programme became integrated into a broader community movement by the Mother's Club at the village level. This experiment has been a great success in South Korea. We can also create such clubs having influential members. We can bring these members in the communication network with the help of a four-step strategy mentioned below :

(a) provide the opinion leaders with the information necessary for a full understanding of the reasons for family planning including its relationships to national and particularly local development.

(b) invite their suggestions for local activities.

(c) involve them in the purview of radio and television programmes.

(d) invite them to open discussion about family planning in the community whether formally or informally.

Mrs. Helvi Sipila has also stressed that the association of women will surely help in checking the menace of population explosion. A study of the inter-relationship of the status of women and family planning was conducted in accordance with economic and social council resolution. The report affirmed.

(a) The right to decide freely and responsibly on the number and spacing of their children is a fundamental right of individuals which facilitates the exercise of other human rights especially by women.

(b) Adequate information, education and services enabling individuals to exercise this right are essential prerequisites for ensuring their complete integration in social and economic development at all levels.

(c) Family Planning which should constitute an integrated and essential part of development plan and programme in countries suffering from over-population can only succeed in concert with other measures which also improve the status of women.

Thus it can be said that the best contraceptive in the world is the involvement and the overall improvement of the status of women.

Coordination with Allied Agencies

Inter-organisation coordination is desirable when the activities of the various organisations concerned are of a complementary nature. The Family Planning Department, State Family Planning Bureau and District Family Planning Bureau are achieving useful coordination with other allied ministries/departments at different levels in the formulation and implementation of the programme. But it is suggested that the meetings and the documentation service dealing with coordination may be reduced to a level essential for programme development. The personal discussion with the family planning programme officials reveals that a great part of their time is spent in these secondary activities and ultimately this affects their primary responsibility. So, only that much coordination is to be achieved which ensures the yardstick of cost-benefit analysis.

Built-in Device to Gain Confidence of the People

The success of the programme depends upon the built-in confidence and faith of the people in the responsiveness and effectiveness of the family planning organisation at all levels. This needs to be assured at all levels.

Use of Modern Management Methods

No matter how excellent the original planning is, an implementation scheme may be designed to develop a certain amount of detail for its effective performance. The management must work to ensure that all the component activities and tasks are accomplished according to the implementation schedule. The effectiveness of national planning and population programme can be increased through the sound use of modern management techniques. The management can take the aid of the various techniques for this purpose, e.g., 'Systems approach' of operational research, systems analysis, programme budgeting, computer-based information system; techniques concerned with the productive use of resources such as work study, network analysis and cost analysis and organisational and behavioural methods concerned with personnel selection, training, motivation, communication, adaptation to change, working in groups, the organisation development, etc. Out of these some can be adopted with great easiness. Let us discuss MIS and MBO.

(i) *Management Information System.* At present, the reporting system prevalent in the Family Planning Programme is not adequate as some information is collected by Demographers (Assistant Directors of Statistics), some by mass-media and communication officers without going much into the causes of low performance and their remedial measures. Therefore, there is a need of a MIS for the identification and clear definition of problems, for the designing of intervention strategies for sound decision-making as well as for the monitoring of the process of change and evaluation of outcomes as part of the cyclic process of planning.

(ii) *Management by objectives.* A policy on population control should be well understood by the entire personnel in the organisation. Even, they may be involved in the policy formulation and execution of the programmes. It would mean the imposition of the standards of performance on one self. Moreover, the administration must share the information with all the field staff about the success and failure of the programme.

Incentive Systems

At present, different kinds of incentives are provided to the people to undergo sterilisation etc. This has resulted in many malpractices. All these incentives in the ultimate analysis cannot be effective in the success of the family planning programme and has created many wrong practices and false reporting. In this way time and money is spent on undesirable cases. There is a great need of supervision to assess the reliability and fitness of the reported cases.

Research and Evaluation

The researches so far conducted have not devoted sufficient attention to fields of organisational structure and functioning of family planning programme and modern methods of administrative management. The WHO Regional Committee for South-East Asia laid great emphasis on administrative problems. We must encourage health administrators in collaboration with university teachers of Public Administration to take up such problems of research. Evaluation machinery needs strengthening at all levels. Independent evaluation may be undertaken to ensure that qualitative aspects of the programme have not been ignored by the States. It is suggested that a particular problem in the field of FPP, in the form of 'Research Project' may be entrusted to university departments to have objective evaluation by disinterested experts in the field. Training and educational requirements for the personnel associated with this programme probably exceed those of any other government programme of the social type. Such training is essential to all categories of personnel especially the workers of lower levels. Training of peripheral workers has been in-service rather than pre-service. Even in-service training has taken its own slow course. Most of the time the workers were not spread for training as some intensive Family Planning drive was always on. Fresh matriculates with rural background without professional skill have blundered in the motivational programme. There is a need to train the field workers in the concrete situation rather than imparting theoretical instructions.

Tax Benefits

The following tax benefits may be given to attract investments for family planning programme.

(a) to develop an incentive package to enable the private sector to set up factories for manufacturing family planning devices such as oral contraceptives and others;

(b) reduce the tax rates of single persons in order to encourage them to delay marriage;

(c) allowing employers or donors to deduct the following expenses on their income taxes:

- Expenses on the provision of family planning services to employees as a part of health care services under the Labour Protection Law.

B. Population Education

(a) Promote the teaching of population education as an independent subject at all educational levels or as part of the regular curricula to meet the needs of each age group.

(b) Create a better understanding of population education by organising population education workshops for family planning administrators at various levels.

(c) Support research studies and evaluation so that the findings can be applied to further the development of population education.

(d) Encourage educational institutions and relevant agencies to carry out studies and research in order to develop appropriate techniques for implementing information, education and communication services on population activities.

Conclusion : We should not be pessimistic. We should hope that the present momentum built-up since the sixth plan would continue. We should not hesitate to bring about innovative changes to make the programme realistic. We cannot afford to allow the programme to go slow as the programme is a source of strength to all other schemes of socio-economic development, whatever may be their immediate goal. Prime Minister Indira Gandhi, has rightly said on September 30, 1983, at New York, while receiving the United Nations Population Award :

> It is said that prosperity is a good contraceptive. But the effects of development are submerged unless we bring about a low birth rate. Family Planning is an input for development, an indispensable exercise in human capital formation. Education, better capacity for producing and earning a higher rise in per capita income are possible only when population growth is curbed.

11

Utilisation of Health and Family Planning Services Among Rural Women

If Indian women are to be freed from their low status as 'expendable assets' they must be released from the bondage of repeated and frequent child births and must be provided a say in the matter of the size of their families. Ensuring adequate medical facilities to protect them during and against maternity is also essential. All the demographic indicators suggest that child bearing in India, for the majority of women, is more of a health hazard than a natural function. It is the high maternal mortality rate which raises the overall death rate for females and accounts for the low sex-ratio. Thus, technologies related to birth and birth control are a great liberating influence for women. But the access of these services to women is affected by a number of socio-cultural factors. Access has often been identified solely with availability. It has generally been seen as a one way process of supplying adequate resources to a consumer's market and simultaneously educating the market to accept the service provided. But there are certain social constraints in rural societies which prevent women from availing themselves of even the existing services. Even if the medical services are provided to the community, these may not be available to women, whose utilisation of these services may be affected by the beliefs of that particular community about the health needs of women and the knowledge and awareness of women themselves

Acceptance of family planning has been considered as one of the important indicators of improvement in the status of women. Margaret Sanger, aptly called the mother of family planning, stated that "family planning is fundamentally and vitally a women's cause. Unless their human right to decide freely and responsibly on the number and spacing of children and to have the means to do so is recognised, they can not exercise and enjoy real equality with men and will continue to be disadvantaged in their attempt to benefit from other reforms." Although a large number of studies have been conducted on issues related to family planning only a small percentage of them have covered rural areas. In a survey of studies related to family planning between 1951-68, it was found that out of 249 studies conducted, only 24.1 per cent cover rural areas and 1.2 per cent were conducted in Punjab (including Haryana) which reflects the utter ancity of research and research material on this issue in this region. An attempt has been made in this paper to find out the access of women to health services relating to pre-natal care, child birth and family planning; various factors affecting it and the attitude towards family planning.

METHODOLOGY

This is a cross-section study of two-sets of villages, one where certain forces of change are present to a greater extent and other where these forces are present to a lesser degree. Two districts were selected from the State of Haryana, one advanced (Karnal) and the other not so advanced (Bhivani) in respect to agricultural and socio-economic development. One block from each district was selected using the same criterion.

In the present paper, the advanced villages of the advanced district have been denoted as region 'A', advanced villages of backward districts as region 'B'. Region 'C' denotes backward villages of advanced districts and the 'D' region stands for backward villages of backward district.

Access to Family Planning Services

If the masses of the Indian women are to be freed from their low status as 'expendable assets', some of the obvious and immediate answers lie in releasing them from the bondage of repeated and frequent childbirth, providing them with some choice in the size of their families and in ensuring adequate medical facilities to protect them during and against maternity. Propagators of the family planning movement in India have been keen to emphasise the improvement in the status of women as one of the direct consequences of acceptance of family planning. An attempt was made to find out the access of women to family planning and the various factors affecting it; the attitude towards family planning and the existing fertility patterns.

An analysis on the adoption of family planning (Table 11.2) revealed that 39.7 per cent of respondents have adopted family planning. A regional comparison indicated that the maximum adoptors of family planning were from region A (56.6 per cent), followed by region B (37.3 per cent), C (26.6 per cent) and region D (12.7 per cent). Thus, women from the progressive villages were making use of these innovations more extensively than those from the backward villages. Family planning coefficient (the number of couples protected by family planning divided by total number of couples in reproductive age group (15-49) came out to 45. The maximum family planning co-efficient was in region A (61.9) followed by region B(45.8), region C (27.5) and least in region D (15.2).

The adoption of family planning measures was found to be significantly related to the age of the respondents. The highest number of adoptors were in the age group of 31-40 years (63.6 per cent) followed by age group of upto 30 years (42.3 per cent), 41-50 years (22.4 per cent) and least number of adopters were in the age group of 51-60 years (4.1 per cent). In the age group of upto 30 years, many respondents were too young and had no children or had one or two children. So number of adoptors in this age group was lesser as compared to age group 31-40 years in which maximum number of adopters were found. After the age of 40, the number of adopters declined considerably. Thus, younger women were found to eb increasingly adopting the family planning methods.

The educational levels of the respondents were also found to be significantly related to the adoption of family planning (Table 3). The largest number of adopters were those educated upto matric and above (80.8 per cent) followed by those educated till the primary school level and the minimum number of adopters were those who were illiterate (32.7 per cent). Thus, education was a factor which facilitated the adoption of family planning.

Table 2

ADOPTION OF FAMILY PLANNING MEASURES ACCORDING TO REGIONS AND AGE GROUPS

Variable		*Adoption*		
		No	*Yes*	*Total*
Region				
	A	66	86	152
		(43.4)	(56.6)	(37.9)
	B	84	50	134
		(62.7)	(37.3)	(33.4)
	C	44	16	60
		(73.4)	(26.6)	(14.9)
	D	48	7	55
		(87.3)	(12.7)	(13.7)
X^2=39.39,** C= .29				
Age (Years)				
	20-30	86	63	149
		(67.7)	(42.3)	(37.2)
	31-40	43	75	118
		(36.4)	(63.6)	(29.4)
	41-50	66	19	85
		(77.5)	(22.4)	(21.2)
	51-60	47	2	49
		(95.9)	(4.1)	(12.2)
X^2=65.15,** C=.37				
Total		242	159	401
		(60.3)	(39.7)	(100.0)

Table 11. 3

ADOPTION OF FAMILY PLANNING MEASURES ACCORDING TO EDUCATION AND EXPOSURE OF RESPONDENTS

Variable	*Adoption*		
	No	*Yes*	*Total*
Education			
Illiterate	203	101	309
	(67.3)	(32.7)	(77.1)
Primary school level	29	37	66
	(45.9)	(56.4)	(16.5)
Matric and above	5	21	26
	(19.2)	(80.8)	(6.5)
X^2=32.39,**C= .27			
Level of exposure			
Low	156	61	217
	(71.9)	(28.1)	(54.1)
Medium	55	62	117
	(47.0)	(53.0)	(29.2)
High	31	36	67
	(46.3)	(53.7)	(16.7)
X^2=26.63,**C= .24			
Total:	242	139	479
	(60.3)	(39.7)	(100.0)

The level of exposure of the respondents to different information sources has also been seen to affect the adoption of family planning, as these two factors are significantly related at one per cent level of significance. The maximum number of adoptors were from the high exposure level (53.7 per cent), followed by those having a medium level of exposure (53 per cent) and finally a low level of exposure (28.1 per cent). The socio-economic status and income level of the family were also found to be related to the adoption of family planning measures. The caste factor was not found to be related with the adoption of family planning measures.

Age was the most significantly related variable with the maximum value of C=.37, followed by education (C=.27), level of exposure (C=.24), socio-economic status (C=.24) and income level (C=.21). Caste as a factor did not matter in the adoption of family planning measures by the respondents.

Although only 39.7 per cent of the respondents had adopted family planning a majority of the respondents (96.3 per cent), expressed their approval of family planning. Thus the attitude of the majority of respondents towards family planning was favourable. The respondents were asked why they had not adopted family planning measures even though they approved of it. Various reasons were given by the respondents.

A majority of the respondents (25.2 per cent) maintained that they were not aware about the methods before as they were popularised only recently with the government laying great emphasis on such programmes. As these respondents had passed their reproductive age they felt it was no longer useful. About 48.9 per cent of the respondents were still young, and had less than the desired number of children. About 24.6 per cent of the respondents said that their husbands were not in favour of family planning, while 22.7 per cent faced opposition from the elders of family who were not in favour of family planning. A large number of respondents (20.7 per cent) believed that family planning measures affect health and 19.6 per cent of them did not have any son which they attributed to be the cause for the non-adoption of family planning. Fear of infant mortality was stated to be the reason by 10.5 per cent of the respondents.

Although a majority of the respondents approved of family planning, a number of factors were found to be hindering the adoption of family planning like the opposition from husbands and other elders of the family, the notion that health would be adversely affected, the desire to have a son, the fear of infant mortality and the lack of knowledge about family planning methods. The preference of male children is very predominant and needs to be changed. The reduction of mortality among children through the provision of health facilities and by educating women about the health needs of mother and child would be a great step towards reducing the fertility. There should be incentives for those women who accept family planning in the form of a token or certificate so as to ensure a higher priority in health care facilities for both mother and their children.

Thus it is clear from the above discussions that the usage of health facilities for pre-natal and natal care is very low, reflecting the poor health status of the rural women. A majority of rural women still rely on the village mid-wife. The programme of training the village mid-wife already in force, would need to be actively expanded assist as it will constitute a step towards modernising rather than moving away from the traditional health care system. Even *vaids* and *hakims* with inadequate qualifications could be taught first aid, nutritional principles and elementary immunisations and provided with an adequate stock of medicines to treat common ailments. They form part and parcel of the community and have been traditional institutions.

12

Family Planning Programme versus Maternal and Child Health Services : The Emerging Trend in India

INTRODUCTION

The Indian health care system has essentially three components, namely, curative health, preventive health, and maternal and child health (MCH) services including family planning (FP) programme. The health care system operates in rural areas through a network of Primary Health Centres (PHCs) and Sub-Centres and in urban areas through a number of hospitals and family welfare centres. Between rural and urban areas of the country, the health care system differs not only nature but also in extent. Curative services are concentrated more in urban than in rural. Nearly three-fourths of the medical facilities (including specialised care) are concentrated in urban where only one-fourth of the Indian population lives. At the same time, three-fourths of the rural population is left with the remaining one-fourth of the medical care. (Srinivasan, 1987 : 14). However, the rural has the advantage of more extension (out-reach) services programmes than the urban. But what extent the extension service programmes reaches the people appears to be unsatisfactory. Health indicators such as crude death rate and infant mortality rate reveal that the rates are higher in rural than in urban which is an indication, apart from the differences in socio-economic status, of the higher availability and/or utilisation of health care facilities in rural.

The health delivery system in the rural areas of the country has undergone a number of changes at least since Independence. Of which, the major changes were the establishment of PHCs and sub-centres during early Independence, the integration of health and family welfare services during late 1960s and introduction of multipurpose health workers scheme during middle 1970s. Along with these changes, the infrastructure facilities also witnessed large scale improvements. The number of PHCs established at the end of first five-year plan (1956) was only 725 and it increased to 4631 by third five-year plan (1966), and to 7210 by the end of sixth five-year plan (1984). Correspondingly, the number of sub-centres also increased from 22,826 in 1969 to 74,307 by the end of sixth five-year plan (1984) (MW, 1985:

540). During 1986, there were 12,979 health centres (including PHCs, subsidiary health centres and upgraded PHCs) and 88,967 sub-centres functioning in the rural areas of the country (MHFW, 1987: 263)

At current population, on average, a sub-centre was serving a population of about 10.3 thousand in 1981 and it reduced to 6.5 thousand in 1986. However, there appears to be State to State variations in the population coverage by a sub-centre. Among the major States in India, the population per sub-centre in 1986 was as high as 8.5 thousand in Bihar and as low as 4.1 thousand in Gujarat.[1]

In rural areas of India, the PHC is the lowest administrative unit and the sub-centre is the peripheral service delivery unit for various health and family welfare programmes. But, except for treatment of minor-ailments by the peripheral unit, medical services are provided only at PHCs and in some States at subsidiary health units as well. Further, the availability of specialised medical services in PHCs is limited as compared to the medical facilities available in urban hostpitals.

Under the multipurpose health workers scheme, a sub-centre has a team of one male health worker and one female health worker, and they are supervised by male health assistant and female health assistant, respectively. Programme Officers at PHCs and at higher levels also guide in the activities of the workers. The job responsibilities of the male and female health workers are more or the less same as far as family planning activities are concerned. Otherwise, female workers have greater responsibilities in maternal and child health programmes and male workers have greater responsibilities in the national health programmes like Malaria. Whether the multipurpose health workers scheme is the operation or not, in most States, at least the female side is functioning almost at par with multipurpose health workers scheme.

Hence, in the rural areas of India, the primary providers of maternal and child health and family planning services are the same : the PHCs along with the network of sub-centres. In addition, other government agencies like social welfare and community development and a number of voluntary agencies are also involved in these programmes either directly or indirectly. However, it appears that most of these agencies are involved more on family planning than on MCH. Even within the health sector, it appears that the activities are directed directly on family planning than working through health and MCH services.

This article analyses the relative developments in MCH and family planning programmes in India including their integration, and the consequent impact of these programmes in realising the objectives or goal.

THE RELATION BETWEEN MATERNAL AND CHILD HEALTH AND FAMILY PLANNING

The Year-book on Family Welfare Programme in India observes that "One of the important aspects of family planning programme is the promotion of health of mothers and children as it creates a sense of security in the minds of parents that the children born, will live a healthy life which in turn will contribute greatly to the acceptance of small family norm as a way of life. With this objective in view, special schemes under family planning programme have been sponsored by the Ministry of Health and Family Welfare. Under the basic MCH services, the health care of the mothers and children is provided as non-plan activity of the States and Union Territories" (MHFW 1987 : 19)[2] Further it is claimed under the heading "Policy on family welfare programme", as "Family Planning Services are offered through the total health care delivery system" (MHFW,1987 : 8). It speaks for itself the realisation of the importance of MCH services in the promotion of family welfare programme in India.

Again, the approach of the fifth five-year plan (1974-78) was to integrate Health and Family Planning Services, MCH and nutrition services in such a way that the package of services was offered to the people enabling them to accept family planning in the context of better health expectancy and services (Kakar, 1982). Naturally this stress has continued in the later five-year plan also. The Alma Ata Conference on Primary Health Care considered "Maternal and Child Health including family planning" as a single component of primary health care. This was in realisation of the close inter-relationship between MCH and family planning services. The MCH services promote family planning and in turn family planning promotes better health of mothers and children. The recent population and health policies of India also envisage the integration of health, particularly MCH, and family planning as a package of services.

Much has been said in the demographic literature on the impact of infant and child mortality on fertility. It has been demonstrated that, the lower the infant and child mortality, the lower the fertility. In other words, the better the infant and child survival, the earlier the couples accept family planning with less number of children. Further, the MCH services not only promote of better survival of infants and children but also help to motivate mothers for FP right from ante-natal period.

KNOWLEDGE AND UTILISATION OF MCH SERVICES AS COMPARED TO FAMILY PLANNING SERVICES

A review of literature indicates that MCH services particularly mother care services are not given sufficient attention to, as compared to family planning services. For example, an All India Survey conducted by Operational Research Group during 1980-81 revealed that only about 18 per cent of the currently married women in the reproductive ages did avail MCH services. To our surprise, as many as two-thirds (64 per cent) of the women informed that they were unaware of the MCH service facilities (MW,1985:569).[3] At the same time, almost all women were aware of one or the other modern methods of family planning. Further, the contraceptive prevalence (modern methods only) was substantially higher, ever use 32.5 per cent and current use 28.1 per cent (Khan and Prasad, 1985 : 317). In India, the experience is that if at all couples practise family planning it was only after having a few children and as such all ever and current users of FP can be assumed to have experienced at least one child birth. Hence, the substantial differences between MCH services utilisation and contraceptive prevalence rates indicate that MCH services fall much below family planning services in India.

A few base-line surveys conducted during 1980-81 in the States of Rajasthan and Madhya Pradesh by National Institute of Health and Family Welfare, New Delhi and in the

State of Bihar by International Institute for Population Sciences, Bombay also revealed similar findings, For example, in Bihar where the survey was conducted in rural and urban areas of six districts, the rural findings showed that the proportion of currently pregnant women registering her name in any medical/health clinic for medical check-up was 7.0 per cent in HQ villages (here a HQ village is a village with a medical institution like a PHC, a Dispensary, or a sub-centre) and 4.8 per cent in non-HQ villages. Those women in third trimaster registering was 8 per cent in HQ villages and 5.5 per cent in other villages. However, the registration in urban areas was as high as 26.8 per cent. The data clearly show that even in villages where some medical institution exist, the ante-natal registration was negligible. When the registration itself is negligible it is superfluous to say much about other pre-natal and natal services like TT administration, FST distribution and conduction of trained delivery. When it is the case, the FP acceptance measured in terms of current use of contraception 9 per cent in HQ villages and 7.2 per cent in other villages. Though the overall level of FP acceptance is very low, but, as compared to MCH services, the contraceptive use level is higher. Further, women having the knowledge of at least one method of family planning was almost universal (IIPS,1982).

A similar finding was reported in respect of Rajasthan also. In 6 districts of Rajasthan where the survey was conducted, the pregnant women registered with any MCH centre was 7.3 per cent and that visited by health staff was 12.3 per cent. In rural area, the registration of their name in a MCH Centre was only 6 per cent in HQ villages (definition same as above) and 3 per cent in other villages. Again, about 97 per cent of the deliveries in the rural areas took place in homes, and that attended by ANM even in the HQ villages, where they are expected to stay and provide services, was only 5 per cent; another 8.5 per cent of the deliveries was attended by trained *Dais*. Otherwise, the bulk of the deliveries were attended by untrained *Dais* and neighbours. As far as family planning is concerned, at least 60 per cent of the married women in the age group 15-49 had knowledge of at least one method in any area studied. Further for the urban and rural areas combined, about 21 to 24 per cent of the couples had ever used a FP method, the current contraceptive prevalence level was 19.3 per cent (Talwar and Bhatia, 1985). These findings clearly show that MCH services fall back FP services.

Two other studies conducted by IIPS (1986) during 1982 or later in two better developed States, namely, Maharashtra and Gujarat also came out with similar findings. It is to be noted that Maharashtra tops most other States in India in family planning achievement.

One important point to be noted in respect of these studies is that the denominator figure for ever/current use of contraception refers to all married women in the broad reproductive age groups 15-49, whereas the denominator figure for ante-natal registration is confined to the expectant mothers, who constitute about only one-tenth of the married women in the age group 15-49. To that extent, the maternal care services are confined to a small rather than all married women in the reproductive ages. The substantial difference between percentage of pregnant women registered for ante-natal services and the percentage of women ever currently using contraception shows that what has been done to the small group of pregnant women has not been done, while much more has been done in family planning to the vast majority of the married women in the reproductive ages.

IMPROVEMENTS IN HEALTH INFRASTRUCTURE, FAMILY PLANNING PERFORMANCE AND MCH SERVICES IN INDIA, 1981-86

In the following paragraphs, an attempt has been made to study the trend in the improvements in infrastructure facilities in rural health care services in India and the relative improvements in MCH and family welfare services during the period from 1981-82 to 1985-86. The base period 1981-82 appears to a good choice because national goals and targets for AD 2000 for most development programmes particularly Health, MCH and FP were made during early 1980s. Further, the targets for various health programmes are based on the principles of 'health for all by AD 2000'. Hence, the analysis of the trend during the initial 5-year period will provide a useful insight into the development of MCH and FP services and will suggest corrective measures for the effective implementation of the programmes.

The variables considered in the trend analysis are as follows : With respect to infrastructure, two variables, namely, the amount spent on health (including sanitation and water supply) and number of health sub-centres, are considered. The number of PHCs as an index of infrastructure is not considered as it differs between States, depending both on the extent of upgraded PHCs and Community Health Centres which are superior to ordinary PHCs and on the subsidiary health centres and Primary Health Units which are inferior to PHCs. In this context the number of sub-centres is a good index of infrastructure facilities in rural areas because not only it is more or less standardised across States in India, but also most heath and FP programmes are implemented only through these units, of course, routed through PHCs. As such, with respect to provision of health and FP services in rural areas, sub-centres are more important than PHCs.

Variables under MCH include yearly achievement in TT immunisation for pregnant mothers, coverage of pregnant mothers for TT immunisation and coverage of infants for DPT immunisation. It is to be noted that the number of pregnant women given medical check-up was not available and in its absence, TT immunisation for pregnant women is a good proxy variably for pre-natal care. Percentage of deliveries received trained attendance (i.e. occurred in institutions and conducted by trained midwives) is not considered because it was felt the TT immunisation is a rather better index as the former depends more on people's economic status and cultural practices, and the latter depends more on the service facilities available to them. With respect to child care, DPT immunisation is a good variable because it is the only immunisation for infants continuously in the regular programme for a long time. Programmes like polio, BCG and measles are either administered by special teams and only recently included in the regular programme of the PHCs.

With respect to family planning, yearly achievement in tubectomy sterilisation and couples protection rate (CPR) are considered. Achievements in other FP methods like IUD, oral pills and condoms are not considered as they are relatively meagre in number, fluctuate from time to time, and also the achievement, except IUD, is estimated based on the amount of contraceptive supply rather that the actual number of users of the method.

Further, three variables, namely crude birth rate number of living children at tubectomy acceptance and infant mortality rate are also included in the study to indicate the impact of MCH and FW programmes in realising the desired goal.

The coverage of ante-natal mothers for TT immunisation and coverage of infants for DPT immunisation are arrived at as follows : Coverage is defined as the achievement in a programme to the expected beneficiaries for the programme, expressed as percentage. Accordingly, TT coverage is the TT achievement during a year to the expected number of live births during that year. It is to be noted that the expected beneficiaries of TT are the expectant mothers in the third trimester which included the live births and the still births. As such, the estimate of TT coverage would be slightly on a higher side and not expected to be an under-estimation. This was purposively done to show the difference between MCH services utilisation and family planning performance more clearly. A crude birth rate (CBR) of 33 for all the years from 1981-82 to 1985-86 (as the figure did not vary during the period) and the population projected (medium) for all India were used to estimate the expected number of births for each year. The same expected number of births was used to estimate the infants eligible for DPT immunisation. A 6-month old infant is expected to receive all the three doses of DPT and hence a (0-6) month mortality rate of 100 was assumed in the estimation of children eligible for DPT immunisation.

For comparison purposes, the values of the variables for each year were converted into an index number. The index number is defined as the value of the variable during a year to the value of the variable in the base year. i.e., 1981-82. However, for CBR, IMR and number of living children at acceptance, as they decline in response to improvements in the services, the reciprocal of the above index number is presented for easy comparison. Hence, an increase in the index number corresponding to any variable means improvement in the variable. It is to be noted that the meaning and interpretation of the index number is very similar to the 'percentage increase' in the normal usage.

Among the variables considered in the analysis, the " Sub-Centres" refer to rural and to beginning of the reference period, and all other variables refer to rural and urban combined, and to during or to the end of reference period. It is expected that the achievement in MCH programmes might be substantially higher in urban area than in rural area. As urban-rural break-up on MCH services are not available this could not be demonstrated but the indications are obvious from the previous section.

With respect to health facilities, the number of sub-centres is increased by 62 per cent. The more than 60 per cent increase in the sub-centres and, may be, a similar increase in the associated infrastructure, during a short period of 5 years is really a tremendous achievement for a country like India.

With respect to family welfare, not only health sector but other sectors are also involved in providing education and motivation. All such efforts, including the recent advancements in the laparoscopic technique of female sterilisation, have almost doubled the family welfare achievement measured in terms of female sterilisation. It is almost true even if we combine both male and female sterilisations. The couples protection rate (which adds all methods after making allowance for deaths, drop-outs, and crossing reproductive age) however showed a 50 per cent increase during the 5-year period. These indicate that there has been a substantial achievement in the family welfare programme which is almost very close to the increase in the infrastructure facilities.

Coming to MCH, the trend is of low elb. Even in terms of absolute performance, the data on TT for ante-natal mothers showed only 46 per cent increase over the 5-year period as against 92 per cent for tubectomy for the same period. It is to be noted that both tubectomy sterilisation and TT for ante-natal mothers refer directly to married women in the reproductive age group, more specifically 20-34 age group who were potential child bearers. Of course, TT refers to pregnant woman and tubectomy refers to women who have given birth recently. As such, women eligible for both tubectomy and MCH (for the recent years) refer to more or less the same cohort, but the data indicate that women are provided more with family planning services than with MCH services. The relatively low improvement in TT performance may be an acceptable trend if the TT performance is already high and FP performance hitherto very low and that further increase would be slower for TT than FP. But the estimated coverage of ante-natal mothers for TT at the beginning of the period was only 31 per cent and that of family planning performance measured in terms of CPR was 24 per cent. It is to be noted that if services are provided, almost cent per cent coverage of ante-natal mothers for TT is possible in a short duration than coverage of couples for family planning and as such the 34 per cent coverage in TT immunisation during 1981-82 cannot be considered as high achievement. Further, for FP adoption, couples should be satisfied with their desired family size (because the method promoted is sterilisation) and many other social, economic, cultural and health factors. At the same time, pregnant women for TT need not be satisfied with anything of this. It appears that no study in India has brought out any adverse effect or objection to receive MCH services, except probably for their ignorance, from any section of the community. Hence, even under these favourable conditions for MCH services, the coverage of pregnant women for TT immunisation increased only by 34 per cent as against 50 per cent increase in couples protection rate.

The working group on health for all by A.D. 2000 constituted by the Government of India had recommended certain targets to be achieved by 1985, 1990 and A.D. 2000. Here, target means coverage of target groups and not merely target-achievement in the conventional usage. Correspondingly, the targets for couples protection rate for the above periods are also presented as recommended by the working group on Population Policy and Working Group on Population stabilisation and MCH care (DFW, 1987).

Table 12.1 as of 1986, the trend shows that we are closer to achieving the CPR target of 36.6 per cent fixed for 1985, but far behind in achieving MCH measured in terms of TT immunisation for pregnant mothers. The target for TT coverage was 60 per cent, but the coverage was only 42 per cent. The situation appears to be still worse in providing medical check-up to pregnant women and in conducting trained delivery. However, coverage of children for immunisation especially DPT for infants was very closer to the target fixed. This is probably due to the campaign approach adopted in some States to perform child immunisation.

The higher progress in family planning, as compared to maternal care services, indicates the undue emphasis given to family planning. Further, the progress in MCH services is not even comparable to the improvements in the infrastructure facilities. As such it appears that the large scale infrastructure facilities created are not utilised to produce appreciable result.

Table: 12.1

TARGETS FOR SELECTED MCH ACTIVITIES AND FAMILY PLANNING FOR DIFFERENT PERIODS UP TO AD 2000

	Indicator	*Target/Coverage*		
		1985	*1990*	*2000*
1.	Percentage of pregnant mothers receiving ante-natal care	50-60	60-75	100
2.	Percentage of pregnant mothers receiving TT immunisation	60	100	100
3.	Percentage of deliveries by trained personnel	50	80	100
4.	DPT immunisation for infants	70	85	85
5.	Polio immunisation for infants	25	40	85
6.	Couples protection rate	36.6	42	60

This shows that creation of any amount of infrastructure facilities may not make any appreciable improvements in the utilisation of services unless they are properly activised to provide the services. This calls for proper management of the infrastructure facilities already created with necessary additional input/facilities to perform the programme more effectively.

FAMILY PLANNING AT THE COST OF MCH SERVICES

Whether family planning needs to be routed through MCH or not, both the programmes are implemented through the same agency and same functionaries. Multipurpose programmes (many programmes by a single worker) some times improve performance faster in each programme than it would have been implemented vertically (separate worker for each programme) and some other times all the programmes suffer, or some programmes improve faster than other programmes. It all depends upon the style of implementation : the integrated approach followed, balance of implementation of different programmes; monitoring of the programmes, etc. Most of the times, the programmes performance goes towards the desire of the higher officers who control the programmes. If the workers are insisted on one programme and not on the other programmes, the tendency of the workers is to side-track to satisfy the officers.

Though not much research is done on this area, the recent trend is that emphasis attached to FPP is much more higher than any other health programme. In the recent years almost all categories of health staff, irrespective or programme and as revenue, rural development, social welfare and education are also given specific targets in FP to achieve and the progress evaluated periodically. Though targets are assigned for other programmes also, they are seldom noticed in the evaluation and review of the programme performance. This is more so when review is conducted by district heads and State level officers, who are always satisfied with cases (meaning sterilisation achievement) than any other programme. Further, the process and the quality of achievement is of no concern to them. Workers are often taken to task for not achieving family planning targets, but this is not the case for other programmes. So the workers also give importance to family planning at the cost of other programmes for which they intended to. Probably the worst hit is the MCH programme particularly Maternal care services. The female health workers who are responsible for MCH also deployed more in family planning because of their vulnerability to this programme. It might be likely that the performance of the female workers are the highest but relevant statistics are not available to study the pattern. Though research findings are scarce, it appears that neither the female health workers nor their supervisors are conducting MCH clinics in villages or at least in their HQrs. Many workers are not even staying in their HQrs. The fact that the service institution like a PHC or a Subsidiary Health Unit/Primary Health Unit is located in one village, some times in a remote village, which are expected to cover 50 to 100 villages, fail to cover at least a few villages round about. Hence, in the hunt for FP cases, other programmes particularly MCH programmes are forgotten or left only in the subconsciousness of both the providers of the services and the evaluators of the programmes.

IMPACT OF FAMILY PLANNING AND MCH PROGRAMMES

The impact of family planning programme is measured in terms of reduction in fertility and of health including MCH is measured in terms of reduction in mortality. Family planning related fertility measures are mainly Crude Birth Rate, total marital fertility rate and average living children at acceptance. The MCH related mortality rates are mainly maternal mortality rate, infant mortality rate and childhood mortality rate. Based on the availability of estimates of these rates, CBR and Average Living Children at Tubectomy acceptance were considered to assess the impact of FP achievements, and IMR to assess the impact of MCH services. It is to be noted that sterilisation accounts almost 90 per cent of the performance in family planning, measured in terms of couples protection rate (MHFW, 1987:204). Again among sterilisation, tubectomy (including Laparoscopic technique) accounts for about 80 to 85 per cent in the recent years (MHFW, 1987:150). Hence the average living children at tubectomy acceptance appears to be an appropriate index to evaluate FP impact.

With all difficulties in the data, the Crude Birth Rate which was 33.9 declined hardly by 1 point during the 5 year period, whereas our expectation is at least 1 point for every two years. It is to be noted that the CBR target for AD 2000 is 21 as per the latest population policy and this calls for a reduction in CBR of at least 0.5 points per year from the current level. The average living children at acceptance was as high as 3.7 and it declined hardly by 0.2 points during the 5 year period. Further, even after 35 years of FP programme in India, not even 25 per cent of sterilisation adoptors did follow the small family size norm of 2 or less living children. The proportion of sterilisation adoptors having 2 or less living children at acceptance (for those accepted during this period) was only about 20 per cent (MHFW, 1987 : 236). With respect to IMR, there appears to be some decline between 1981 and 1984, apart from the sudden decline during 1985. Even with the sudden decline during 1985, the decline in the IMR during the 5-year period was 13 per cent and that of fertility was hardly 5 per cent. The slower rate of improvement in MCH services has produced greater impact, as compared to the rate of improvement in FP programmes and its consequent impact on fertility. It is to be noted that the rates presented here are combined for both rural and urban areas. Though the rates for rural are higher than for urban, the trend over the period is as almost the same.

DISCUSSION AND CONCLUSION

During the recent years there has been a large scale increase in the infrastructure of health delivery system in India, especially in rural areas. The Indian approach to family planning is stated to be integrated with health particularly with maternal and child health services. Improvements are taking place both in MCH and in family planning. The improvements in family planning, though sort of expectation, at least closely followed the improvements in infrastructures. But the improvements in MCH services particularly maternal care services appear to be not only far behind the expectation, but also far below the improvements in infrastructure facilities and in family planning achievement. As a result, infant mortality rate continues to be high and almost stagnant for years together. Consequently, though there is relatively better performance in FP, its impact on reducing fertility and achieving small family size norm is negligible. One reason for this state of affairs is that the family planning programme covers only the elderly women who had a large family size. Another reason is that the programme did not realise the importance of spacing of children in achieving reduction in fertility and in population growth. For, the proportion of couples protected due to temporary methods, is only about 10 per cent. Probably India is the only country in the world which is dependent almost fully on sterilisation in their FP activities.

The low achievement in temporary methods of family planning, the very high family size at the acceptance of sterilisation and low performance in MCH, indicate that not only FP operates independent of MCH services but also unable to produce any tangible impact. In high family size at sterilisation adoption indicates that people still desire large family size and it may be that reduction in family size is difficult without substantial reduction in infant and child mortality. Or it may be that women in India marry very early and before attain physical maturity they bear a large number of children. After having a number of children, they realise the consequences of having it rather than they plan it. At last, they do accept family planning, probably, to avoid any further unwanted child bearing. If these women are educated early in their age on the importance of child spacing and the adverse consequences of large family size, and further they are assured of survival of their children, they would have come forward to accept spacing methods initially and later permanent methods, with less number of living children. Definitely this strategy is easy to adopt through MCH services than directly, because, FP is adopted immediately after or within a short period after a child birth, and hence education on FP combined with MCH services will be an appropriate motivation factor.

Though all these strategies are accepted in principle and adopted in our policies, they are not implemented in our programmes. We are over enthusiatic in achieving family planning targets rather than family planning impact. In this process, workers are instigated to achieve family planning, and under this grip other programmes suffered. At the end, neither we could achieve (with impact) family planning not other programmes particularly maternal and child health.

On the whole the analysis suggests the FP is to be implemented whole-heartedly within the broad health programmes particularly MCH services, to make any substantial impact on fertility. Otherwise we may achieve family planning performance and not family planning impact. The availability of infrastructure, if not satisfactory, is definitely not inadequate to make an integrated approach to this problem. What is needed is an optimistic approach to these programmes particularly on the part of the programme officers, and implement and review the programmes accordingly. Unless and the programme planners and programme officers considers these issues seriously, the national goal is difficult to be reached.

References

1. DFW, 1987, *The Methodology of Setting Targets for Family Planning Programme —A Resume,* circulated by Department of Family Welfare, Ministry of Health and Family Welfare, Government of India, New Delhi
2. IIPS, 1982, *Report on the Baseline Survey on Fertility, Mortality and related factors in Bihar,* International Institute for Population Sciences, Bombay.
3. IIPS, 1986, *News letter,* International Institute for Population Sciences, Bombay 27.2.
   Kakar, D.N., 1982, "The Development of an health care system in India : An appraisal", *Journal of Family Welfare,* 28.2
4. Khan, M.E. and Prasad, C.V.S, 1985, "A Comparison of 1970 and 1980 Survey findings on family plannings in India", *Studies in Family Planning,* 16.6
5. MHFW, 1981, *Report on the Working group on Health for All by A.D. 2000,* Government of India, Ministry of Health and Family Welfare, New Delhi.
6. MHFW, 1987, *Family Welfare Programme in India: Year Book* 1985-86, Government of India, Ministry of Health and Family Welfare, New Delhi.
7. MW, 1985, *The Child in India : A Statistical Profile,* Government of India, Ministry of Welfare, New Delhi.
8. ORG, 1983, *Family Planning Practice in India : Second All India Survey,* Operation Research Group, Baroda.
9 Sriniwasan, K., 1987, *Developmental and Demographic Changes in Independence,* JSS Institute of Economic Research, Dharwad.

Notes

1. Worked-out based on the sub-centre statistics and the population estimates (medium) of MHFW (1987) and as assumption of 25 per cent of population is urban, (Uttar Population in 1981 was 23.3 percent).
2. This statement is repeatedly found in the previous issues of the Year-book.
3. The information was stated to be taken from ORG, 1983, p. 55.

13

Underutilisation of MCH and Family Planning Services—A Case Study of Andhra Pradesh

INTRODUCTION

The Family Welfare Programme continues to occupy an important position in our socio-economic development plans. Its central role in human resource development and improving the overall quality of life of people needs no reiteration. Its form part of the 20-point programme which calls for the promotion of "Family Planning on a voluntary basis as a people's movement." Improvement of the delivery of medical care to pregnant women (MCH services) and young children is a high priority in health ministries throughout the developing world, but progress has generally been disappointingly slow. Providing family planning information and services can help improve the success of maternal and child health programmes by enabling couples to avoid high-risk pregnancies and births.

As the popular family planning methods currently available require clinical intervention and as health sectors has been closely involved in the programme. Family planning would continue to be integrated with a package of health services through an ever expanding out-reach system.

One of the important aspects of the Family Welfare Programme is the promotion of health of mothers and children. It creates a sense of security in the minds of parents that the children born, will live a healthy life which in turn will contribute greatly to the acceptance of small family norm as a way of life. With this objective in view special schemes have been sponsored by the Ministry of Health and Family Welfare. Under the basic Mother and Child Health (MCH) Services, the health care of mothers and children is provided as non-plan activity of the States.

But the question of 'underutilisation' will arise, when the objectives and policies do not work as expected. Eventhough the Government of India is one of the Government to profound an official programme first from the beginning of the planning era in the country in 1951-52, still we are on the way to reaching the goals.

The Indian Family Planning Programme is by now a well established part of the country's governmental apparatus. It is administered through as many as 5,428 Rural Family Welfare Centres at the Primary Health Centre level: 18,618 Rural Family Welfare Sub-centres and 2,500 Urban Family Welfare Centres. The number of couples currently protected, up to March 1984, was estimated at 40.41 million forming 32.7 per cent of the estimated 123.7 million eligible couples in the country. Taking into account the use-effectiveness of various methods, which taken as 100 per cent for sterilization and oral pills, 95 per cent for IUD and 50 per cent for conventional contraceptives, the number of couples effectively protected up to March 1984 was only 36.44 millions forming 29.2 per cent of the total eligible couples, the target is 60 per cent of eligible couples by A.D. 2000.

Coming to child health services, we can say that achievement of immunisation programme ranges only between 70-80 per cent in 1983-84, except Polio. Regarding MCH beneficiaries, only 25.37 million women are benefited out of 123.7 million eligible couple by 1983-84, and the corresponding number of children is 73.16 million. By 1985, the population of children below 16 years has increased 296 million, from 230 million in 1971. Percentage of one-year old children fully immunised by 1984-85 are 65 against TB. 51 against DPT and 37 against Polio. The proportion of pregnant women received tetanus injection is 33 per cent. Only 33 per cent of births are attended by trained health personnel by 1983. If we see the results of 'the Base Line Survey on Fertility, Mortality and Related Factors'(IIPS, 1986) in Maharashtra, the utilisation of health services is poor in that State, the reasons are : 'no need', 'no body fell ill', and 'minor ailments are treated at home'. As for the immunisation of the children in this study area, less than one-third had received B.C.G., D.P.T. and oral Polio vaccine.

Similarly, most of the informants in Uttar Pradesh were ignorant of the needs and sources of pre-natal and post-natal precautions such as vaccinations, protection against nutritional anaemia, iron folic tablets and vitamin tablets (J.W.F. Vol. XXVIII, No. 1, 1986 : 1-9).

In the same way with regard to family planning, the recent World Fertility Survey (J.W.F., Dec. 1986 : 3) findings have indicated that in most developing countries a sizeable proportion of couples who are not interested in an additional child were not practising family planning. A similar situation prevails in India too.

In some of the developing countries, even though the women want no more children they are not using contraceptives, (Deborah Maine, 1981 : 42-44). The proportion of women who say that they do not know where to get contraceptive device or supplies. In general, countries where large proportions of women do not know where to get contraception are the same countries in which large proportions of women who want no more children are not using any method.

However, it is important to remember that many of these women do not have easy access to contraceptive supplies of information. And also, the time and expense to travel to the family planning site, having services available at a time a day when women can get away from their family duties and many other factors may influence utilisation of MCH and Family Planning services.

A CASE STUDY OF ANDHRA PRADESH

Objectives (of the paper) :

1. to know the extent of underutilisation of family welfare services,
2. to know the causes of underutilisation of family welfare schemes,
3. to know the residential (Rural/Urban) variation of the underutilisation of family welfare services, and
4. to know the differences of underutilisation among responsible, moderately responsible and not responsible parents.

This study is conducted in Prakasam district of Andhra Pradesh, Ongole taluk of Prakasam district is selected for actual sample survey. The sampling technique used in this study is cluster Random Sampling Technique. In the 1st stage, the taluk is divided into two groups, e.g., urban and rural to facilitate the comparison. For urban area, the Ongole town is chosen. With the help of field map of Ongole town, it is divided geographically into four divisions and from each division some wards are chosen at random for collecting the data. From the selected wards of each division 50 currently married women in the reproductive age group with or without children are selected for the study. Thus, the total sample in the urban area is two hundred (200). Similarly, for the rural area, the Ongole taluk is divided into four geographical areas with the help of the taluk map of the census. One village is selected at random from each geographical area. Like that four villages are selected in the rural areas of Ongole taluk for rural study based on geographical stratification. From each village one hundred (100) currently married women in the reproductive age group with or without children are selected for the study. Thus the sample size in the rural areas is 400, the total sample of study is 600 in this study. With the help of a scoring technique, the respondents are classified in three categories : (1) not responsible parents, (2) moderately responsible parents and (3) responsible parents. Different variables are considered to determine the status of responsible parenthood separately for the women with children and without children.

The minimum and maximum score for each variable/item is zero (0) and two (2) respectively. The score value is assigned depending upon the answers provided by the respondents for each twenty-four questions concerned. This can be explained clearly in the following way with an example. The question posed to the respondent is "what is the ideal interval between marriage and 1st conception." The answer may be less than one year, one year, two years, three years and so on. The score value given to these answers are given below :

Ideal interval	*Score value*
< 2 years	0
2 years	1
3 years	2

Thus, for each question these are the different score values. Since only ten questions (items) are considered for the respondents with no children, the minimum and maximum score value for these ten items are zero and 20 respectively. Similarly, for the 24 items that are considered for the respondents with at least one child, the ranges of score values is zero to fortyeight. Based on these score values, the respondents are classified into : (1) not responsible parents, (2) moderately responsible parents and (3) responsible parents. The procedure for classifying is as follows :

1. Not responsible parents : Women whose score value is equal to or less than 49 per cent of the total score.

2. Moderately responsible parents : Women whose score value which lies between 50 per cent to 59 per cent.

3. Responsible parents : Women whose score value is equal to 60 per cent and above.

This status of responsible parenthood is cross classified with demographic, socio-stratification variables, health variables and family planning variables.

RESULTS AND DISCUSSION

In general, the responsible parenthood is more among responsible parents in this study, regarding the MCH and Family Planning services also both in urban and rural areas. But utilisation of anti-natal, post-natal services available to mothers and immunisation of children is not satisfactory.

Coming to MCH services, from Table 13.1, 79 per cent of pregnant women have had regular health check-up during their pregnancy period. It was 78 per cent in rural area and 81 per cent in urban area. The women who have had regular health check-up during pregnancy is high (99%) among responsible parents as against moderately responsible (89%) parents and not responsible parents (61%) in total sample. This same trend is observed in urban and rural samples also. The women who have had regular check-up during the pregnancy period are 55 per cent of not responsible mothers, 35 per cent of moderately responsible mothers and 98 per cent of responsible mothers in urban area. In rural area it was, 62 per cent of not responsible mothers, 92 per cent of moderately responsible mothers and 100 per cent of responsible mothers. If we see the reasons for not having regular health check-up during pregnancy period, highest percentage (15%) as "not necessary." It was 16 per cent in rural area and 13 per cent in urban area. And also this reason is expressed highly (30%) among not responsible women, it was 29 per cent in rural and 34 per cent in urban samples. But it is only 9 per cent and 5 per cent among moderately responsible women in urban and rural sample, respectively, whereas it is only 2 per cent and nil among responsible women. The other reasons stated are "no habit of going to the hospital, no help at home, due to fear and no answer." "Ignorance and poverty" are expressed by 2 per cent of rural women only.

Table: 10.1

NUMBER AND PERCENTAGE DISTRIBUTION OF NOT RESPONSIBLE PARENTS, MODERATELY RESPONSIBLE PARENTS AND RESPONSIBLE PARENTS BY THE REASONS FOR NOT GOING REGULAR CHECK-UP AT THE TIME OF PREGNANCY

Status of parenthood	*Reasons for not having check-ups*							*Total*
	Having checkup	*No help in house*	*No habit to go to hospital*	*Not necessary*	*No ans-wer*	*Due to fear only*	*Ignorance poverty*	
Urban								
1.	(55.3) 26	—	(10.6) 5	(34.0) 16	—	—	—	(26.70) 47
2.	(84.6) 55	(1.5) 1	—	(9.2) 6	(3.1) 2	(3.1) 2	—	(36.98) 66
3.	(98.4) 63	—	—	(1.6) 1	—	—	—	(36.36) 65
Total	(80.7) 144	(0.57) 1	(2.84) 5	(13.07) 23	(1.14) 2	(1.14) 2		177
Rural								
1.	(62.3) 104	(0.6) 2	(4.2) 7	(28.7) 48	—	—	(3.6) 6	(50.00) 167
2.	(92.3) 120	—	(3.1) 4	(4.6) 6	—	—	—	(38.92) 130
3.	(100.0) 37	—	—	—	—	—	—	(11.08) 37
Total	(78.14) 261	(0.6) 2	(3.29) 11	(16.17) 54	—	—	(1.80) 6	324
Total								
1.	(60.7) 130	(0.9) 2	(5.6) 12	(29.9) 64	— —	— —	(2.8)	(41.96) 214
2.	(88.7) 175	(0.5) 1	(2.1) 4	(6.2) 12	(1.0) 2	(1.0) 2	— —	(38.24) 195
3.	(99.0) 100	—	—	(0.9) 1	—	—	—	(19.80) 101
Total	(79.02) 403	(0.39) 3	(3.14) 16	(15.10) 17	(0.39) 2	(0.39) 2	(1.18) 6	

1. Not Responsible parents.
2. Moderately responsible parents.
3. Responsible parents.

About 30 per cent of pregnant women have taken tetanus injection during their pregnancy period. High per cent (39%) of urban women took tetanus injection as against rural (12%) women during their pregnancy period. It was high among responsible women (38%) as against to moderately responsible women (23%) and not responsible women (12%) in general (Table 13.2). But in rural areas high percentage (16%) of moderately responsible women took tetanus injection, where as it is high (52%) among responsible women in urban area. If we see the reasons for not taking tetanus injection during their pregnancy period, are : "no body gave"(56%), no answer (22%) and don't know (1%). The reason 'no body gave' is expressed by 84 per cent of rural women whereas it is only 4 per cent of urban women. Similarly high percentage (55%) of urban women expressed the reason as "no answer" as against 5 per cent of rural women. This results shows the "need of supply of services" in rural area, and may be "unawareness or disinterest" in urban area. Because, it is observed that, status of urban women is little higher to the rural women and they would like to take to rich medical services. Whatever may be the reason stated, the per cent of women who did not take tetanus injection is high among not responsible women than moderately responsible women and responsible women.

Table: 13.2

NUMBER AND PERCENTAGE DISTRIBUTION OF NOT RESPONSIBLE PARENTS, MODERATELY RESPONSIBLE PARENTS AND RESPONSIBLE PARENTS BY THE REASONS FOR NOT GETTING TETANUS INJECTION DURING PREGNANCY

Status of parenthood	*Reasons for not getting tetanus injection*				*Total*
	Taken	*No body gave*	*Don't know about that*	*No answer*	
1	2	3	4	5	6
Urban					
1.	(25.5) 12	—	(6.4) 3	(68.1) 32	(26.70) 47
2.	(35.4) 23	(4.6) 3	(1.5) 1	(58.5) 38	(36.93) 65
3.	(51.6) 33	(6.3) 4	— —	(42.2) 27	(36.36) 64
Total	(38.64) 68	(3.98) 7	(2.27) 4	(55.11) 97	176

Contd.

1	2	3	4	5	6
Rural					
1.	(7.8) 13	(85.6) 143	—	(6.6) 11	(50.00) 167
2.	(16.2) 21	(81.5) 106	—	(2.3) 3	(38.92) 130
3.	(13.5) 5	(81.8) 30	—	(5.4) 2	(11.8) 37
Total	(11.8) 39	(83.53) 279	—	(4.79) 16	334
Total					
1.	(11.7) 25	(66.8) 143	(1.4) 3	(20.1) 43	(41.96) 214
2.	(22.6) 44	(55.9) 109	(0.5) 1	(21.0) 41	(38.24) 195
3.	(37.6) 38	(33.7) 34	—	(28.7) 29	(19.80) 101
Total	(20.98) 107	(56.08) 286	(0.78) 4	(22.16) 113	510

1. Not responsible parents.
2. Moderately responsible parents.
3. Responsible parents.

Table : 13.3

NUMBER AND PERCENTAGE DISTRIBUTION OF NOT RESPONSIBLE PARENTS, MODERATELY RESPONSIBLE PARENTS ANDRESPONSIBLE PARENTS BY THE REASONS FOR NOT TAKING IRON FOLIC TABLETS DURING PREGNANCY.

Status of parenthood	*Reasons*			*Total*
	Taken	*No body gave*	*Don't know about that*	
1	2	3	4	5
Urban				
1.	(29.8) 14	—	(70.2) 33	(26.70) 47
2.	(33.8) 22	—	(66.2) 43	(36.93) 65

Contd.

1	2	3	4	5
3.	(51.6) 33	(3.1) 2	(45.3) 29	(36.36) 64
Total	(39.20) 69	(1.14) 2	(59.66) 105	176
Rural				
1.	(7.2) 72	(86.8) 145	(6.0) 10	(50.00) 107
2.	(14.6) 19	(82.3) 107	(3.1) 4	(38.92) 130
3.	(13.5) 5	(81.1) 30	(5.4) 2	(11.08) 37
Total	(10.98) 36	(84.43) 282	(4.79) 16	334
Total				
1.	(12.1) 26	(67.8) 145	(20.1) 43	(41.96) 214
2.	(21.0) 41	(54.9) 107	(24.1) 47	(38.24) 195
3.	(37.6) 38	(31.7) 32	(30.7) 31	(19.80) 101
Total	(20.59) 105	(55.69) 284	(23.73) 121	510

1. Not responsible parents.
2. Moderately responsible parents.
3. Responsible parents.

Similar trend is observed in respect of the use of iron folic tablets during the pregnancy period in this study (Table 13.3). Iron folic tablets are taken by only 21 per cent of women, it is high (39%) in urban area as against 11 per cent in rural area. Among the users also responsible women are high (38%) than moderately responsible (21%) women and not responsible (12%) women. This same trend is there in urban and rural areas also. The women who have had iron folic tablets during the pregnancy period are, 30 per cent of not responsible mothers, 34 per cent of moderately responsible mothers and 52 per cent of responsible mothers in urban area, and in rural area it was 7 per cent of not responsible mothers, 15 per cent of moderately responsible mothers and 14 per cent of responsible mothers. As in the case of tetanus injection, the reason for not taking iron folic tablets is states as "no body gave" by 56 per cent of women it is 84 per cent in rural area and 1 per cent of urban women. But the reason "don't know" is expressed by 60 per cent of urban women as against only 5 per cent of rural women.

Table : 13.4

NUMBER AND PERCENTAGE DISTRIBUTION OF NOT RESPONSIBLEPARENT, MODERATELY RESPONSIBLE PARENTS AND RESPONSIBLE PARENTS BY THE ACTUAL IMMUNIZATION GIVEN TO THE CHILDREN

Status of parenthood	*(First Child) Immunisation*				*Total*
	Nil	*DPT,BCG, Polio, smallpox*	*Only small pox*	*All*	
1	2	3	4	5	6
Urban					
1.	(46.8) 22	(14.9) 7	(8.5) 4	(29.8) 14	(26.70) 47
2.	(16.9) 11	(13.8) 9	(10.8) 7	(58.5) 38	(36.93) 65
3.	(6.3) 4	(9.4) 6	(3.1) 2	(81.3) 52	(36.36) 63
Total	(21.02) 37	(12.50) 22	(7.39) 13	(59.09) 104	176
Rural					
1.	(50.3) 84	(10.2) 17	(6.6) 11	(32.9) 55	(50.00) 167
2.	(29.2) 38	(10.8) 14	(10.0) 13	(50.0) 65	(38.92) 130
3.	(21.6) 8	(13.5) 5	—	(64.9) 24	(11.08) 37
Total	(38.92) 130	(10.79) 36	(7.19) 24	(43.11) 144	334
Total					
1.	(49.75) 106	(11.2) 84	(7.0) 15	(32.2) 69	(41.96) 214
2.	(25.1) 49	(11.8) 23	(10.3) 20	(52.8) 103	(38.84) 195

Contd.

1	2	3	4	5	6
3.	(11.9) 12	(10.9) 11	(2.0) 2	(75.2) 76	(19.80) 101
Total	(32.75) 167	(10.87) 55	(7.25) 37	(48.63) 248	510

1. Not responsible parents.
2. Moderately reponsible parents
3. Responsible parents.

If we come to the child health services, from Table 13.4, performance of immunisation is not satisfactory. Among eldest children, only 49 per cent of children got immunisation against all diseases. In rural area it was 43 per cent and in urban areas it was 59 per cent. It is high (75%) among responsible parents than moderately responsible parents (53%) and not responsible parents (33%). Similarly it is observed in urban and rural areas (Table 13.4). About 33 per cent of sample children were not give immunisation against any disease, it is 21 per cent in urban area, and 40 per cent in rural area. This is more (50%) among not responsible parents than moderately responsible parents (25%) and responsible parents (12%).

When the mothers were asked the reasons for not giving immunisation to children, 20 per cent of mother said "don't know", it is 11 per cent in urban area and 24 per cent in rural area (Table 13.5). The other reasons are : "not available at that time (9%), no body gave (8%) and others (7%)". Under "Others" the main reason stated is "due to illness of child."

With regard to family planning services, all respondents are aware of different family planning methods both permanent and temporary in this study. But the adoption of temporary birth control methods in the past—prior to the survey—is quite poor both in urban and rural areas. In urban area only 6 moderately responsible mothers have used temporary methods out of 65, it is 19 out of 64 among responsible mothers. Adoption of temporary methods it is high among responsible mothers with <2 living children. Only one not responsible mother with 3-4 living children used temporary methods in rural area (Table 13.6). But, the adoption of birth control methods at present—at the time of survey—is little high comparatively to the past. Adoption of temporary birth control methods it is only 3.9 per cent. It was 3.7 per cent with <2 living children and 3.9 per cent with 3-4 living children and 5.1 per cent with 5+ living children. This trend is same in rural area also, i.e., 2.2 per cent with <2 living children, 2.5 per cent with 3-4 living children and 3.7 per cent with 5+ living children, in total the adoption of temporary methods it is 2.4 per cent in rural area. In urban area it is more (6.8%) than in rural area. In urban area, 7.3 per cent with <2 living children, 6.1 per cent with 3-4 living children and 8.3 per cent with 5+ living children adopted temporary birth control methods. Use of temporary methods it is more among responsible mothers (8.9%) than moderately responsible mothers (3.6%) and not responsible mothers (1.9%). More number of responsible mothers using temporary methods in urban area, whereas it is moderately responsible parents in rural area. About 78 per cent of mothers with 3-4 living children adopted sterilisation, whereas it is 64 per cent with 5+ living children and 38 per cent with <2 living children. Highest per cent of mothers adopted sterilisation with 3-4 living children even in urban and rural areas also. In urban area it was 37 per cent with <2 living children, 78 per cent with 3-4 living children and 67 per cent with 5+ living children. In urban area it was 40 per cent with <2 living children, 77 per cent with 3-4 living children and 58 per cent with 5+ living children. The adoption of sterilisation is highest (73.3%) among responsible mothers comparatively to moderately responsible mothers (63.1%) and not responsible mothers (41.1%). In urban area it was 65.6 per cent among responsible mothers, 64.6% among moderately mothers and 40.4 per cent among not responsible mothers. In rural area it was 86.5 per cent among responsible mothers, 62.3 per cent among moderately responsible mothers, and 41.3 per cent among not responsible mothers. When the mothers were asked the reasons for not adopting birth control method, 21 per cent of mothers stated as "the desire for more children." It was 15 per cent in rural and 25 per cent in urban. This reason is expressed by high (25%) of not responsible mothers as against 21 per cent of moderately responsible mothers and 15 per cent of responsible mothers. In rural area also this type of trend is observed. In rural area, 27 per cent of not responsible, 25 per cent of moderately responsible and 11 per cent of responsible mothers expressed the reason as "desire for more children." But surprisingly, in urban area, "desire for more children is low (12%) among moderately responsible mothers. But about 17 per cent of not responsible and responsible mothers expressed this reason. The other reasons stated are :"now planning to adopt sterilisation (3%), fear of illness and death (2%) and necessary (10%) etc. (Table 13.7).

In this study mothers were asked whether they continue to have a child if a doctor tells that this might be undesirable for child's health/mothers health (herself) (Table 10.9) out of 187 own-adoptors 145(78%) are willing to stop conception according to the doctor's suggestion. It is 85 (70%) out of 122 non-adoptors in rural area, and, it is 60 (92%) out 65 non-adoptors in urban area. And also this opinion is highest (93%) among responsible parents as against to moderately responsible parents (77%) and responsible parents (74%). This same type of differentiation is observed among three categories of urban parents in this study. In urban area, 81.8 per cent of not responsible mothers, 95.5 per cent of moderately responsible mothers and 100 per cent of responsible mothers are willing to stop conception according to the doctors suggestion. But in rural area it was 71.8 per cent of not responsible mothers, 66.7 per cent of moderately responsible mothers and 60.0 per cent of responsible parents. Because, in rural area, 27 per cent of not responsible mothers, 33 per cent of moderately responsible mothers and 40 per cent of responsible mothers are unable to give their definite opinion regarding this aspect, they simply said "don't know." But in urban area, one each among not responsible and among moderately responsible mothers are in this indefiniteness.

Table : 13.5

NUMBER AND PERCENTAGE DISTRIBUTION OF NOT RESPONSIBLE PARENTS, MODERATELY RESPONSIBLE PARENTS AND RESPONSIBLE PARENTS BY THE REASONS FOR NOT GIVEN IMMUNISATION TO THEIR CHILDREN

Status of parenthood	*Reasons for not given immunisation to children*					*Total*
	Immunisation given	*Don't know*	*Nobody gave*	*Not available at that time*	*Others*	
1	*2*	*3*	*4*	*5*	*6*	*7*
Urban						
1.	(36.2) 17	(27.3) 13	(8.5) 4	(17.0) 8	(10.6) 5	(26.70) 17
2.	(72.3) 47	(7.7) 5	(6.2) 4	(12.3) 8	(3.1) 2	(36.93) 65
3.	(87.5) 56	(3.1) 2	(3.1) 2	(1.6) 1	(4.7) 3	(36.36) 34
Total	(68.18) 120	(11.36) 20	(5.11) 9	(9.66) 17	(5.69) 10	176
Rural						
1.	(38.3) 64	(28.7) 48	(12.0) 20	(13.8) 23	(7.2) 12	(50.00) 167
2.	(60.8) 79	(22.3) 29	(6.9) 9	(4.6) 6	(5.4) 7	(38.92) 13
3.	(75.7) 88	(8.1) 3	(2.7) 1	—	(13.5) 5	(11.08) 37
Total	(51.20) 171	(23.95) 80	(8.98) 30	(8.68) 89	(7.20) 84	334
Total						
1.	(37.9) 81	(28.5) 61	(11.2) 24	(14.5) 31	(7.9) 17	(41.96) 214
2.	(64.6) 126	(17.4) 34	(6.2) 12	(7.2) 14	(4.6) 9	(38.24) 195
3.	(83.2) 84	(5.0) 5	(3.0) 3	(1.0) 1	(7.9) 8	(19.30) 101
Total	(57.06) 291	(19.61) 100	(7.65) 39	(9.02) 46	(6.67) 34	510

1. Not responsible parents.
2. Moderately responsible parents.
3. Responsible parents.

TABLE 13.6

NUMBER AND PERCENTAGE DISTRIBUTION OF NOT RESPONSIBLE PARENTS, MODERATELY RESPONSIBLE PARENTSAND RESPONSIBLE PARENTS WITH THE STATUS OF FAMILY PLANNING ADOPTION IN THE PAST — TEMPORARY METHODS

Status of parenthood	*Nil*			*Used*		
	<2 *Living Children*	3-4 *Living Children*	5+ *Living Children*	<2 *Living Children*	3-4 *Living Children*	5+ *Living Children*
Urban						
1.	(100.0) 21	(100.0) 20	(100.0) 6	—	—	—
2.	(92.0) 23	(91.2) 31	(100) 5	(8.0) 2	(11.8) 4	—
3.	(63.9) 23	(77.8) 21	(100.0) 1	(36.1) 13	(22.2) 6	—
Total	(81.7) 67	(88.9) 72	(100.0) 12	(17.9) 15	(12.3) 10	—
Rural						
1.	(100.0) 78	(98.5) 67	(100.0) 21	—	(1.5) 1	—
2.	(100.0) 75	(100.0) 50	(100.0) 5	—	—	—
3.	(100.0) 32	(100.0) 4	(100.0) 1	—	—	—
Total	(100.0) 185	(99.2) 121	(100.0) 27	—	(0.8) 1	—
Total						
1.	(46.3) 99	(40.7) 87	(12.6) 27	—	(0.5) 1	—
2.	(50.3) 98	(41.5) 81	(51.3) 10	(1.0) 2	(2.1) 4	—
3.	(54.5) 55	(24.8) 25	(2.0) 2	(12.9) 13	(5.9) 6	—
Total	(49.4) 252	(37.8) 193	(7.6) 39	(2.9) 15	(2.0) 10	—

1. Not responsible parents.
2. Moderately responsible parents.
3. Responsible parents.

Table : 13.7

NUMBER AND PERCENTAGE DISTRIBUTION OF NOT RESPONSIBLE PARENTS, MODERATELY RESPONSIBLE PARENTS AND RESPONSIBLE PARENTS ACCORDING TO THE REASONS FOR NOT ADOPTING ANY FAMILY PLANNING METHOD

Status of parenthood	Reasons							Total
	Not applicable	More children desire	Now planning	Fear of death and ill health	Not necessary	Due to ill health and lack of help at home	Others	
Urban								
1.	(53.2) 25	(17.0) 8	(4.3) 2	(6.4) 3	(17.0) 8	—	(2.1) 1	(26.70) 47
2.	(67.7) 44	(12.3) 8	(4.6) 3	(1.5) 1	(7.7) 5	(4.6) 3	(3.1) 2	(36.93) 65
3.	(70.3) 45	(17.2) 11	(4.7) 3	(1.2) 1	(1.2) 1	(3.1) 2	(3.1) 2	(36.36) 64
Total	(64.77) 114	(15.34) 27	(4.55) 8	(2.84) 5	(7.95) 14	(2.84) 5	(2.84) 5	176
Rural								
1.	(43.1) 72	(26.9) 45	(3.0) 5	(3.6) 6	(16.2) 27	(4.8) 8	(4.2) 7	(50.00) 167
2.	(63.1) 82	(25.4) 33	(3.1) 4	—	(7.7) 10	(0.8) 1	(0.8) 1	(38.92) 130
3.	(86.5) 32	(10.8) 4	—	(2.7) 1	—	—	—	(11.08) 37
Total	(55.69) 186	(24.55) 82	(2.69) 9	(2.10) 7	(11.08) 37	(2.70) 9	(2.40) 8	
Total								
1.	(45.3) 97	(24.8) 53	(3.3) 7	(4.2) 9	(16.4) 35	(3.7) 8	(3.7) 8	(41.96) 214
2.	(64.6) 126	(21.0) 41	(3.6) 7	(0.5) 1	(7.7) 15	(2.1) 4	(1.5) 3	(38.24) 195
3.	(76.2) 77	(14.9) 15	(3.0) 3	(2.0) 2	(1.0) 1	(2.0) 2	(2.0) 2	(19.80) 101
Total	(58.82) 300	(21.37) 109	(3.33) 17	(2.36) 12	(10.00) 51	(2.74) 14	(2.55) 13	510

1. Not responsible parents.
2. Moderately responsible parents.
3. Responsible parents.

Table : 13.8

NUMBER AND PERCENTAGE DISTRIBUTION OF NOT RESPONSIBLE PARENTS, MODERATELY RESPONSIBLE PARENTS AND RESPONSIBLE ACCORDING TO THEIR OPINION IN CONTINUING PREGNANCIES IF A DOCTOR TELLS THAT THE MOTHER'S HEALTH WOULD SPOIL IF SHE CONTINUE

Status of parenthood	*Not applicable*	*No*	*Don't know*	*Yes*	*Total*
1	2	3	4	5	6
Urban					
1.	(53.2) 25	(2.1) 1	(6.4) 3	(38.3) 18	(26.70) 47
2.	(66.2) 43	(1.5) 1	—	(32.3) 21	(36.93) 65
3.	·(67.2) 43	—	—	(32.8) 21	(36.36) 64
Total	(63.07) 111	(1.14) 2	(1.70) 3	(34.09) 60	
Rural					
1.	(53.3) 89	(0.6) 1	(12.6) 21	(33.5) 56	(50.00) 167
2.	(70.0) 91	—	(10.0) 13	(20.0) 26	(130) 130
3.	(86.5) 32	—	(5.4) 2	(8.1) 3	(11.08) 37
Total	(63.47) 212	(0.30) 1	(10.78) 36	(25.45) 85	334
Total					
1.	(53.3) 114	(0.5) 2	(11.2) 24	(34.6) 74	(41.96) 214
2.	(68.7) 134	(0.5) 1	(6.7) 13	(24.1) 47	(38.24) 195
3.	(14.71) 75	—	(2.0) 2	(23.48) 24	(19.80) 101
Total	(74.3) 323	(0.59) 3	(7.65) 39	(28.43) 145	510

1. Not responsible parents.
2. Moderately responsible parents.
3. Responsible parents.

In general there is a opinion that elders or in-laws influence is there on couple in adopting sterilisation. Fortunately in this study this influence is quite less, *i.e.*, only two mothers in urban area are discouraged by their elders in adopting sterilisation.

CAUSES

Several psychological, cultural, and economic and organisational explanations are there for this relatively poor acceptance of birth control and health services.

Psychological Causes

1. Due to illiteracy and lack of proper family life education, mothers feel shy or embarrassed to go for health check-up and to accept conventional contraceptives.
2. The most important one is fear of side-effects due to sterilisation and other temporary methods. Couples should be instructed 'how to use', 'when to use' etc. and how to avoid complication if any.
3. And also fear of adverse effects due to sterilisation — that there would be pain etc., and they cannot work for family and for themselves.
4. *Fear of death*—due to unskilled operations, and operations hurriedly to reach the target, acceptors may have complications which sometimes may leads to death. This type of cases may be very few, but in rural areas due to ignorance and illiteracy it will be more effective on their minds. And also 'adoptors' are the main source of family planning information in most of the rural areas.
5. The reasons stated above are applicable to children also, for not accepting immunisation and other MCH programmes.

Cultural Causes

1. Going to the hospital during pregnancy for health checkup often is not appreciated by some of the women, they simply say "not necessary"; only at the time of serious conditions they would like to go to the hospitals.
2. Regarding family planning acceptance first they will delay on account of desire for more children, sons; after that, they will think that they may not conceive—no need to go in for operation, natural sterility will be there.
3. In some of the villages before three months of delivery people do not like to go to the hospital at all even when ill. Because they believe that in the early days of delivery mother and child should not come out of the rook as some evil spirits (*Druishti*) will trouble them if they are exposed.

Economic Causes

1. Anxiety of lack of help at the house to the mother and children is expressed in rural poor small families if the mother has undergone sterilisation.
2. Due to poverty, both wife and husband have to go out to work; otherwise they have to starve; with this feeling also many are not accepting birth control methods.

If we go through any rural family welfare survey results the above said causes will be noticed, some may not be expressed by many. With author's survey experience, author has noticed those as very important for not achieving the goals of family welfare programmes. Some sterilisation failure cases also author has found in author's survey experience. This unusual things will spread over other rural areas very easily. People will have the opinion that there is no use of operations except morbidity and mortality. They did not know that this caused by unskilled health personnel.

Organisational Causes

1. Extension educators and welfare workers are not always welcome by the people due to their half hearted services.
2. The community leaders are not fully convinced and give only immaterial support to the programme.
3. Extension educators who are graduates and post-graduates and finding no promotions, get frustrated and leave the job after some time.
4. Other personnels are part-time, private practitioners, who are visiting clinics at a particular period to perform prescribed quota. That time may not be convenient to the adoptors. This discourages acceptors and also makes it difficult for the doctors to complete their quota.
5. The doctors remuneration is proportionately reduced to dissatisfaction. They put this work to some other any doctors available and not making a part-time appointment.
6. Drawing rural clients to urban centres, makes it impossible to render post-operative services to visitors from outside area.
7. Sometimes a group of health personnel used to come to the villages to do some operations and go. They will not be available for follow-up services.

Like this due to so many factors MCH and Family Planning services are underutilising.

Suggestions

The following remedial measures are suggested to improve the utilisation of MCH and Family Planning services :

1. An indepth analysis may be made to identify and analyse the causes for poor performance with a view to instituting remedial services.
2. To ensure the quality of performance under all circumstances and to remove fears associated with side effects and failures, council should emphasise the importance of post-operative care of sterilisation case and adequate follow-up of users of specific methods.
3. Constant training and re-training of medical and para-medical workers in family planning methods and techniques is necessary to improve the quality of performance which leads to reach the goal of Family Welfare Programme.

4. All types of mass-media should be mounted to every nook and corner of all the villages to create awareness of the Family Welfare Programmes.
5. Incentives should be in the form of beneficial to the whole family or to the children, e.g., educating children, good free food and medicines to the mother and children till she recover from the operation, employment facilities, etc.
6. The council should have a fresh look at the entire communication machinery at the Central and State levels to restructure the same.
7. Continuous and close contacts be promoted among Researchers, Programme Planners and implementors to identify constraints in the way of effectively implementing the programme and achieving desired results.
8. Community health workers from doctors to village health workers should be duty-minded, they have to serve with heart and soul. For that their remunerations must be reasonable and satisfactory. Money should not related to the work. For that there is a need constitute or re-vitalise village health committees. These committees would be in a position to promote Family Welfare education in the community as also earliest community participation in the programme.
9. There is a need to give wide publicity to the provision of the MTP Act, particularly in the rural areas. Medicines and follow-up health services after MTP and sterilisation should be improved.
10. Immunisation programme should be strengthened a lot. Health personnel should be educated and trained properly and carefully.
11. Appointments and medical personnel and others should be on the basis of their sense of dedication to the programme and well being of the people.

References

1. *An Analysis of the Situation of Children in India*, UNICEF, 1935.
2. Deborah Maine, *Family Planning : Its Impacts on the Health of Women and Children*, 1981.
3. Department of Economic and Social Affairs, United Nations, *The Population Debate, Dimensions and Perspectives*, Papers of the World Population Conference, Bucharest, 1974, Vol. 1, Population Studies, No. 57, 1975.
4. IIPS News letter, *Fertility, Mortality and related Factors*. 1986.
5. *Journal of Family Welfare*, Vol. XXVIII, No. 1, 1986, 1-19.
6. *Ibid.*, December 1986, p. 3.
7. Ministry of Health and Family Welfare, *Family Welfare Programme in India, Year Book 1981-82*, Government of India, New Delhi, 1983.
8. *Ibid.*, 1983-84.
9. *The State of the World's Children*, UNICEF, 1987.
10. V.T. Kothari and R.S. Pandya, *Family Planning in India*, pp. 134-36.

14

Changing Trends in Medical Social Work

Since its origin, the profession of social work has been moulding itself into many forms as a response to the many demands made to provide services to various kinds of population groups and to the newly emerging social problems. In the beginning, social workers worked in generic social welfare setting. Later, they started conceptualising their role in different functional settings. Medicine has provided one such setting for the social workers.

It was only with the emergence of new theories which moved away from the doctrine of specific etiology that the psycho-social aspects of health were begun to be recognised. Earlier, the need for specialised personnel dealing with specific psycho-social problems was never felt. The multi-casual conception of disease, which advocated that illness was the result of an interaction of many factors, changed the perception of health problems. Further, the development in the behavioural and social sciences scientifically proved the belief that patients need to be treated as total organisms in a complex social setting.

This resulted in a growing awareness among the medical professionals about the limitations of clinical and individual orientation to patient care. There has been an increasing realisation of the need to supplement the strictly medical approach with a non-medical approach for better results and the need to look at the patient's treatment in a more holistic fashion so that his medical treatment is followed up by a rehabilitation programme through an inter-disciplinary approach. In fact, medicine became "a form of applied sociology, since to understand the illness of a patient it is important (indeed necessary) to locate the patient in a social and personal environment" (Turner, 1987)

Social work which had been already identified as a helping profession with a concern for interpersonal and social problems, has responded to this need and thus set the ground for the development of a specialised area called medical social work to make provisions for social inputs in the field of medicine. This had led to the emergence of the medical social worker as an important functionary in the medical setting.

Medical social work can be defined as an approach of professional social work for the prevention of physical, psychological and social dys-function which results in the disability of people affected by sickness. Here the social worker is identified as a person who helps the individual and his family to change the crisis situation of hospitalisation into a growth experience by activating the social networks.

The field of medical social work has gained impetus due to two factors. The first is the changing trends in the nature of disease. From 19th to the 20th century there was a change in the pattern of diseases from acute and contagious to long-term chronic disorders, needing special social and psychological help. The second is the changing trends in health care.

For a long time, however, medical social work remained a clinical profession catering to the needs of the patients of different medical institutions. In a "hospital (where) tangible results are of paramount importance, the results of the work of the medical social worker cannot be perceived directly" (Warde, 1987) (Warde Sulabha Madhukar). This led to the medical social workers making a desperate attempt to have tangible work roles which resulted in their spending "time on more visible activities like doing out material aid, arranging queues and so on preventing them from sufficiently clear and aware of their true professional strength and worth "(*Ibid*). For a long time the role of social workers suggested the "image of smoothing over, filling in gaps, and raising the quality of service on an individualised basis—a not unimportant task. But (they) have been slow to grasp the potential for social work to lead, develop and promote institutional and service delivery change". (Rapport, 1970).

There is growing realisation among the medical social workers on the institutional constraints involved in trying to bring out the full potential of the social workers' professional knowledge and skills. At the same time studies by Goffman (1961) brought out clearly the negative impact of institutionalisation on the patients and there was a growing demands for the decarceration of patients.

Under these circumstances a new trend has emerged in the care of the sick with an "emphasis no longer on the individual alone but also on the community. (In) this new approach of community health, the entire community is taken into consideration in planning and programming preventive, curative and rehabilitative services. (Warde, *op. cit*). This resulted in the creation of Community Health Centres, the integration of health programmes with socio-economic development programmes, the recognition of the importance of community participation for the successful implementation of health programmes, the adoption of the health programmes to the local socio-cultural conditions and social advocacy. All these have emerged as potential areas for the medical social worker's intervention. Because of its knowledge of the psycho-social dynamics of sick and healthy people and also because of its expertise in community organisation, medical social work provided to be well suited for meeting the challenges that arose due to these changing trends.

This approach is very necessary in developing countries like India where the health problems need a community approach. Because of the magnitude of problems created by illness like leprosy, malaria, small-pox, tuberculosis and filariasis the government has to necessarily develop national programmes. If these programmes have to be successful, community acceptance and participation is a must. Otherwise, they tend to fall in achieving the objectives. Again, a medical social worker has a major role to play in the successful implementation of these programmes. But virtue of his training he can act as an educator and an enabler and could enlist community participation.

At present, the medical social workers have started perceiving their role in a developmental perspective that is "to assist micro community to build its own resources through community cooperation and through action which serves the interest of all its groups.." (Desai, 1981). They have also now realised that the medical social worker is primarily "a practitioner whose main concern is to remove the psycho-social dys-function of individuals, families, groups and communities (and) like the policy maker, community organiser and social planner he (must be) related to those dys-functional forces in society which interfere with psycho-social functioning and (should seek) to have them ameliorated.

Keeping the above in view, social work inputs in medical settings are mainly related to social change perspectives. They are (Kochar, 1985) :

1. The knowledge that under special circumstances, changes due to unbalanced development depose the poverty groups to additional health hazards emerging from the developmental process itself.

2. Poverty groups exist in a social matrix which tends to isolate or ignore them. Health and developmental programmes get trapped in the complex social dynamics in rural communities thereby depriving them from resources or services meant for them.

3. Certain habits, practices, beliefs and social situations act as strong barriers to positive health and developmental change. Health benefits some times depend more on collective and cumulative action rather than action at the individual levels.

4. Effective implementation of disease prevention and control programmes require changes in traditional health practices, illness behaviour, changes in ecology, adoption of new techniques and other changes. All these changes are structurally. and functionally interrelated. Change is one aspect is often linked to change in some other aspects also. Health changes do not occur in socio-cultural isolation. Similarly, new health techniques are not introduced in a cultural vacuum.

Thus, it can be summarised that medical - social workers, in response to the changing social realities, are showing an inclination to move away from the traditional enabling and facilitating roles in secondary settings to those areas of practice where they can "lead, develop and promote institutional and service delivery change " (Rapoport, Op.cit).

However, they are also aware that in this process of change they cannot ignore the tasks which are remedial and for those whose functioning is already impaired (Report of Second Review Committee on Social Work Education, 1981). What they are trying to do is a "rearrangement of (their) priorities so that the primary problems affecting the larger segment of our population receive greater emphasis than the residual problems" (*Ibid*).

References

1. Desai. A.S. "Social Work Education in India—Retrospect and Prospect." In Nair T.K. *Social Work Education and Social Work Practice in India* Association of Schools of Social Work in India, Madras, p. 212, 1981.

2. Goffman, E. *Asylums*, Penguin Books, Harmondsworth, 1961.

3. Kochar Vijay, "Health and Social Change among the poverty groups : An outline " In : *The Proceedings of the Seminar on Changing Trends in Health Care and Implications for Social Work Education*, Bombay : Tata Institute of Social Sciences, 1985, pp. 18-19.

4. Rapoport, Lydia, "Education and Training of Social Workers for Roles and Functions in Family Planning," In Kendall Katherine, A (ed) Population Dynamics and Family Planning—*A New Responsibility For Social Work Education*, Council on Social Work Education, New York, p. 134, 1970.

5. Report of the Second Review Committee on *Social Work Education in India—Retrospect and Prospect*; University Grants Commission, New Delhi, p. 42, 1981.

6. Stream, H.S., *Clinical Social Work—Theory and Practice*, The Free Press, New York, p.37, 1978.

7. Turner, Bryan S., *Medical Power and Social Knowledge*, Sage Publications, New Delhi, p. 5, 1987.

8. Warde, Sulabha Madhukar, "Social Work in Medical Setting", In Ministry of Welfare, Government of India; *Encyclopaedia of Social Work in India*, Vol. III ; Director, Publication Division, Ministry of Information and Broadcasting, Government of India, New Delhi, p. 176,1987.

15

Sociology of Health Policy in India

Medical planning in India has a number of objectives. Among the three important objectives are : (a) keeping up with modern development in the field of allopathic and other medicines, (b) making medical care and medical education relevant to India's needs, and (c) increasing the access of the masses to the modern and other medicines. The progress made in the health planning in all its aspects has been periodically reviewed by several committees appointed by the Central government since Independence. The purpose of this chapter is to review, briefly, certain important aspects of health planning of the country on the basis of valuable guidelines suggested by various committees. The second section contains a series of alternative viewpoints for a health policy which is more relevant to the local conditions and has a wider access to the people. The last section contains the mini conclusions drawn by this paper.

REPORTS OF THE HEALTH COMMISSION AND COMMITTEES

The process of health planning in India began with the work initiated by the well known Bhore Committee in 1946. The Bhore Committee reviewed the state of health care in the mid 1949s and suggested valuable guidelines for its future development. In the following years, several other committees were set up by the Central government to review the implementation of various aspects of health policy in the country. The committees that deserve mention are : Mudaliar committee (1961), Chadah committee (1963), Mukherjee committee (1965), Jungalwala committee (1967), Jain committee (1968), Kartar Singh committee (1973) and Shrivastava committee (1975). Besides these committees, some studies on health policy were conducted by autonomous institutions like the ICSSR and the ICMR. The important recommendations by these various committees can be thematically grouped under the following : (a) to improving the existing structure of health care delivery system, (b) to improving the supporting services for a proper and quick delivery of medicare facilities, and (c) to improving the quality of the delivery system thereby improving the health standard of the masses. We shall discuss the important features of some of these committees, starting with the Bhore committee, and then go on to how health care planning has undergone changes in its structure, personnel and in its access of the populace. The review mostly highlights the modern system of medicine.

THE BHORE COMMITTEE (1946)
(THE HEALTH SURVEY AND DEVELOPMENT COMMITTEE)

The Government of India appointed the Bhore Committee in October, 1943 to survey the state of the health organisations in the country and to make recommendations for their future development. The committee submitted its report in 1946. It was published in the year that India gained its Independence. The committee had to confine itself mainly to statistics of ill health and death in the absence of data on positive health. The Committee reviewed the nation's health (British India) under :

1. Public health,
2. Medical relief,
3. Professional education with special reference to professional training of hospital social workers,
4. Medical research, and
5. International health.

The proposals for the health programmes were formulated and their contents remain valid even today. They are : (i) no one should fail to secure adequate medical care because of an inability to pay for it; (ii) the health programmes from their inception must lay emphasis on preventive work; (iii) health services should be placed as close to the people as possible; (iv) the doctor of the future—the basic doctor as the report called him—should be social physician; (v) medical services should be free to all without any exceptions and the contribution from those who can afford to pay should be through general and local taxation; (vi) full-time salaried staff should be employed by government to ensure that doctors served in areas where they were most needed; (vii) greatest attention should be paid to environmental sanitation, nutrition and health education.[1]

To achieve the above objectives the committee has suggested both, short-term and long-term measures. The short-term measures consist of the setting up of primary units covering a population of 40,000 and secondary units with as many as 16 doctors covering a population of 600,000 at a sub-district level. It requires two medical doctors and 36 non-medical staff per primary unit. The long-term measurers suggested include the setting up of a district headquarters be staffed with 269 medical officers and 1,398 non-medical staff; the raising of the bed-population ratio to 2 per thousand, and the establishment of more medical colleges having training centres for nurses.[2] The Bhore Committee also suggests the setting up of primary units covering a population of ten to twenty thousand which could be manned by six medical officers and 78 non-medical staff per unit. Secondary units have been conceived of at the sub-divisional staff level with as many as 140 medical officers and 358 non-medical staff. It also suggested the raising of the bed-population ratio from 0.24

per 1000 to 1.03 at the end of 10 years, providing for travelling dispensaries to supplement the health services rendered by primary health centre and the promotion of hygiene.

THE MUDALIAR COMMITTEE (1961)

The Government of India, Ministry of Health set up a committee in June, 1959 to undertake a review of the developments that had taken place during late 1940s and 1950s. This committee was essentially formed with a view to formulate new health programmes in the country for the third and following Five Year Plans. The terms of reference of this committee were :

1. The assessment of developments in the field of medical relief and public health centres, and submission of Health Survey and Development Committee Report.
2. Review of the aspects relating to health projects in the Second Five Year Plan and,
3. Formation of recommendations for the future health development projects in the country.

The committee known as the Health Survey and Planning Committee (Mudaliar Committee) submitted its report in October 1961.[3] The major recommendations of the committee in respect to the future organisation of health in the country are as follows : (i) the consolidation of advances, efforts and achievements made during the first two five year plans in the field of health; (ii) equipping district level hospitals with specialist services; (iii) regionalising health services by setting up of regional structures between the state and district headquarters; (iv) ensuring that each primary health centres does not serve more than 40,000 people, (v) improving the quality of care provided by the PHC; (vi) the integration of medical and health services as suggested by the Bhore committee, and (vii) the constitution of an all-India Health Service on the lines of the Indian Administrative Service.

The Mudaliar Committee analysed the extent to which the Bhore Committee targets had been realised. The committee noted that though there had been a large increase (from 7,400 in 1946 to 12,000 in 1958) in the number of hospitals and dispensaries, it was still proving difficult to provide proper health care services to the people due to the 'large increase in population', and because of an unbalanced distribution of the trained personnel. The Bhore Committee desired a ratio of one doctor for 2,000 population by 1971. In 1960, only one doctor for 4,850 population and one nurse for 14,300 population could be achieved. The realisation of the doctor-population ratio goal was slowed down because of the planning commission's decision to sanction a PHC per community development block with the population varying from 60,000 to 70,000. Since, most villages were still about 8.6 miles away from the nearest hospital the Mudaliar Committee strongly recommended the re-adaptation of the Bhore Committee short-term plan for the establishment of PHCs for a population of 40,000 and a staff of two doctors and 36 non-medical staff per unit. In addition the committee suggested the setting up of taluka level hospitals manned by 3 doctors each and a district level hospital providing speciality services in atleast nine areas.

The future of the country's well-being depends on the all-round development of the rural areas. But these have not benefited eighty per cent of the population living in rural areas[13]. The PHC, started way back in 1932, should have been the major vehicle for the delivery of health care services to the rural population. However, a committee which was constituted by the government of India recommended that additional staff be recruited for the various agencies administering the health services in the country to overcome the shortcomings in the existing infrastructure. The suggestions were—I. At the level of the PHC—one basic health worker for a population of 1,000, one health inspector for every four basic health workers, one clerk and one laboratory technician. II. At the level of the District Health Organisation-upgradation of the post of administrative officer sanctioned under the FPP, one health supervisor for every PHC subject to a maximum of one per district, one public health engineer for 2 or 3 districts and one sanitary inspector. III. At the level of the district hospitals—one administrative officer. IV. In urban areas—one basic health worker for a population of 15,000 and one health inspector for 5 basic workers.

The scheme for establishing the PHCs was launched in India in 1952. By March 1978, 5400 PHCs and 38,115 sub-centres had been established in 5228 blocks. Out of these, 4,568 PHCs are being served by two doctors per centre, while the remaining 771 PHCs are without any doctor[14]. The PHC has not made the kind of impact expected of them. The basic objectives of these health centres are to create delivery system of health service which reaches out to the grassroots level in rural areas[15]. Of the 4,500 PHCs 700 are without any buildings while 2,620 have not staff quarters[16]. Of the 39,000 sub-centres functioning today, 15,000 have no buildings[17]. This shows how inadequate these services are in terms of staff and facilities.

Thus, this committee deals with the 'basic health services' which should be provided at the block level and the measures required at higher levels of administration.

THE JUNGALWALA COMMITTEE (1967)

The committee on integration of health services was appointed in 1964 under the chairmanship of Dr. N. Jungalwala, who was then the Director of the National Institute of Health Administration and Education, New Delhi, to examine the various problems including those of service conditions[18]. The major recommendations made by the committee included the integration of organisations and personnel in the field of health from highest to the lowest level through a unified cadre, common seniority, recognition of extra qualifications, equal pay for equal work, special pay for specialised work and no private practice but good service conditions. The committee did not spell out steps or programmes for the integration recommended by it but left the matter entirely in the hands of individual states. It, however, defined the integrated health services as a (i) service with a unified approach for all problems instead of a segmented approach for different problems. (ii) a system of medical care for the sick and conventional public health programmes functioning under a single administrator and operating in a unified manner at all levels of hierarchy with due priority to each programme[19].

Thus, this committee tries to integrate the personnel of the health organisations by defining their work and service conditions. To review the development of the health infrastructure and manpower, government of India once again set up a committee in 1968.

THE JAIN COMMITTEE (1968)

The Government of India appointed the Jain committee in 1968 to review the development in the health infrastructure and health manpower[20]. This committee observed that for the period 1961-66 the doctor-population ratio has remained more or less stationery at 1:16,000 in 1961 and 1:11,000 in 1966. According to this committee "inspite of the considerable progress made during the last twenty years since Independence, the country has remained short of medical men, nurses and other para-medical personnel. This deficiency makes the work of establishing comprehensive health services extremely difficult." This committee noted that the recommendations of the Mudaliar Committee could not be accepted (by the Central Council of Health in 1962) due to the shortage of trained personnel and funds. The development of PHCs was, therefore, to continue as envisaged by the Planning Commission. The committee remarked that 'complete' integration of medical and health services even in the PHCs was still to be achieved[21].

The national programmes in the field of Health and Family Planning and Nutrition have been in operation in the country for many years. In general these programmes are run independently of each other by their respective staff. There had been little or no coordination between the field workers or supervisory personnel of these programmes. They are separate and independent functionaries. This state of affairs came into existence because the various health programmes and the family planning programme were launched at different times and each was conceived as a vertical project to be run with its own staff. A debate on whether the same objectives could be achieved by coordinating these programmes and pooling personnel spurred the organisation of the committee on multi-purpose workers under the Health and Family Planning Programme.

COMMITTEE ON MULTI-PURPOSE WORKERS UNDER HEALTH AND FAMILY PLANNING PROGRAMMES (1972-73)

The first meeting of the executive committee of the Central Family Planning Council held on 20th September, 1970 recommended that steps should be taken for the integration of medical, public health and family planning services at the peripheral level. It was also suggested that a committee should be set up to examine and make detailed recommendations on the (i) structure of integrated services at the peripheral and supervisory levels; (ii) feasibility of having multi-purpose/bi-purpose workers in the field; (iii) training requirements for such workers; and (iv) utilisation of mobile services units set up under family planning programme for integrated medical, public health and family planning services[22].

After its suggestions on the feasibility of having multi-purpose workers in the health care delivery systems and their expected training requirements, another committee known as Kartar Singh Committee was set up to pursue the recommendations made by executive committee of the Central Family Planning Service (1972).

THE KARTAR SINGH COMMITTEE (1973)

The government of India constituted a committee in October 1972 on "Multi Purpose Workers under Health and Family Planning" under the chairmanship of Kartar Singh, the then Additional Secretary Ministry of Health, Government of India. The committee's terms of reference were to study and make recommendations on :[23]

1. the structure for integrated services at the periphery and supervisory levels;
2. the feasibility of having Multi-purpose workers in the field;
3. the training requirements for such Bi-purpose workers; and
4. the utilisation of public mobile units set up under family planning services operations in the field.

The Kartar Singh Committee submitted its report in September 1973. The multipurpose health worker scheme of the committee was a significant development favouring grass-root level integration of several vertical health programme. The main recommendations of the committee were : (i) 'the Auxiliary Nurse Midwives be replaced by newly designated Female Health Workers' and the existing basic health workers, malaria eradication assistants and family planning health assistants be replaced by 'Male Health Workers' (ii) the programmes for having multi-purpose workers be first introduced in areas where malaria is in the maintenance phase and small pox has been controlled and later in other areas, (iii) for a proper coverage there should be one PHC for a population of 80,000 (iv) each PHC should be divided into 16 sub-centres each having a population of about 3000-3500 depending upon topography and means of communication (v) each sub-centre should be staffed by a team of one male and one female health worker, (vi) there should be some to supervise the work of 3-4 male health workers and a female health supervisor to supervise the work of four female health workers. The post of lady health visitor should be re-designated as female health supervisor, and (viii) the doctor incharge of a PHC should have charge over all the supervisors and health workers in his area.[24]

Certain practical difficulties surfaced at three levels, namely, at the administrative, training and at the level of attitude during the actual implementation of these recommendations. For many other reasons too the scheme of multi-purpose health workers could not gain momentum. The failure of these schemes could be attributed to (i) the quick change over of doctors at various centres; (ii) the failure on the part of the state government to sort out basic bureaucratic details like pay scale of these workers, what kits they were to carry with them and how they were to be replenished. Despite these major shortcomings, the government expected to complete the training of multi-purpose workers by 1983.[25]

THE SHRIVASTAVA COMMITTEE (1975)

The Government of India in 1974 appointed the Shrivastava Committee known also as the "group of medical education and support manpower" under the chairmanship of J.B. Shrivastava, the then Director General, Health Services, Government of India, to review the progress in the field of medical education and identify the reasons for its failure to make an impact on the health needs of the masses.[26] The terms of reference of the group were :

1. to design a suitable curriculum for training a cadre of health assistants who could be made conversant with basic medical aid, preventive welfare activities so that

they could serve as an effective link between the qualified medical practitioners and multi-purpose workers, thus forming an effective team to deliver health care, family welfare and nutritional services to the people.

2. to suggest suitable ways and means for implementation of the recommendations of the earlier committees on medical education especially the medical education committee (1968) and the medical education conference (1970) and to suggest steps for improving the existing medical educational process so as to provide due emphasis on the problems particularly relevant to national requirements, and

3. to make any other suggestions to realise the above objectives and matters.

After examining various reports and papers relevant to the subject the recommendations of the group were : (i) to evolve a nation-wide network of efficient and effective services suitable for our conditions, limitations and potentialities; (ii) to take steps to create a bands of para-professional or semi-professional health workers from the community itself to provide simple protective, preventive and curative services which are needed by the community; (iii) these workers should interact as mediators between the community and PHC, and should be trained and equipped to give simple specified remedies for day to day illness. Health assistants should work as intermediaries between the health workers and the PHC. The health assistants should be located at the sub-centres. Like the health workers, they should also be trained and equipped to give specific remedies for simple day-to-day health problems. While they have a supervisory role over the health workers; they should also function as health workers in their own areas and carry out the same duties and responsibilities but as a higher level of technical competence; (iv) the PHCs should be provided with an additional doctor and a nurse to look after the maternal and child health services; (v) the possibility of utilising the services of senior doctors at medical college should be explored; regional medical college hospitals should each develop direct links with the community around them, as well as with one another within a total referral services complex; (vii) the government of India should constitute a medical and a Health Education Commission for co-ordinating and maintaining standards in medical and health education based on the pattern of the U.G.C.

This committee opined that "it will be financially impracticable to increase the number of primary health centres, except perhaps marginally." The committee advocated the creation of a "Health Assistant" cadre to affect curative programmes amongst others, and suggested that ultimately there should be one health assistant (male/female) for every two health workers (male/female). It envisaged that by the end of the sixth plan there should be one male and one female worker for every 5000 population. The committee recommended the creation of local para-professional workers in the community itself to provide simple specified medicines for day-to-day illness'. Thus, a major contribution of the Shrivastava Committee was the involvement of the community health workers. There was approximately 1.40 lakh community health volunteers in the field as on 1st April, 1980. By 1985, the Government of India hopes to have 3.60 lakh community health volunteers.

The Government of India is fully aware that an in-depth evaluation of the centrally sponsored Community Health Volunteer scheme is necessary to make the programme effective. The decision to recruit para-professional from the community itself, like the Chinese model of barefoot factors, indicates that the policy shift was made with the hope of creating an active community participation.

After the Shrivastava Committee's action plan and the creation of the village level workers by the government there were more changes implemented. Compulsory sterilisation and family planning camps during Emergency rule, in the country led to widespread hostility among the people leading to the overthrow of the Congress party by the Janta regime and this resulted in altered approach in health services. Besides giving importance to family planning, Mr. Raj Narain, the then Health Minister encouraged to the scheme of the village level workers as suggested by the Shrivastava committee. The recommendations of a Shrivastava committee and the inspiration from the Chinese Scheme of barefoot doctors formed the basis for the introduction of the Community Health Volunteer (CHV) scheme in India by Mr. Raj Narain. This scheme, now renamed as Village Health Guide scheme, provides for one village guide for a population of 1000.[27] The need to revive the earlier multi-purpose worker scheme for the effective functioning of the primary health centre was underlined. Besides, large mobile vans fully equipped for the village-level health services were operated under the instructions of the health minister with a view to create mobile clinic services. These were under the control of the government and municipal hospitals. An objective analysis, however reveals that these mobile clinic services extended through the preventive and social medicines departments of hospitals in urban areas and slums have not made any positive impact.[26]

HEALTH FOR ALL BY THE YEAR 2000 A.D.

The low access to the basic health care facilities is a common phenomenon in most of the developing countries. In order to provide minimum basic health facilities, it was decided by the Health Assembly of the WHO to launch a movement known as 'Health for All by the Year 2000 A.D.' In 1978, the Alma Ata conference reaffirmed Health for All as the major social goal of all governments. In 1981, a global strategy for this programme was adopted by the WHO, which was later endorsed by the United Nations Central Assembly. India is a signatory to those declarations and has made efforts to extend health facilities to the vulnerable sections of its society." Health for All has been defined as attainment of "a level of health that will enable every individual to lead a socially and economically productive life."[29] To achieve the goal of 'Health for All by the year 2000 A.D.', the Ministry of Health and Family Welfare, Government of India convened a national conference to discuss national strategies and action plans. The Planning Commission appointed a working group on 'Health for All' to suggest and monitor the progress of this programme on a regular basis. The working group submitted its report in 1981. The goals recommended by the working group are[30] :

(a) reduction of infant mortality from the present level of 125 to below 60 by 2000 A.D.

(b) to raise the expectation of life at birth from the present level of 52 years to 64 by 2000 A.D.

(c) to reduce the crude birth rate from the present level of 33 per 1000 population to 21 by 2000 A.D.

(d) to reduce crude death rate from the present level of 14 per 1000 population to 9 per 1000 by 2000 A.D.

(e) to achieve a net reproduction rate of one by 2000 A.D.

(f) to provide potable water to the entire rural population by 1990.

The concept of 'Health for All by 2000 A.D.' implies a substantial change in basic health policies and in the approaches to health care. In order to provide minimum health facilities, the Government of India along with state government have increased the allocation to the health sector and have started some additional programme to boost its success in this field. The Minimum Need Programme which was first launched in the Fifth Five Year Plan was reformulated in 1978 to provide minimum facilities to the poor which includes education, health, food, water and to the centre for a population of 5000, one PHC for 30,000 people and one community health centre with specialisation in four areas for a population of 1,00,000 has been targeted. The Sixth Plan provision for the minimum need programme for the state amounted to Rs. 5807 crore which was increased to Rs. 1008.72 crore in the Seventh Plan.[31] In order to achieve the goal of this programme, the concept of PHC, that is, the active participation of the people—individually and collectively was promoted. Primary health care includes these eight elements—promotion of food supply and proper nutrition; an adequate supply of safe drinking water; basic sanitation; education; methods of preventing and controlling the maternal and child care including family planning, immunisation against major infectious diseases, prevention and control of locally endemic diseases, appropriate treatment of common diseases and injuries and the provision of essential drugs.

Thus, the important operational components of primary care should be formulated as[32] :

(i) it should be need-based.

(ii) it should be accessible to all.

(iii) it should conform the cultural and the economic set-up of community.

(iv) it should involve people actively and ultimately make them self-reliant in health.

(v) it should have appropriate linkages with other health services.

(vi) it should be accompanied by necessary socio-economic development of community.

The measures undertaken by the government for providing health care include the introduction of the rural health scheme based on the principle of placing people's health in people's hand. Under the rural health scheme, there are two functionaries at the village level, namely, a village health guide and a trained *dai* who are entrusted with the delivery of primary health care. Special emphasis was laid under this programme on the health status of mothers and children which stipulated an acceleration of programmes for the welfare for women and children and nutritional programmes for pregnant women, nursing mothers and children. The national health policy also gave great importance to maternal and child health programmes by extending more services in rural and urban areas, through primary health centres, rural family welfare centres, sub-centres urban family welfare centres, and post partum centres. Stress was also laid on the control of communicable diseases. The immunisation programme also considered as important with its objectives to reduce the incidence of diptheria, whooping cough, tetanus, poliomyelitus childhood, tuberculosis and typhoid fever.

On the whole, it appears that there has been a tremendous investment in widening the health infrastructure which include within its purview a variety of programmes and view health and humans a vital components of overall socio-economic development. For the realisation of the various objectives, the policy lays down that specified goals are to be achieved by 1985, 1990, 1995, and the year 2000.[33]

AN ALTERNATIVE STRATEGY

A group set up jointly by the ICSSR and ICMR with Dr. Ramalingaswami as the chairman, came up with an alternative strategy to achieve health for all citizens. It suggested certain steps for restructuring the health cares services infrastructure based on the principle of promoting the preventive and curative aspects of health. This group felt that, "the growth of health care services in the country has been haphazard and unrelated to the needs of poor and rural people who stand most in need of health care." This group remarked that several assumptions on which the present system is based are wrong. For instance, there is no distinction between planning for 'health' and that for 'health services' so that little or no attention has been paid to the social, economic, political and cultural dimensions of health. Health is regarded as responsibility of the Ministry of Health, whereas it ought to be a national responsibility of all concerned, that is, the people. The Western model of health services adopted is wholly inappropriate being top-heavy, over-centralised, heavily curative in its approach, urban and elite oriented and costly and dependency creating[34]. Therefore, the group recommends that "the Government of India should, in consultation with all concerned, formulate a comprehensive national health policy on health dealing with all its dimensions, that is, philosophical, cultural, socio-economic, nutritional, environmental, educational, preventive, and curative. The coordinated and planned implementation of this policy should be result of the cooperation among individuals, families, local communities, health personnel and state and central government[35]."

The recommendations of the study group are more practical and provide details of health services upto the village level. It points out that most common illnesses can be self-cured and need only symptomatic treatment with simple remedies, be it herbal, indigenous or allopathic medicine. A majority of these illnesses are communicable. These diseases can be controlled by preventive measures, can be readily diagnosed and treated with the help of cheap and highly effective drugs. The group, therefore, proposed that primary health services should be extended to the community through a trained and involved community health volunteer preferable male and female, for a population of 1,000. It should then aim at offering supplementary services for guidance and training and also lend support to the preventive and curative activities provided by the sub-centres which have total of five beds to deal with common medical and surgical problems including intravenous, dehydration, deliveries, minor injuries and to provide facilities for family planning. The group has recommended the elimination of the PHC category as it feels that it is an institution of semi-professional and paramedical personnel who deliver poor medical care extend no preventive and promotive health care.

The referral services needed for medical and surgical cases and which cannot be tackled at the sub-centres level will be provided at the community health centre, according to the group. This will operate for a population 100,000 and will have medical staff with specialisation in various fields. The Community Health Centre (CHC) will monitor, guide, supervise and coordinate all preventive, promotive, and curative health services. The CHC will have medical officers including those with specialisation. The doctors working at the CHC will work in an environment that will meet their personal needs such as proximity to educational and other facilities. They are likely to be happier in such places. The doctor will also not be isolated from his colleagues who have specialised in other fields and will have access to the latest developments in these areas, the group maintains.

To lift the status of preventive and promotive aspects of medical services from their present level, the working group has suggested that greater emphasis be given to departments of preventive and social medicine, which are currently underdeveloped. By improving the status of women we can hope to better the quality of population, the group says. In the field of Health, the drug industry is encouraging a curative bias in the country. Keeping this damaging influence of the drug in mind no attempt should be made at expanding this industry either at the private sector level or the public sector level, the group lays down. Thus, the group provides details on the services needed and on the components needed for improving the health of the people such as education, environmental conditions, level of nutrition and employment.

AN OVERALL VIEW OF THE PRECEDING REPORTS

The Health Services and Development Committee known also as the Bhore Committee (1946) pointed out the link between the socio-economic conditions and health of the people. It also suggested the establishment of PHCs for providing health care. The Health Survey and Planning Committee (Mudaliar Committee) in its report (1961) pointed out that the doctors were concentrating on curative work and suggested that they should instead share responsibilities with the auxiliary health personnel. The committee also recommended that vertical programmes be scrapped. The Chadah Committee took care of malaria vigilance in addition to family planning services at all levels. In 1965, the Mukherjee Committee recommended the extension of the educational approach to the family planning programme in place of the clinic-dominated functioning in the field. The Jungalwala Committee (1967) recommended the integration of organisations and personnel in the field of health through a unified cadre, common seniority, recognition of extra qualification, equal pay for equal work and no private practice but good service conditions.. In 1968, the Jain Committee suggested the need to integrate the medical and health services in the field of the PHCs. The Committee on the multi-purpose workers (1973) pointed out, among other things, the unsatisfactory functioning of the PHCs and noted that 60 per cent of the time of the medical officers at the PHCs were not accounted for. It recommended an integrated approach to the PHC services with the health supervisors providing guidance to the multi-purpose workers. The Kartar Singh Committee defined the feasibility of the multi-purpose workers and their training requirements. To make the death services community based, the CHV scheme recommended by the Srivastava Committee (group on Medical Education and Supporting Manpower, (1975) was launched on October 2, 1944. 'Health for All by 2000 A.D.' was a substantial shift in the basic health policies practised was a healthy improvement in the approach to health care and, in laying stress on the provision of minimum basic health facility to each and every citizen. The alternative strategy also suggested health for all based on the principle of integrating promotive, preventive and curative aspects.

In the above pages, we have highlighted the significant aspects of the official reports available on the health committees and commission. Since we are concerned with the health situation in independent India, we started off with the Bhore Committee report (1946) and ended with the report on alternative strategy (1981).

The Bhore committee identified two aspects of social policy which was subsequently accepted and pursued in fee India. These related to the social role of medicine and the doctor, as well as the quality of the training and personnel.[36] The first recommendation of the Bhore Committee underlines that every person suffering from a disease should get immediate medical attention irrespective of his socio-economic status. Oommen (1955)[37] commenting on the same theme says : "health problems should not remain the private worry of diseased individuals but should be recognised as a public issue to be tackled by the government." Another recommendation of the committee was "the doctor of the future should be a social physician.."[38] It may be viewed that a social physician is one who has an altruistic outlook towards the community he serves. In fact, this is the real task of a doctor, the report enumerates. In the country like ours, there is a need for health professionals to serve in rural areas rather than concentrate in the urban sectors. The government should draft a policy that motivates trained physicians to work in rural areas.

To review the health scene between the second and third five year plans, a period spanning almost fifteen years, the Mudaliar Committee was appointed in 1961. This committee found that though noteworthy progress had been made in many directions, even the short-term targets of the Bhore Committee were far from accomplished and this committee revised the targets in a more realistic manner. While working in the area of communicable diseases, it was realised that the health services for maternal and child welfare were fragile and their reach was limited. This committee spoke against the revival of short term courses even as a traditional measure. The committee found that the medical profession and all the associations connected with professional bodies were against it.

There were two reasons for this :

> (i) the proper development of the country in the field of health can take place only if the doctors posses the minimum qualification. (ii) India is no longer alienated from the international health scene and is participating in all problems of international health. The world health organisations has laid down certain minimum standards of qualifications. In view of India being an active member and, participating in all

public health measures at the international level we think that it will be unfortunate if at this stage a recourse is taken in short-term measures.

The Mudaliar Committee defended its position by forwarding two arguments. First, the committee felt that its recommendations for training several categories of para-medical personnel would justifiably meet the demand and, therefore, the need for short-term medical course would be redundant. Second, those with short-term training are usually the ones who go to rural areas. This would amount to an different treatment accorded to rural areas in matters relating to health care.

An analysis of the recommendations of the Bhore Committee and the Mudaliar Committee relating to the policy of training medical personnel indicates that these were based on the following considerations : (i) a concern for qualitative medical services; (ii) a belief in facing resistance from the medical profession; (iii) an anxiety to maintain international standards in medical education; (iv) the belief that para-medical personnel can serve as a functional alternative to medical personnel in some contexts; and (v) a concern for maintaining parity in the quality of medical services between rural and urban areas.[39]

After the Bhore Committee and the Mudaliar Committee, came the Jain Committee (1968) to review the situation of the health infrastructure and health manpower. This committee noted that the recommendations of the Mudaliar Committee could not be accepted mainly because of the shortage of trained personnel and funds. Therefore, the Planning Commission envisaged the development of PHCs. The Jungalwala Committee (1967) recommended the integration of health services. Over a period of time, the government of India has come to recognise "the urban orientation of medical education in India which relies heavily on curative methods and sophisticated diagnostic aides, with little emphasis on the preventive and promotional aspects,"[40] or the needs of the country, primarily because of the emphasis on community health rather than institutional care. A committee of allopathic experts known as the Srivastava Committee (1975) attempted to evolve a framework for organising a "nationwide network of efficient and effective health services for the country.[41]" The committee advocated the principle that "...health services should be provided within the community itself.[42]" It may be explained that the concept that the community level health workers should essentially provide the links between the people at large and the multi-purpose workers functioning at the sub-centre and doctors at the PHC level was behind this rationale. The committee admitted that the modern system of medicine (that is allopathy), although manned by the fully trained and competent persons, lacked the emotional, psychological and social angle in its interaction with the community. In contrast, the practitioners of indigenous system, while not sufficiently trained or competent according to the committee, had the necessary rapport with the community. To remedy the situation, the committee recommended the creation of a cadre of para-professionals to be designated as health assistants who could provide the essential and day-to-day health and medical services with an emphasis on promotive and preventive functions.[43]

The committee, however, concludes that "...what we need even for rural areas is a better trained doctor..." and it found "....no justification to make any change in the present policy of producing an adequately trained general practitioner, both for rural and urban areas[44]."

It is a fact that India lives in its villages (eighty per cent) hence, the delivery of health services in those areas is of paramount importance. However, the reports and recommendations of various committees on developing a community based delivery system failed to make an impact on the ultimate consumers of the health services that is the people of the rural areas. The only targets reached by the health sector were the production of doctors and urban hospitals. Therefore, the Government seriously considered an alternative machinery and constituted a committee on multi-purpose workers under health and family planning programmes (1972-73) followed by the Kartar Singh Committee (1973). A few other committees have been appointed by government of India to review the National Malaria Eradication Programme (the Chadah Committee, 1963) and the Family Planning programme (the Mukherjee Committee 1965).

It has been seen that the various reports lined up different programmes of action and are different in their emphasis. Top priority has been given to the control of communicable diseases, medical education, training of health personnel, medical research, services for promoting health of children and mothers, nutrition, and national malaria eradication. It was this urgency in the situation that prompted the government to evolve the National Health Policy. The NHP aims at taking the health services to the door-steps of the people and ensuring a fuller participation of the community in the health development process. It has been recognised that if the quality of the lives of the people is to be improved their health status must be raised. In this perspective, health development is to be viewed as an integral part of the overall human resources development. Consequently, a coordinated approach is sought to be established among all the health related programme, for example, protected water supply, environmental sanitation and hygiene, nutrition, housing and education.

There have been some new strategies recommended by social scientists and by those medical scientists who are keen to promote a social sciences perspective. The Ramalingaswami Committees health policy document entitled, *'Health for All'* is a comprehensive report. The committee notes that in the last thirty years, the reproduction of institutions based on western models, services and values have increased tremendously. It pleads for the abandoning of these western models of health-care services which have been actually imposed on us[45] and also impress the fact that health for all cannot be achieved through a linear expansion of the existing system or by tinkering with it through minor reforms. The committee advocated nothing short of a radical change and called for a comprehensive national health policy.[46]

The above reviews of the health planning process in India clearly indicates the enormous efforts made by the various committees to chart out the growth of health manpower in India. The work of these committees have, however, been subject to serious data limitations. Information on different categories of health personnel, their profiles and distribution (especially in respect to professionals outside the public sectors) has been rather scanty. The various committees and even institutions like the ICSSR/ICMR group have been focusing on their attention providing expert opinion rather than garnering hard statistical data. No committee has been able to take into account the contribution of non-governmental health institutions and that of professionals in rendering health care services. Also, perhaps more importantly, the committees have been unable to assess the health care needs of the people through field surveys and ascertain the extent of utilisation on health care institutions and practitioners.[47]

No concerted effort has yet been made to develop a health care system that encompasses both theory and practice. Today, we need a comprehensive National Health Policy for the developmental health programmes. This policy should be essentially Indian and distinct from the western and Chinese models and strategies developed in other countries. The new model should attempt to integrate health plans with the socio-economic development. It implies that the human environment has to be conducive to health, that food should be available to all and that everyone should have the means to get sufficient food. Other implications are also involved that people must be aware of health as a right and a responsibility and they must be willing to participate in plans and programmes to promote their own health and the health of the community as a whole.

The National Health Policy lays down an integrated and comprehensive approach as envisaged above for the development of health services in the country, including family planning services. The policy is aimed at providing 'health for all' by 2000 A.D. through primary health care approach as recommended by the Alma-Ata declaration. The stress in the National Health Policy is on the provision of preventive, promotive and rehabilitative health services to the people representing a shift from medical care to health care and in short, from the urban to rural population. This includes substantial augmentation and provision of primary health care facilities and family welfare services on a universal basis in every village, town and urban community; acceleration of programmes for the welfare of women and children, including family planning; control of leprosy, tuberculosis and blindness and nutrition programmes for pregnant women, nursing mothers and children, especially in the more remote, hilly and backward areas. Quantitative targets have been fixed for each of these areas. At this point, it is clear that if the adequacy of care, that is, the distribution of health services, could be improved, these should result in considerable savings to the economy of the nation, not only in strict economic terms, but also in a general social and psychological sense of well-being of the society. Improvement in the health status of the population, then may be less dependent upon increasing the amount of health services than it is on re-organising them to improve their availability and accessibility.

Given the health planning structure in the country as inherited from the 1950s, it is unlikely that the alternative strategies suggested will be incorporated in the health planning in the country. The health care plans for the near future is to be centred around the expansion of the existing facilities to the areas/groups who have no access to them. In view of this one has to find ways and means to improve the existing health delivery system for the masses. Even in this area a number of problems are faced by the people which include doctor's attitudes, organisational difficulties, people's beliefs, cost effectiveness and in-accessibility of life saving drugs. However, the existing literature on health care has either neglected these or hardly highlighted them while framing the policies in the health field for the masses.

References

1. Ramalingaswami, P. and Ramalingaswami V., *"India"*, in Wilson D and Melachian, G. (ed) *Health Service Projects and International Survey*. The Lancet, The Nusfield Provisional Trust, London, 1973.
2. Government of India, *Report of the Health Survey and Planning Committee*, Ministry of Health, Government of India, New Delhi, 1962.
3. Government of India, *Report of the Health Survey and Planning Committee*, Ministry of Health, Government of India, New Delhi, 1962.
4. Yesudin, C.A.K. *"Health Manpower Planning in India"*, *The Indian Journal of Social Work*, Vol. XLV. No.1, April, 1981.
5. Goel, S.L. *Health Care Administration : Policy Making and Planning*, Sterling Publishers,New Delhi, 1981.
6. Government of India, *Report of the Health Survey and Planning Committee*, Ministry of Health, Government of India, New Delhi, 1961.
7. Government of India, *Report of the Health Survey and Planning Committee*, Ministry of Health. Government of India, New Delhi, 1963.
8. Government of India, *Report of the Health Survey and Planning Committee*, Ministry of Health, Govt. of India, New Delhi, 1966.
9. Government of India, *National Health Policy*, Lok Sabha Secretariat, New Delhi, 1985.
10. Shah, Gita, *"Changing Focus of Health Policy in India"*, *The Indian Journal of Social Work*, Vol. XLV, No. 1, April, p. 102, 1984.
11. Government of India, *Handbook on Social Welfare Statistics*, Government of India, Ministry of Social Welfare, New Delhi, 1981.
12. Shah, Gita, *op. cit.*, p. 103, 1984.
13. Anita, N.,*'The Dilemma of Primary Health Care,'* in proceedings of the Conference on *Evaluation of Primary Health Care Programmes*, Indian Council of Medical Research, New Delhi, 1980.
14. Goel, S. *Health Care Administration : Ecology Principles and Modern Trends*, Sterling Publishers Pvt. Ltd. New Delhi, 1980.
15. Shah, Gita, *op. cit.*, 1980.
16. Saigal, *Indian Express*, Chandigarh, 28th August, 1978.
17. *Ibid.*
17. *Ibid.*
18. Government of India, *Report of the Health Survey and Planning Committee*, Ministry of Health, Govt. of India, New Delhi, 1967.
19. Goel, S.L. *op. cit.*, 1981.
20. Government of India, *Report of the Health Survey and Planning Committee*, Ministry of Health, Government of India, New Delhi, 1968.
21. Government of India *op. cit.*, p. 8, 1985.
22. Govt. of India, *Report of the Health Survey and Planning Committee*, Ministry of Health, Government of India, New Delhi, 1972.

23. Government of India, *Report of the Health Survey and Planning Committee*, Ministry of Health, Govt. of India, New Delhi, 1972.

24. Government of India, *Report of the Committee on Multi-purpose Workers*, Ministry of Health, Govt. of India, New Delhi, 1973.

25. Shah. Gita, *op. cit.*, p. 104, 1984.

26. Government of India, *Reports of the Health Survey and Planning Committee*, Ministry of Health, Govt. of India, New Delhi, 1974.

27. Yesudin, C.A.K. *op. cit.*, 1989.

28. Shah. Gita, *op. cit.*, pp. 105, 1984.

29. Government of India, *Health For All by 2000 A.D.* Report of the Working Group, Ministry of Health and Family Welfare, New Delhi, 1981.

30. *Ibid.*

31. *Ibid.*

32. Trivedi, C.R. *Swasth Hind*, September, 1985.

33. Government of India, *National Health Policy*, Lok Sabha Secretariat, p. 13, New Delhi, 1985.

34. ICCSR and ICMR, *Health for All : An Alternative Strategy*, Indian Institute of Education, Pune, p.10, 1981.

35. *Ibid.*, p.14.

36. Oommen, T.K., "Health and Society in India: Towards a Sociological Understanding", *Relevant Sociology*, Vol. II, No. 1, May, pp. 4-5, 1985.

37. *Ibid.*, p. 5.

38. Government of India Ministry of Health, *Report of Health Survey and Planning Committee*, (Aug. 1959-Oct.1961), Vol.1, p. 20, New Delhi, 1962.

39. Oommen, T.K. *op. cit.*, p. 6, 1985.

40. Quoted in Oommen's Article, *op. cit.*, p. 6, 1985.

41. Government of India, Ministry of Health and Family Planning, *Health Services Medical Education*. Report of the group on Medical Education and Support manpower, p. 2, New Delhi, 1975.

42. *Ibid.*, p. 11.

43. Government of India, *op. cit.*, p. 26, 1975.

44. Oommen, T.K. *op. cit.*, p. 9, 1985.

45. Indian Institute of Education, *Health for All : An Alternative Strategy*, Report of a Study Group set up jointly by the Indian Council of Social Science Research and the Indian Council of Medical Research, Distributed by Voluntary Health Association of India, p. 262, New Delhi, 1981.

46. Oommen, T.K. *op. cit.*, p. 10, 1985.

47. Yesudin, C.A.K. *op. cit.*, 1984.

16

Social Perspectives of Health and Health Care

SOCIOLOGY, MEDICINE AND PUBLIC HEALTH

The history of medicine is as old as civilisation. Every society through experience has evolved ways to cope with illness and physical disorders. These ways are cultural specific and vary greatly from the society to another. The roots of modern medicine lie in the age old magical rites and antiquated practices. Medicine in the beginning of civilisation consisted of what Sigerist (1960) calls "a mishmash of religion, magic and empirically acquired ideas and practices...". In primitive society, the treatment instead being rational was primarily magical in character and accompanied by prayers, manual rites or dances. Religion exerted a profound influence on medicine and its beliefs and practices were an important part of the treatment (Banks, 1953). In order to control the disease and cure the patient, religious leaders and saints as well as traditional healers were called upon, particular god or deity associated with the disease was worshipped and its blessings obtained and visits to sacred places were made (Hasan, 1967). The oriental health practices combined in them religious, cosmological theories and speculative thought associated with Ayurvedic medicine and acupuncture. The principles of such pre-scientific medicine, according to Pytlik *et al.* (1978) continue to fascinate many today, not only because they sometimes bring unexplained relief from suffering and chronic illness but also because they actually anticipate recent discoveries about the inter-relationships between mind and body—attitude and physical health.

Distinctions have, however, been made between primitive medicine and folk medicine. The former is viewed as non-scientific and as being largely dependent upon supernatural explanations of disease and as looking upon magic as an essential ingredient of therapy. Folk medicine, on the other hand, is defined as medical beliefs and practices which were widely shared among people as opposed to knowledge as an exclusive property of the practitioners. Both medicines, however, have many things in common : the belief that the nature of disease depends largely on the culture; treatment as well as preventive measures are logically related to beliefs about causation; sick people follow the same behaviour pattern to cope with illness that is, self treatment, seeking others' advice or seeking help from professional healers.

Even before sociology emerged as an independent discipline, scholars made attempts to study incidence and prevalence of illness in relation to the socio-cultural framework of society and the psychology of the patient. The authors of ancient and medical times tried to relate health problems to the prevailing social, political and economic conditions. The anthropologists' interest in primtive-medicine and in the relationship between prayers and rituals and the prevention and cure of disease is also quite old (Ackerknecht, 1942). The association of certain diseases and disabilities with particular occupations can be seen in the accounts of ancient Egypt and Greece.

The sociological interest in the problems of health is a recent development. A systematic investigation of such problems began only in the eighteenth century (Sigerist, 1960; Straus and Clausen, 1963) with the shift in the emphasis of medicine from communicable diseases to chronic and degenerative disorders. With the advent of the germ theory and bacteriological approach to medicine, the spread of communicable diseases could be controlled with remarkable success and the help of social sciences was not called for much. Rapid industrialisation, urbanisation and technological advancement, however, made the social environment full of stress and strains giving rise to chronic and degenerative diseases. This development brought a drastic shift in the approach to disease-control offering an unique opportunity to use the knowledge of social science to improve health. This also led to a shift in the goals from disease-control to attainment of positive health as defined in terms of physical, mental and social well-being. Besides, a clear distinction between prevention and treatment also emerged and several social problems like alcoholism and drug abuse also came within the scope of public health (Suchman, 1968).

The need for a social science base in medicine and health began to be increasingly recognised and this fact was repeatedly acknowledged in the medical circles. Rudolf Virchow for instance, asserted that "medicine is a social science in its very bone and marrow." L.J. Handerson termed the practice of medicine as "applied sociology". Knowles (1979) also noted, "I believe that medicine is a social science as well as a physical and biological science and that it needs the social sciences and the effects of their study as never before in history". Lamenting on the importance accorded to social sciences in public health programmes, Mountin (1951) noted "public health is an applied technology resting on the joint pillars of natural science and social science... until both the pillars of natural and social science are strong, the arch of public health will not be firm." This understood the growing recognition of the need to use sociological theory, knowledge and methodology in public health. Those negating its importance met with repeated warnings : "... public health workers cannot ignore the social sciences; if they do, it is at their own peril" (Robinson, 1963).

There are at least three ways, according to Suchman (1968), in which the knowledge of sociology can prove helpful in implementing public health programmes: (i) recognition of the significance of social forces in health that is, change in cognitive processes; (ii) need to deal with such social forces as beliefs, values and motivation that is, change in effective processes; and (iii) taking into account such forces in organising and administering public health programmes that is, change in behavioural processes. He also maintains that "effective public health action will come about only when social factors are accorded the same type of recognition, that is now given to the germ theory in relation to communicable diseases. A lack of concern for basic social causes will mean that public health will continue to deal with these problems not on the level of prevention... but on the haphazard, ineffective level of containment or maintenance".

Though sociologists are accused of not having paid as much attention to the public health dimension of our social system as they have to religion, economy, education and government, and sociology of health still being in its infancy, despite Suchman found almost all areas of sociological fact and theory relevant to medical and health care. These include knowledge of cultural forces influencing meaning and definitions of health and disease and acceptable methods to control the disease; social forces which affect not only occurrence of health problems but also the structure and function of community and group reactions to such problems; psychological forces determining individual's response to health and disease and efforts to improve health and control disease and economic and political forces affecting the supply, demand and cost of health facilities as also strength and form of health administration.

Even in the early stages of medicine, the close connection between disease and social environment was accorded recognition but it is only recently that the social scientists have noted the limited application of sociology and the paucity of data. Many physicians still doubt whether the sociologists can contribute anything relevant to medicine. Sociologists have also ignored this field till the World War II. The factors that have contributed in bringing the two disciplines closer to each other are listed (Coe, 1978) as under :

1. The basis of epidemiology was broadened from the study of distribution of communicable diseases among the population to the study of ecology (distribution in the population) of any disease or physical handicap. The interest in the causes of diseases has also expanded to include differential effects on different population in different environment.
2. The increased interest in the control of chronic diseases paved the way for the increased emphasis on the concept of multiple, causation of disease that is, factors other than biological are also regarded as important in determining the diseases.
3. The increased emphasis on the long range participation of every citizen for the prevention of diseases and hence on health education.
4. A growing recognition world-wide to provide adequate medical care and programmes to all communities and all people and hence need to measure needs of medical care available at present and ways to meet the gaps.
5. Stress on the rehabilitation of patients who have suffered disability through illness or accidents in their own social milieu.
6. The emergence of occupational health/medicine as an important science to help cope with the problems caused by industrial toxins.

7. The development of a positive concept of health (as opposed to a negative one merely involving the control of diseases). To include "a state of complete physical, mental and social well-being and not merely the absence of disease and infirmity."

Disease affects everyone everywhere but not always to the same degree or in the same way. The study of how diseases affect human groups and the ways in which groups react to disease provides a substantive ground for the application of sociological knowledge and research techniques, Coe has identified at least four dimensions from this standpoint :

1. Differential distribution of illness in terms of social structure and the differing life style it imposes on people provide clues about the nature and causes of diseases.
2. People view the disease from perspectives of their culture and based on these perspectives, they tend to respond to the disease in predictable way.
3. People develop an array of institutions to treat the diseases that appear in their group.
4. The treatment of disease involves more than the mere application of medical knowledge through medical institutions. They involve physicians, hospitals, pharmaceutical firms and other supporting institutions in the modern complex society and religions rituals, neighbours and kinsmen supporting medical efforts of the healer in the traditional simple society.

The distribution of disease in society, cultural perspectives on disease the role, attitudes and values of health providing institutions and the relationships of treatment and support facilities all form the subject matter of sociology. This has led to the emergence of medical sociology within the broader field of sociology.

In addition, health administrators have been seeking the help of sociologists to evaluate health programmes, to study different dimensions of pathological conditions and to identify ways and means to promote community participation in health programmes (Boek and Hilleboe, 1956). The sociologists, understanding of the people's needs and desires and the community's leadership pattern and power structure can be of great help in enlisting public support, particularly in health programmes affecting sensitive areas of social and individual behaviour. Besides, with the increased specialisation and resultant segmentation and impersonalisation of medical care it is essential for the health personnel to be oriented, as part of their training, to the socio-psychological dimensions of illness, taught the importance of close contacts with patients so that they are able to identify likely sources of resistance and support of the patients and also ways to promote cooperation. However, the greatest obstacle in employing the knowledge of sociology in health is the pressure on health personnel to show results (Foster, 1961). The assistance of social scientists is also being sought in the study of health institutions, their internal structure, work pattern, social interaction and in the utilisation of facilities and services.

Thus, social sciences have been used in almost all aspects of medical and health care. The practitioners use social sciences in programme planning, on its implementation and its evaluation. The teachers use sociological knowledge and to concepts and theories for a better understanding of health problems. The researchers use social research designs for testing hypothesis relating to social causes and control of disease and also as a base for collecting and analysing data. Likewise, courses in public health practice, health care administration, health education and social epidemiology are heavily dependent upon sociological knowledge. Similarly, without appropriate survey or observation techniques, the studies of sociological factors in disease resistance to health innovation and adoption of family planning techniques cannot be effectively conducted.

Besides being useful in the control of diseases and promotion of health, the sociologists growing interest in medical and health problems has proved advantageous to the growth of their own discipline. Many sociologists regard the domain of medical and health as a convenient area for testing out general sociological theories (Merton et al., 1959). For Hall (1951), medicine offers an unique area for sociological studies because research can be focused on three main areas : (i) on institutions where the work goes on (that is hospital), (ii) occupational division of labour, and (iii) social psychology of work (that is, relationships between work and personality organisation).

A matter which is of considerable interest is the distinction made between sociology in medicine and sociology of medicine (Straus, 1957). The former implies the application of sociological concepts, knowledge and techniques in order to clarify medical and socio-psychological problems involved in the solution of health problems. In contrast, sociology of medicine concerns itself primarily with the study of health and medical personnel, their relationships with others, institutions and organisations and their services. However, the distinctions are now getting blurred.

Although the term "social hygienic" was used in 1938 by J.A. Rochoux (1838), the adjective 'social' with 'medicine' was introduced first by Gu'erin in March 1948 (Gu'erin, 1948). He divided social medicine into four parts : (1) social physiology as the study of relation between physical and mental condition of a population, its laws and social conditions; (2) social pathology as the study of social problems in relations to health and disease; (3) social hygiene as the determination of measures for health promotion and disease prevention; and (4) social therapy as the provision of medial and other measures to deal with social disintegration and other conditions that societies may experience.

Opposing the view that medicine as a social science is a vague Utopian dream, Rosen (1977) termed it as a conceptual formulation meant to support a programme of action and identified its three basic principles: (i) that people's health is a society's direct concern and obligation; (ii) that social and economic conditions have an important—often crucial—impact on health and disease, and (iii) that the steps taken to promote health and to combat disease must be social as well as medical. These principles find clear expression in the draft for a Public Health Law submitted to the Berlin Society of Physicians and Surgeons in 1849 (Kroeger, 1937) in which three objectives of public health were stressed : (i) healthy mental and physical development, (2) prevention of all dangers to health and (3) control of disease.

During the middle of the eighteenth century, the terms 'public health', 'social hygiene' and 'social medicine' were used interchangeable, since public health, primarily concerned with improving environmental conditions, shared its goals with social medicine (Rosen,

1958). The public health began to achieve its distinct identity when sanitary reforms were directed to achieve its narrower aims and the attention of medicine was shifted from the control of social and physical environment to the control of communicable diseases following development in medical bacteriology. In the present century, an increasing concern with social aspects of health brough public health once again in to prominence and brought it closer to social medicine as well as to the new discipline of medical sociology (Rosen, 1977). Public health, which is now viewed as an applied medical science and rests heavily on major sociological elements in its practice, deals with prevention of illness or disability in any stage of the condition, within community context, by control of agent, host, and environmental factors with support and cooperation of community groups and individuals (Roney, 1960).

The idea of systematically investigating medical problems in the light of social science was conceived by Alfred Grotjahn (1915). He advanced several principles basic to the study of illness from the social point of view :

1. The social significance of a disease is determined by its frequency of occurrence.
2. The form in which the particular disease occurs most often must be known.
3. The etiological relationship between social conditions and disease may be expressed in four ways : Social conditions may :

   (a) create or favour a predisposition for a disease;

   (b) cause disease directly;

   (c) transmit the causes of disease; and

   (d) influence the cause of disease.
4. Disease originating in or caused by social conditions may in turn influence social conditions, particularly through their outcome.
5. To establish whether the prevalence of disease that is important from a social point of view can be appreciably influenced by medical treatment and whether such therapeutic success is important from a social point of view.
6. Preventing diseases or influencing their course by social measures requires attention to the patients social and economic environment.

To lay stress on the aforesaid principles, Grotjahn evolved the concept of social hygiene and asserted that this should form an essential part of the medical curriculum. He reserved the term 'social medicine' for medical care. However, the scope of social medicine has tremendously broadened in the recent past to include new factors and situations caused by the increasing industrialisation, urbanisation and changing technology that has tended to alter and degrade environmental qualities.

The use of the knowledge of sociology, despite its proven contribution in medical and health care, is constrained by several factors. The main problem lies in the difference in approach and outlook between sociologists and medical personnel (Hyman, 1968), while sociologists tend to generalise their findings, clinical medicine focuses on the understanding of individual cases. The former views all patients alike with respect to their attitudes and behaviour, whereas the latter treats each patient as an unique case (Brown, 1965). The life-death nature of many medical problems calls for quick solutions without the results of prolonged research of the sociologists and in case action is taken on the basis of incomplete data, failure is most likely. Further, sociologists tend to classify patients according to their socio-psychological and physical attributes in matters of rehabilitation but the medical administration tends to provide benefits to all patients regardless of the probability of success and hence may ignore findings of sociological research.

Besides, the theoretical limitation of the subject is also believed to be responsible for its limited use in the medical field. The value of sociological research lies in its identification of the causal factors which the medical practitioner can manipulate. However, sociology offers only a few of such factors many of which cannot be easily manipulated. If the problem lies with the community and its value system, it is almost impossible to change them. Behavioural sciences, in fact, proved more effective in dealing with the problems of individual and small groups (tuberculosis control) than those concerning large complex groups such as pollution control (Foster, 1961).

The effectiveness of sociology in public health is to a large extent closely associated with the effectiveness of the death care delivery system itself. If health care delivery system does not have clearly defined objectives and workable valid programmes to achieve those objectives, sociology will hardly be of any use. The death care system proved to be quite successful in controlling communicable diseases even prior to sociology emerging as an organised discipline; however, it has not proved effective in preventing or controlling the major health problems the world is facing today, whereas sociology has proved to be helpful in dealing with public health problems. The present day health problems are far more difficult to understand and very little is known about them. Their control requires a radical change not only in health care but in medicine as a whole. The sources of many health problems can be traced to social conditions. This is where sociology can prove to be helpful but the contributions of sociology can be effective only if drastic changes are brought about in the fields of medicine and public health. While the apathy of the public regarding the use of health services is known and needs to be overcome, the health personnel also required to approach the people in the people's own frame of reference rather than that of their own or professionals.

CONCEPT OF HEALTH AND DISEASE

The meaning of the term 'health' as a subjective concept varies with individual and group, time and place and socio-cultural contexts. The measures used to define health greatly vary and range from purely biological and physiological to social, cultural and psychological. Whereas in positive terms it is defined as a state of complete physical, mental and social well-being, it is viewed negatively as the absence of disease or ill health. When defined negatively, the indicators selected are objectively defined and measured such as, rates of morbidity and mortality. Any change in these rates is construed as a change in the health status of the people. None of these rates are in fact persisting ones.

The concept of 'health' and 'disease', which are relative and culture-specific, assume different meanings even in the same society. Health, for example, is viewed simply as absence of disease or infirmity. Since such a notion does not provide a total view, WHO defined health as a state of complete physical, mental and social well-being. Health is defined also in purely physical terms, that is, height, weight, appearance. Associated with this is the concept of 'mental health' which has come to assume great importance with the wake in stress and tension resulting from rapid technological and social changes. Mental health as a state free from worries, anxieties, stress, tension and frustration is greatly influenced by the social environment (Basu, 1977). What pleases and keeps one happy differs from person to person and the same holds true of other measures of health.

The concept of disease similarly varies greatly depending upon the type of society, culture or individual. Usually, it is defined as a deviation from the normal functioning which may adversely affect the future health status (Mechanic, 1962). Since a diseased person is unable to perform his normal social responsibilities, his behaviour is viewed as deviant and hence dysfunctional by the society which undertakes to cure him as early as possible to make the person normal.

The notion of disease was never governed by the 'objective facts'; rather it depended on the decision of the society (Martin, 1968). The diseases and illness were believed to be caused not only by the individual's bio-physical conditions but also by supernatural beings, violation of religious rules, disobedience and the resultant wrath of the god or goddess and the sins committed by the person in the life or in the past lives. The internal disorders are believed to be the result of three humours (Tridosha) of human body, namely, wind, bile and flasom (Fillozat, 1964; Hasan, 1967). Such notions about diseases have been the root cause of many irrational beliefs and practices in treatment which tend to make the task of health care quite difficult.

Most groups recognise a sick-role. If a sick person is not able to perform his normal role, some alternate arrangement is made by the group. Thus, the sick role is a social role which has certain rights and obligations as well as complimentary roles. One of the rights enjoyed by the sick person is that he or she is excused from normal duties and he or she is also allowed to interfere with the performance of others, roles as well. The patient also has a claim upon others for assistance and care. However, this role also imposes certain obligations on the sick person; it is concerned with the patients, speedy recovery through competent technical help and cooperation and this obligation is aimed at preventing the patient from 'enjoying' the state of being sick or from receiving 'secondary gain' (Parsons, 1951).

A distinction has also been made between disease and illness; while former is medical in character, the latter is basically social. "Contrasted with disease, which is a concept of biology and more specifically of pathology, illness is defined as a phenomenon which is apparent to the individual in terms of an altered state of perception of self... a disease can occur in individuals without any awareness of feelings of sickness and without anyone else knowing them to be other than in a 'normal' state thus, a disease process may take place within individuals without recognisable symptoms ever being produced... it is also possible that persons may feel sick-even so miserable that they are incapacitated without any of the organic processes of disease being manifested" (Coe, 1978).

Illness is viewed as a personal as well as social phenomenon. Coe observes "...as long as what we feel is not communicated to others or what we do is not observed by others, illness remains a personal event...illness becomes a social phenomenon when it becomes visible to others and when this leads to modification of the social interaction pattern between sick person and other people." Thus sickness as a social event is known through direct observation by others and by the patients, communicating his feeling to others.

The domain of health and illness is full of contrasts for each society has evolved its own mechanism to cope with the problems of health and illness and the ways in which these have been defined (Morris, 1973). Every society experiences illness and prescribes treatment compatible with its own social and cultural background. Illness is viewed as a departure from normalcy over which one does not have any control but the response to which is governed by societal values and customs. This explains the different perceptions, interpretations and modes of treatment of the same disease in societies with different socio-cultural background. So is the case with the varied effects on individual, family, society and economy commensurate with the intensity, duration and severity.

Problems relating to health and disease are neither viewed with the same seriousness nor call for equal health care. There exists a wide variation in medical care, depending on the nature and seriousness of the illness. While some are not prepared to accept the seriousness of a health care problem, others define the problem in terms of insuring against 'catastrophic' illness and the treatment sometimes swallows the whole of the patients' income. Still other see the problem as one of the insuring 'medical care for all' in order to cover those who need medical care most but do not get it.

SOCIO-CULTURAL APPROACH TO HEALTH AND DISEASE

The advances made in medical science in the past few decades have undoubtedly made a great dent in prolonging lives, improving health care and lowering disease and death rates. However, the improvement in the field of health and disease-control is not entirely due to the advancement in medicine. The reduced incidence of several diseases can also be attributed to the gradual improvement in the standard of living. While antibiotic drugs still continue to be necessary to control normal diseases, many other health hazards and diseases such as hypertension, cancer and mental illness are now being caused by industrialisation, urbanisation, technological change (with its impact on occupational and geographical mobility) and stressful environment (resulting from competitiveness, smoking and improper diets). The old epidemiological approaches seeking bacterial or viral explanations for new diseases are no longer of much help in controlling the new set of diseases. The attention therefore, has now shifted to the etiology of diseases which lays emphasis on behaviour patterns, lifestyles and cultural factors to unearth the cause of diseases and their likely control or prevention. The social-epidemiological approach to the health problems calls for the identification of whole process of causation for understanding the etiology of disease so that the events leading to the disease can be traced. For centuries, now it has been established that lifestyle, customs and traditions, beliefs and practices, vocation and profession have serious consequences on the health of an individual. With the increasing attention towards prevention rather than therapy, it is now recognised that many chronic diseases can be efficiently prevented and controlled by a timely change in behaviour, lifestyle and dietary pattern.

Social-epidemiological studies have made efforts to identify socio-cultural factors associated with the incidence and prevalence of diseases and also those factors associated with preventive and therapeutic care (Suchman, 1965). Despite several attempts at ascertaining the causation of the disease, no simplistic conception of one disease-one cause has emerged. In fact, a number of factors have tended to contribute to the development of each disease.

Though environmental factors are largely responsible for the prevalence of genetic disorders, yet their prevalence in one specific group rather than among others indicates a genetic susceptibility of the host. The class of psychosomatic or sociosomatic diseases may have genetic components but are produced primarily in groups faced with stressful situations. In both genetic and sociosomatic diseases, the commonly known vector and agent are missing since there is no virus, bacteria or chemical involved. Graham and Reader (1977) have attempted classification of disease according to social groups or behaviour pattern associated with them. Thus, many diseases occur more frequently among a particular socio-economic, racial, religious or ethnic group than among others. Many diseases are known to be caused by smoking, coronary disease, peptic ulcer and cancer of the bladder, mouth and lungs. Diseases are also classified according to sociological variables such as social mobility, alienation, anomic and over-work. For example, mobility, is found to induce coronary diseases, hypertension, peptic ulcer and arthritis. The classification based on newer conceptions of disease-causation has also been useful. The concepts of water-borne diseases sheds light on the etiology of diseases and has encouraged programmes on pure drinking water systems to control such diseases. This suggests that the knowledge of other factors is necessary to control diseases and, according to Graham and Reader, these are very frequently social factors. This is amply demonstrated by the elaborate review of studies on different diseases associated with the socio-economic status, ethnicity and religion, familial characteristics, socio-cultural and socio-psychological processes including cultural changes, mobility and migration, status inconsistency and life changes and events. The study group of ICSSR-ICMR (1981) took cognisance of the relationship between health of the people and the surroundings and considered health care services necessary but not sufficient. It noted : "Health is a function not only of medical care but of the overall integrated development of society cultural, economic, educational, social and political. Health also depends on a number of supportive services nutrition, improvement in environment and health educational."

Socio-economic status or social class has been correlated with several diseases particularly those resulting from industrialisation, modernisation and urbanisation. The inverse relationship often reported between the socio-economic status and the rise of disease led to the policy decisions in favour of increased health services for the poor and improvement in the standard of living. Social factors particularly those involving class seem to affect diseases at three levels: (i) physical level in which the social class environment consisting of nutrition and housing is viewed as responsible for infectious diseases; (ii) psycho-social level in which diseases are attributed to the prevalence of mental stress and strain resulting from specific environmental factors, and (iii) cultural level where different diseases prevalence rates among different social classes are interpreted in terms of attitudes and beliefs towards preventive and therapeutic care. Medical and health personnel have paid attention to the social factors in the same order that is, more to be improvement of physical conditions than to the averting of psychosocial disease-producing characteristics of certain social environments or to the accounting for different attitudes among various cultural groups about seeking medical and health care (Hyman, 1968).

The review of the studies attempted by Graham and Reeder (1579) clearly points out that the socio-economic status is closely associated with hypertension, blood pressure, coronary diseases, different types of cancer, and tuberculosis. The vulnerability to and prevalence of serious illness were found to be greater among the poor. The explanation offered by scholars for this phenomenon includes poor housing, crowded living, low income, lack of education and a strained environment. Among several socio-economic status variables, education is reported to be the most closely related to health.

Another group of studies reviewed by Graham and Reeder concerns itself with role of ethnicity and religion and notes that certain diseases are prevalent more among particular ethnic and religious groups than others. For instance, the Polish-Americans are vulnerable to high risks of cancer of esophagus and lungs, whereas the Italian-Americans are prone to high risks of cancer of the bladder, large intestine and pharynx. The Blacks in the United States were similarly found to have comparatively higher blood pressure levels, and suffered more from hypertension and heart diseases than the Whites. The degree of religiosity was found to have an inverse association with the incidence of myocardial infraction. The distinctive behaviour and lifestyle appear to be responsible for such an association. The relationship between the frequency of church attendance and coronary diseases and mortality has also been recorded. The low incidence of different types of cancers among religious groups in the United States was reportedly due to religious prescriptions against alcohol, tobacco and caffeine.

The behavioural characteristics peculiar to individual families particularly those concerning child-bearing practices tend to protect against or foment certain diseases. The review of Graham and Reeder reveals that the rates of hypertension were highest among single women which decline progressively among women with one child, two children and with three or more children. In certain families diseases may be due to either social or genetic inheritance.

The association of socio-cultural processes with certain diseases was also clearly brought out in there view attempted by Graham and Reeder. It uncovers how the modernisation process in the under-developed countries has led to an increase in mental disorders and heart diseases as individuals were required to adapt to modernised cultural modes involving geographical, occupational and social. The individuals and groups with rapid geographical and social mobility show higher rates of mortality and suffer more from coronary heart diseases than those who are less mobile. The explanation for this is to be found in the lifestyles of people who are mobile which is characterised by intense work pressure, sharp competitiveness, meeting of deadlines, overcommitment to profession/vocation and an excess of drive. The discrepancy in rank and social status has also been shown to cause stress with adverse effects on physical and mental health. The close connection between the events in a person's life and diseases, particularly mental disorders have been demonstrated. The differing rural-urban ratio in the relevance of diseases, infant mortality and morbidity rates has also been explored.

These analyses suggest that many diseases can be prevented if the socio-cultural causes are neutralised or removed and the approach does not remain confined towards therapy only.

The nature, type and conditions of work, are also largely responsible for a variety of health problems. The ICSSR-ICMR study (1981) reveals how the mining, quarrying and mineral-processing industries like the chemical industries expose the workers to different diseases. Besides, inadequate lighting, poor sanitation, inadequate ventilation and mental stress during work have also been pruned to effect the physical well-being of a worker. Some of the health-problems caused by different type of occupations pursued by women have been brought to our notice by the National Commission on Self-Employed Women and Women in the Informal Sector (1988; 136-172).

SOCIAL CONSIDERATIONS IN HEALTH CARE PROGRAMMES

Socio-cultural and psychological factors have also been shown to affect the seeking of medical and health care services. In his 'Foreword' to the Benjamin D. Paul's 'Health, Culture and Community' (1955), Hugh, R. Leavell accepted that, "it is not easy to persuade the public to make full use of the health information at hand, except when people are aroused by some obvious epidemic or other disaster. It is in the 'public' part of public health that we are weak; the 'health' aspects somehow seem simpler for us." As an approach to public health, he further asserted, "we must not only obtain his (individual person) consent but personal habits and ways of living must frequently be altered radically. If changes of this sort are to be brought about, we must apply what is known of human relations."

Benjamin Paul (1955) is equally emphatic in using the public view of health in health programmes. Before asking a group of people to assume new health habits, it is wise to ascertain the existing habits, how these habits are linked to one another, what functions they perform and what they mean to those who practise them." Justifying such an approach he maintains, "what appears from outside as our irrational belief and behaviour becomes intelligible when viewed from within. Perceiving the connections between items of belief and behaviour as the people themselves perceive them enables us to make better sense of the seemingly capricious pattern of acceptance and rejection of successful and unsuccessful educational efforts."

Illness in all cultures is a psychological crisis for the individual and a social crisis for his family. The way the illness is classified determines the question of seeking a specialist's help, the type of specialist's to be approached, the manner of behaving during a session with the specialists and the way of using his advice. The illness itself is defined as much by that particular culture's definition of it as by the intrinsic nature of the ailment. The social dimensions of an ailment and its therapy become more apparent when a physician, who is alien to a particular culture, tries to treat the disease and prescribes a treatment that differs from the expectations of the patient and his society. The study of two communities by Carstairs (1955) clearly brings out the different perceptions in prognosis and healing and deals with the problem of transmitting health knowledge and medical care. In a traditional society, he says, first the roots of illness both in the realm of human conduct as well as in cosmic world are traced. To set the patient right morally as well as medically, the healer then serves as a link between the mortal man and the purposeful cosmos. For a Western physician, physical weakness signifies malnutrition and anemia and calls for prescriptions of iron tonics and vitamin concentrates. But for the local people of a traditional society, physical debility is connected with moral weakness and transgressions of the ethical code for which the ideal remedy would be pilgrimages, ritual baths to wash away one's sins and atonements rather than tonics.

Viewing the phenomenon of illness from the standpoint of social structure, Marriott (1955) noticed three concentric realms in the social world of the villagers: the intimate realm of family and kinship; the realm of village and caste and the remote realm of the outside world. Despite good intention, he says, the doctor practising Western medicine is perceived as a member of an outside world and, therefore, regarded with suspicion and his prescriptions are ignored, whereas indigenous folk medicine—magical, sacred and secular—flourishes in the community. Even from the point of view of the number of patients, expenditure, frequency of sue, the patronage of indigenous treatment surpasses that of western medicine. Besides, several ideas and practices have come to be associated with Western medicine namely, personal privacy, individual responsibility, reliability of certain techniques and of inter-personal trust, and these are not seen as compatible with the traditional social organisation of the Indian village.

Providing an insight into the determinants of behaviour which lead to the acceptance or rejection of health practices, the Health Belief Model (HBM) postulates that people seek health care only if they possess the minimum level of motivation and knowledge; view themselves as vulnerable and the conditions as threatening; feel convinced of the efficacy of health intervention and perceive few difficulties in undertaking the recommended action (Rosenstock, 1974). This being the case, though socio-economic and demographic factors affect the health motivations and perceptions, they do not directly influence the health action. Rather it is determined by one's readiness to be concerned about health problems; perceptions of vulnerability to illness; perceptions of the severity of illness or its after affects; belief about the relative efficacy of alternative actions; belief about potential physical, economic and psychological costs of such actions and the critical incidents which may trigger a response (Becker, 1977).

The 'illness behaviour' is determined by the culture which ranges from doing nothing at all to extensive and prompt use of health care. Several events take place between the state of good health and sickness. While the symptoms of a disease affect everyone its perceptions, interpretations and treatment differ greatly with age, sex, race, class, ethnic group, level of education and also with the degree of susceptibility and severity.

Many health practices considered sound from a medical standpoint have proved unfunctional and many undesirable practices have proved functional for the patient and his community. By neglecting this essential truth one could ask affecting negatively the patient as well as, the society. This point is well illustrated by Mead (1960) who in relation to child birth says : "In the first place we treat childbirth not as a natural event of great significance but as an illness. We place the expectant mother in a hospital, otherwise assigned to the care of the ill; induce weakness and dependency in her by the use of drugs, straps, and soon isolate her from her husband and other children just we isolate the sick and the dying... The classification of childbirth with illness has a great variety of repercussions although our culture..." The disabling consequences of the entry into the sick role have been highlighted by many such sociological studies.

Many well-meaning health programmes have met with failure mainly because the health personnel have not taken into congnisance the perceptions of the client population. These failures have been termed as 'fallacies' by Polgar (1962, 159-205): (i) the "fallacy of empty vessel" which assumes that the local people do not have any health measures and has resulted in a failure to take into account the positive features of what already exist; (ii) the "fallacy of separate capcual" which makes health workers build programmes in terms of their own beliefs and practices; (iii) the "fallacy of single pyramid" which assumes that local people form a homogenous group; and (iv) the "fallacy of interchangeable faces" which ignores individual differences and personal relationships.

Polgar has also identified the major problems from which most health programmers suffer. He lists them under—(a) 'cultural gap' that is differences in culturally determined values and assumptions about the cause of illness; (b) 'status gap' that is, the gap between health functionaries and the people and between community leaders and common men, and (c) "urban adjustment gap" caused by migration of rural folk into cities. From a social science perspective, the health care should logically address itself to the following uses :

1. "What appears from the outside as an irrational belief and behaviour becomes intelligible when viewed from within. Perceiving the connection between items of belief and behaviour as the people themselves perceive them enables us to make better sense of the seemingly capricious pattern of acceptance and rejection of the successful and unsuccessful educational effort." Hence, there is a need to reeducate the community to accept new health values and practices.

2. The behaviour of an individual regarding the illness "is determined as much by cultural definition as by the intrinsic nature of the ailments... But what seems natural is one social milieu often appears unnatural in another." Hence, the need for health services to fit themselves to the public need instead of attempting to make the client fit the established tradition of the professional health service.

3. "The controversial issue of birth control" outcome of the decline in infant mortality and early death from communicable diseases, "rests on conflicting basic values

and is thus not subjected to scientific adjudication." Hence, there is a need to overcome widely held notions of virility, fidelity and male authority for achieving success.

4. The caste and class cleavages and conflicts among the local population and the resultant division in community interests have exerted adverse effects on several health programmes." The organisational devices that facilitate health action in one social setting may be constructive in another." Hence, there is a need to secure the cooperation of community groups through the application of the knowledge of social science.

One of the major challenges of the health programmes in the developing world is to maximise the communist participation and acceptance. This can be successfully achieved by using the findings by community organisations, interest groups, social groups and inter personal relationships and individual's perceptions, expectations and behaviour.

Pressure groups and organised special interest groups operating in the health care arena tend to exert a significant and powerful influence on the acceptance or rejection of health policies and programmes, pressure groups are of different types namely, 'religious' (that affect birth control programmes); and 'economic' (that hinder pollution control measures); and 'educational' (that oppose sex or veneral disease education in schools/ colleges). The desirable health measures in areas of smoking drugs, foods addictives, dairy products and insecticides are strongly opposed by vested interests in each field. Public opinion on such uses needs to be subjected to sociological research so that the analysis could prove helpful to the health administration in identifying areas of support and opposition and in initiating corrective measures.

Inter-personal relations and members of social groups, classes and associations are known to be powerful influence agents in the acceptance or rejection of several health practices and programmes. Such social group influences tend to work independent of the knowledge of the disease or their control measures (Cornley and Bigman, 1961). The main motivating factors in determining the response to health innovations are external such as, one's role expectations by others, what pleases other members of the group or how other members of the group would respond.

Further, the health habits and perceptions are deeply ingrained in one's personality and cannot be easily altered. According to Rosenstock (1961), a positive response of the individual to the disease control measures is determined by the belief (i) that he is susceptible to it; (ii) that its occurrence is a serious problem; and (iii) that the effective and acceptable means to control the disease exist and are available.

The use of traditional healers and magico-religious leaders is widely prevalent among the local population and faith in such agencies is found to be inversely related to the use of medical and health care facilities. The unfavourable attitude towards hospitals is more common among the illiterate and isolated communities than others. This can be observed more clearly in the care and treatment of expectant and lactating mothers, infants and in diseases believed to be associated with supernatural powers. An understanding of these and similar behaviour is necessary for ascertaining correct responses to health care.

Persons' (1951) characterisation of illness in sick-role highlights the determining role of 'significant others' in the patient's choice of the sick-role and other roles. Greenblatt *et al.* (1955) identified several areas of sociological intervention in the patient care : greater appreciation for the low level of social interaction, marked social and psychological distance between health personnel and patients, attributes/ traits of patients attracting or repelling health care personnel, ward society involving patient leaders, satellites and isolates and the role of relatives and friends in the treatment. It is now increasingly felt that the values and personality of the mental patients are influenced by all types of social interaction and not merely by contact with psychiatrists and hence, greater stress is being laid on social treatment or what is known as "social recovery" method derived from sociological principles (Cumming et al., 1956). The increased use of peaer group therapy and the assumption by patients of active and utilitarian roles within hospitals have tended to reduce the disabling effects of stay in the hospitals. The efforts to promote social interaction have tended to reduce boredom and bring a sense of normal social life. Likewise, the emotional and physical deterioration of the patient in the hospital despite successful treatment has been found to be mainly due to the unsatisfactory interaction between the patient and the health personnel. Whereas the patient is in acute need of personal attention, its absence causes emotional strain; hospital culture promotes impersonal, formal relationships and the patient is not expected to express his feeling freely and frankly (Brown, 1965). The population, which is accustomed to the dedicated and selfless healers devoted to the well-being of the people at a considerable personal sacrifice, does not find such an atmosphere conductive to early recovery and health care (Gamson and Suchman, 1963).

Mental illness is emerging as a greatest single health problem in the modern world. This is also rooted in the socio-cultural and psychological factors. For example, studies showed greater likelihood of the problem among men than women, among single persons than among married, among urban-dwellers than among ruralities and among the poor than among rich. The pressure of ones occupation, loneliness, absence of spouse to provide sympathy and support, of impersonality and anonymity and similar factors have been often attributed to the problem. The treatment of the mental health patients is also influenced by institutional factors which include, besides others, one's class position determining type of treatment, bias of health personnel in favour of institutionalised treatment, lack of psycho-therapists and training facilities and inadequate financial support (Horton and Laslie, 1970).

Many of the problems of mental health and physical disorders are believed to be rooted in emotional disturbances. The deviant behaviour is often accompanied or followed by emotional tensions and anxieties which lead to several physical ailments (Dunbar, 1947). The deviant persons, when emotionally disturbed, are less likely to remain healthy. It is because of emotional involvement that popular participation could not be enlisted in health campaigns for smallpox and rat killing.

Alcoholism and drug addiction, are now being increasingly viewed as major health problems. Though the problem varies considerably from one social group to the other, these are fast becoming part of a cultural pattern. Beginning rather tentatively, the involvement of the individual has tended to increase gradually resulting in complete demoralisation. What is puzzling however, is the fact that the use of these substances has become problem in one group but not in the other. The variation is often attributed to the degree of compatibility with the cultural and social pattern. Where these substances are associated with manliness and virility, the problem, particularly alcoholism, is widespread. Under the impact of modern life styles individuals are being increasingly subjected to great strain and seek escape in alcohol or drugs. The incidence of such problems is far greater in cases of personality disturbances, social isolation and mobility. Cultures that prohibit their use provide protection against involvement.

The main controversy in the medical circles centres around the method of treating such problems. While some argue in favour of legalising them, subjecting them to strict official control, others favour suppression and elimination of the problems. One such group holds such individuals as anti-social and argues for harsh punishment while others treat the problem as, an 'illness' and advocate measures to de-addict the patients. It is the latter view that makes these pathologies health problems.

VALUE PREMISES IN MEDICAL CARE

Socio-cultural conditions not only determine the prevalence of diseases but also greatly affect decisions on whether or not to provide health care. The advances in medical sciences, which have on the one hand exerted a discernable impact on the promotion of health and control diseases, have raised several moral and socio-economic questions pertaining to the use of medical sciences on the other (Pytlik *et al.*, 1978). The demand for highly specialised services in the medical field has resulted in the shifting of health care from home to hospitals. The humanistic aspect in the process has been relegated to the background and the easy personal, informal and intimate doctor-patient rappot has been substituted by an impersonal and formal relationship devoid of real concern to alleviate suffering and distress. In belief, the attention is shifted from the 'patient' to the 'disease' and from 'doctors' to the 'hospitals'.

An important issue highlighted by Pytlik *et al.* pertains to the controversy between medical study as opposed to the welfare of the society. Take the instance of the aged population which is growing in size steadily and showing all signs of increasing further, especially with the infant mortality rate falling sharply. Many of these old people are being kept alive by drugs are otherwise reduced to docile and inactive people. Medical discoveries have similarly made survival and reproduction possible for patients with genetic defects. The doctors are now faced with a peculiar dilemma of either denying the patient treatment or treating the patient only to place on society a growing responsibility of supporting and caring for defective people and allowing them to pass on their defects to future generations. Such decisions are ultimately social rather than medical. This controversy deepens when viewed in the context of organ transplantation : Who among thousands needing transplantation should receive an organ considering the shortage of donors? Who can be allowed to take such decisions which include some and exclude others? How can a doctor be allowed to decide whom to save and whom not to? Further, as the recipient of an organ is under a social and moral obligation to offer something in exchange to the doctor, and as failure to do so invites censure, it is difficult to decide how one can repay in kind. Also, the question of whether close relatives should be excluded from this exchange arises. The social and psychological pressures on the donors complicates the situation further.

Opinion is sharply divided on the question of the distribution of health care. While some argue that medical services should be made available only to those who ask for it, others lay stress on the provision of health services for everyone in need of it. Still others advocate the importance of educating people so that they voluntarily seek treatment, particularly those who do not view ill-health a social problem and attribute it to their own fault. Besides, the present infrastructure of health care facilities prohibit people from asking for the services they need and precludes others because of the prohibitive costs. Medical services hence needs to make room for such people as well.

STATUS OF HEALTH AND HEALTH CARE

"Illness is probably the greatest single cause of human suffering in modern society. It is doubtful if any other single circumstance produces so much poverty and dependency, so much family disruption, or so much economic inefficiency as illness" (Horton and Laslie, 1970: 531). India is no exception in this matter, the situation being quite abject as compared to many developing countries.

There exists a wrong notion that ill-health is due to the lack of medical care or that variations in health levels are due to variations in the available medical care. Health, infact, is a product of numerous variables including heredity, diet, living conditions, personal habits, cultural patterns and of course medical and health care. Each one of these is important in determining one's health status. But it so happens that poor health is invariably accompanied by low levels of medical and health care. In India, a substantial population does not have any access to medical care and others, medical needs are only partly met. The problem is actually two-fold : (i) some people do not have access to medical help when in need, and (ii) others for one reason or another do not seek medical care owing to socio-cultural and economic reasons.

The uneven access of medical and health care facilities can be attributed also to the concentration of facilities in some areas like the metropolitan can large cities with little or no facility available in rural areas. Also, the medical staff serving the rural and poorer population are comparatively less trained and have lesser specialised training as compared to those serving the urban areas and the richer population. It is evident that economic incentives weigh more than the provision of medical facilities for rural areas. Factors like the preference to work with fellow medical staff and in places with better laboratory and specialised services also contribute a great deal to the concentration of the medical staff in certain areas. The physicians' preference for establishing their practice in cities is also well known. One of the major consequences of the existing disparities in the medical and health care facilities is the prevalence of higher rates of illness and death rates in rural areas and among poorer populations. These disparities are the sharpest in cases where the diseases can be prevented or cured through medical care. The diseases include typhoid, whooping cough, dysentry, diphtheria, tuberculosis and those related to pregnancy, pneumonia and diarrhoea. The existing social discrimination among people tends to reduce the availability of medical facilities to weaker and poorer sections. The poorer sections with little or no 'influence' and money suffers from a far greater chance of having insufficient health care facilities than the richer sections of the population.

According to an ICSSR-ICMR (1981) compilation, India has developed a vast network of health care services which consumes about three-fifths of the total investment in health. The per capita government investment worked out to be Rs. 1.50 in 1956; Rs. 3.79 in 1966-67 and Rs. 10.63 in 1975-76. The total number of hospitals and dispensaries in 1979 were 17607; The Primary Health Centres accounted for 5423; the sub-centres numbered 40124, hospital beds totalled 4.49 lakhs; the qualified registered doctors added upto 2.36 lakh; homeopaths numbered 1.51 lakh the ayurvedic practitioners were 1.19 lakh, unani practitioners added upto 10.3 thousand; the sidha practitioners were 1.6 thousand; the nurses numbered 1.20 lakh and there were 1.19 lakh midwives. Besides, there was a total of 1.6 lakh non-institutionally qualified Ayurveds; 20.2 thousand Unanis; 16.6 thousand Sidhas and 55.7 thousand auxiliary midwives. However, the structure of health services remained incompatible to our culture and tradition being west-oriented, urban-based; the PHC continuing to be urban biased, mainly curative in nature and elite oriented.

As in the other sectors of the economy, the health care infrastructure also manifests the caste and class cleavages that are to be found in the larger social system. While most physicians come from upper or upper-middle class, the nurses and the staff belonging to the technical facilities are drawn from the middle socio-economic status groups and the lower level health personnel are generally drawn from the lower-middle stratum. The treatment of the patient is similarly governed not by his disease but by his status in society.

Children below five and women in the reproductive age groups (15-45) who constitute 37 per cent of our population from the largest group vulnerable to diseases. The efficiency of health services for them are closely related to family planning services, infant mortality rates and the status of women themselves. Statistical evidence shows that health services have not able to bring any marked change in this direction. The damaging infant and female mortality rates, the sex ratio, the deteriorating status of women and inept family planning programmes prove this point amply. The attitude of society which view's women basically as mothers or potential mothers has been responsible for the failure of public health programmes as they were only geared towards maternal and child health (MCH). A combination of ineffective programmes and bad nutrition has exposed this section to more diseases.

One of the important hallmarks denoting the state of health of our population is the infant mortality rates. These rates continue to be as high as 105 per thousand and 158 for those under five years of age. Of the 23 million children born every year, 2.5 million die within the first two years; one out of nine dies before reaching age of four and half of them suffer from malnutrition. Only 25 per cent of the children have been covered by the immunization programme. About 13 million of them (3000 per day) die of diseases which could be averted by immunisation. India's performance in bringing down infant mortality rates has been comparatively poor. During 1960-85, these rates were brought down from 165 to 105 in India; from 190 to 89 in Turkey; from 179 to 93 in Egypt; from 160 to 72 in Vietnam; from 150 to 36 in China; from 135 to 49 in Jordon (UNICEF 1987).

UNICEF has attributed the poor performance of India on the health front to the lack of health facilities. Approximately, 62.2 per cent of the total births is attended by untrained professionals, the corresponding proportion for rural areas is as high as 71.5 per cent. Besides, India was spending only 2.4 per cent of its total plan allocations on health as compared to 18.6 per cent in the Federal Republic of Germany; 13.4 per cent in Switzerland; 7.3 per cent in Brazil; 7.0 per cent in Kenya; 5.7 per cent in Iran and 3.2 per cent in Zaire.

Research and evaluation reveal that the status of women's health is not only lower than males but is rapidly deteriorating. The important indicators of this fact are the sex ratio, morbidity and mortality rates, age at marriage, age at child-birth, birth rates and other such data. The unbalanced sex ratio, which stood at 972 in 1901 dropped to 933 in 1981. This can be attributed to the harsh treatment received by women, the preference for a male child over a female child; the poor access of health facilities, and inadequate post-natal facilities. Women and female children have higher death rates upto 35 years of age. The early marriages teenage pregnancies, early child-births and a succession of births have enhanced the chances of maternal and infant mortality. Though the average age of marriages has increased to 17.16 years in 1971 and 18.32 years in 1981, 7 per cent of the girls of 10-14 years of age and 43 per cent of 15-19 years of age were already married in 1981. The death rates of the population has registered a steady decline from 42.6 in 1901 to 12.4 in 1981 and the infant mortality rates dropped from 204 in 1911-1915 to 146 in 1951-1961. However, the birth rate continues to be high. These rates continue to be unfavourable for women as compared to men. Women are highly vulnerable to malnutrition and uncontrolled fertility. While they need additional calories during pregnancy and lactation, the actual intake has been found to be deficient by over 1000 calories.

The explanations for the sharp decline in death rates should not be sought solely from the advances of medical science and improvement in the health infrastructure but a look into the non-medical realm is essential. In the advanced countries, mortality rate came down following a sharp rise in the food production and supplies that helped in averting starvation deaths. It is then not unlikely that effective control of famines since 1920's by transporting food from one region to another through the innovation of railways by the Britishers has contributed greatly in bringing down mortality rates. The support for such an observation comes from higher morbidity rates and higher malnutrition among landless as compared to land-owning classes (Kielman and Oberoi, 1972). The association between mortality and malnutrition is widely known (Chen, 1980). The male-female as well as rural-urban divide are the manifestation of the same reality. In Punjab, there was greater malnutrition among female children (71.4%) as compared to males (28.6%) (Govt. of Punjab 1974). Higher death rates among females as compared to males can be explained by different levels of malnutrition among them.

The tendency to attribute the decline in death rates to the advances in the field of medicine and the expansion of health facilities is also questioned on the ground that the death rates began to decline ever since 1920 when the medical sciences in India were not as developed as it is today and that the crude death rates also registered a sharp decline by the 1960's when the health services were still in the process of being organised and expanded.

Clearly, poverty and malnutrition combined with the inaccessibility of health services have emerged to be the major contributory factors for the poor health of the masses. The fact that the class system has been the key determinant to the accessibility and availability of health services is well recognised today (Banerji, 1981). How class position influences one's health needs hardly any explanation. Obviously, it tends to influence the living and working conditions such as earning capacity, purchasing power, nutritional status and housing and sanitary conditions. Poor living and working conditions are known for their detrimental effects on morbidity and mortality rates. The class status also determines one's ability to face natural calamities like droughts and famines. During such periods, the employment ratio drops and assets are transferred to the rich resulting in the inaccessibility of food and health care; and disease and misery become rampant. In these circumstances, massive investment in production programmes benefiting mostly to the rich are launched and priority is given to specialised health services at the cost of primary health care which tends to make the life of the poor far more miserable.

Further, the socio-cultural explanations for the depressing health scenario is not without substance. Poverty tends to exert a negative influence on the standard of living and make the surroundings conducive for the eruption of diseases; the poor quality of food and low nutrition bring down the resistance to these diseases; illiteracy leads to ignorance about health and disease-causing factors and influences treatment-seeking behaviour. The socio-economic inequalities therefore, leads to the deterioration in health standards and in the ability to control diseases.

Nutrition improvement programmes have provided great support to the health care projects in India. While starvation death figures are insignificant, the morbidity and mortality figures due to malnutrition and undernutrition are quite alarming. Malnutrition, which makes people more prone to infection and decreases resistance to overcome it, is severe among women and children. Besides, the problem of under-nourishment is causing serious concern due to its manifestation in the form of Vitamin-A deficiency, anemia and goitre. The Malnutrition, according to Dr. P.V. Sukhatme, is estimated to be 25 per cent in urban areas and 15 per cent in rural areas. About 45 million children are believed to be undernourished and need an extra 300 calories per day. Over three-fifths of the households consume inadequate diets. The different programmes launched to remedy the situation fall into two broad categories : programmes to remove some nutritional deficiencies (Goitre control, iron deficiency, anemia, Vitamin-A prophylaxis programmes) and supplementary feeding programmes (Applied Nutrition Programmes, Supplementary Feeding and Integrated Child Development Scheme and Mid-Day Meal Programmes.) Being ad hoc in nature and inadequate in scope, these have not been able to make a dent into the serious problem and no marked improvement has been noticed in the nutritional status particularly of women and children.

The problems of malnutrition and undernutrition are to a great extent influenced by food, fads and fallacies. Such beliefs tend to undermine the confidence of the people in the nutritive value of certain foods, encourage them to ignore medical diagnosis, advice and care and mislead them into buying and using foods not needed or even harmful to health. Such beliefs are associated not only with foods supposed to cure a disease or result in rapid body growth and strength or change in complexion but also with food believed to be sacred and auspicious and related to gods and spirits. In fact, food has become a formidable source of joy, pleasure, status, prosperity and strong inter-personal ties.

It is not surprising that people easily succumb to such false notions particularly when there exists widespread illiteracy, poverty and disease, and tend to seek easy and cheaper solutions which lead to dietary deficiencies and malnutrition and undernutrition. The growth of industrialisation and education and the onset of urban influence have significantly and altered the traditional food beliefs and practices and in the process low cost, locally available and nutritionally rich dietary practices have been replaced by costly and less nutritious options based mainly on the status of an individual.

Besides maldistribution of food and poor purchasing power, which are major constraints, unscientific cooking practices, dietary habits, alcoholism and drug addiction and even wasteful expenditures on medical care often reduce the money available for essential foods and in the process women and children are often deprived of their due share. Infact, India represents a dual society where a small group is well fed while the masses are undernourished. The rich sections of society face no shortage of food but suffer from disease which affect the affluent—over eating for instance, as in case of developed countries. In contrast, malnutrition is often noticeable in severe forms among the poor agricultural labourers, scheduled castes and tribes, urban-dwellers and among women and children. The development programmes could not alter the situation much (ICSSR-ICMR, 1981).

As a major support to the health care system, emphasis has also been laid on providing a clean, hazard-free environment which includes the provision of safe drinking water the proper disposal of waste, improved housing, control of pollution and a check on the adverse effects of industrialisation. Among these, the provision of safe drinking water is of great importance for health but while a significant per cent of urban population was covered only one out of ten villages have adequate water supply of accepted quality; over 2.1 lakh villages have adequate water supply but with pollution risks; another 1.85 lakh villages have adequate but unprotected supply sources. There are still 1.53 lakh problem villages. With no check on the poor quality of water, outbreaks of water-borne diseases are frequent. The scheduled castes face the added problem of inaccessibility to common water sources. (ICSSR-ICMR,1981).

Associated closely with the problems of health and disease is the question of size, distribution and quality of our population. In India, the annual addition to population is more than any other country in the world. With only 2.4 per cent of the world's surface area, India's share in world population is one in every seven person. With the present fertility rates, India's population is likely to be 1480 million by the year 2021 A.D. India's population, which stood at 238 million in 1901, has registered a three-fold increase to 685 million by 1981. This is mainly due to the rapid socio-economic development and elaborate health and medical care facilities which have brought about a sharp decline in mortality rates from 42.6 in 1911 to 27.4 in 1951 and 11.1 per thousand in 1986. However, this decline has not been followed by a decline in the birth rates which remained as high as 33.9 per thousand in 1981 and 32.9 in 1985 as against 49.2 in 1911 (Govt. of India, 1988). The high birth rate coupled with a sharp decline in the death rate and the galloping growth in population is posing a serious threat to our well-being. Under the circumstances, birth control measures and family planning programmes assume great importance.

The National Family Planning Programme which started in 1951 with a clinical approach was subsequently expanded into a community oriented service programme which provided family planning services as part and parcel of the overall health package of services including maternity, child health and nutrition. Under the contraception programme, 55 per cent of the couples in the 30-44 age group and 16 per cent of those "below 30" age group were covered. It implies that of the 133 million eligible couples about 50 million have been protected by the contraception programme. By 2000 A.D., the number of eligible couples would rise to 170 millions out which 60 per cent is proposed to be covered by the programme. According to the Government of India estimates, 85 million births have been averted since the inception of the programme (Govt. of India 1988). The inter-state comparison, however, points out that whereas 75 per cent couples in Kerala, 53.6 per cent in Punjab, 53 per cent in Himachal Pradesh and 52 per cent in Haryana were protected, the score in Uttar Pradesh has most deplorable with couple protection rate of only 20.6 per cent (*The Hindustan Times*, dated 5-2-1988). The failure of the family planning programmes has been primarily due to the socio-economic considerations or handicaps involved; religious customs and traditions opposing the idea; perception of child birth as god's gift; male superiority and obsession with sons; perception of a child as an additional source of income; high infant mortality rates acting as a disincentive and the concept of family planning education looked upon as absence (Mohan Dharia, 1989).

The problem has become more acute because of the uneven distribution of population among different regions and groups. The largest pick up on population is observed in the favourable agro-climatic regions cities, and towns. When survival is at stake and competition is sharp, theoretically the fittest would survive according to Darwin's notion of survival of the fittest. However, among humans, survival is not simply governed by biological competition; cultural values, beliefs and attitudes play a significant role and serious efforts are being made as part of health care programmes to reduce the mortality rates among the infants and children—the weakest among the humans. It is however, feared that if the weak are protected through human interference, the quality of population is bound to be lowered.

Apprehensions about lowering of the quality of population through birth control measures are also expressed. As birth rates are generally higher among the rural population as compared to their urban compatriots and among the poorer socio-economic status groups than among the richer ones, (the latter groups are more open to the idea of limiting their families, marrying at later age and making greater use of birth control measures) the share of rural and underprivileged groups in the population is likely to increase which then logically implies a decline in the quality of population. These foreseeable implications have forced some people to advocate compulsory sterilisations to bring the birth rate at par with the death rate. But this option brings with it serious complications at the social, cultural and religious levels. Those who oppose population control measures argue that the decline in fertility can be brought about only through socio-economic progress; the elimination of basic causes of high fertility like poverty and ignorance; through a redistribution of wealth and resources; the provision of employment and means of subsistence; radical changes in widely held beliefs such as that a - woman's status is determined by number of children she bears, that children provide security in old age, that certain fertility control measures are risk, prone and that the modern population control programme is unnatural, immoral and an interference in the personal domain by the government — by ensuring an even distribution of the population and by exercising restraint on the over-consumption of scarce resources by the rich few. India's development policy and programmes are trying to address themselves to both meticulously planned programmes on fertility control as also to the improvement of the living conditions of the masses.

A great significance needs to be attached to the movement known as "Health for All By the Year 2000 A.D." by the Health Assembly of WHO and its reaffirmation by the Alma Ata Conference in 1978. The goal was later on endorsed by the U.N.O. India was one of the signatories to the declaration. In order to achieve the "Health for All", goal the government of India formulated strategies and programmes and the Working Group appointed by the Planning Commission set up goals to be achieved by the year 2000 A.D. which include, besides others, the bringing down of infant mortality rates from 125 to 60; raising expectation of life at birth from 52 to 64; reducing the crude death rate from 33 to 21 per 1000; reducing the crude birth rate from 14 to 9 per 1000; the achieving of a net reproduction rate of 1 and the provision of potable water to the entire rural population by the year 1990 (Govt. of India, 1985). The Ramalingaswami study group set up jointly by ICSSR-ICMR to study and suggest measures to restructure the existing health care services, noted the incompatibility of our health care system which is top-heavy, over centralised, costly and dependency—creating and called for a coordinate, collaborative, cooperative and multi-disciplinary comprehensive approach to health care. The recognition of the validity of the social science approach to health care is evident, in the emphasis being laid on socio-cultural factors, education, environmental and nutritional dimensions along side curative aspects. The arguments in favour of improving the status of women in order to improve the quality of population also goes in favour of this approach. (ICSSR-ICMR, 1981).

These are some issues which are central to any discussion on the sociology of health. The contributors whose names have been included in this volume have tried to address themselves to one or more of the issues and problems identified above. Keeping in view the main focus, papers were tentatively categorised into six parts : (i) Introduction (ii) Health and Disease : Socio-Cultural Determinants; (iii) Health Status and Structural Framework; (iv) Medical Profession and Institutional Setting; (v) Dynamics of Population; and Health; and (vi) Health, Nutrition and Society.

Tracing the historical framework of the health policy in India, B.K. Nagla and Madhu Nagla have provided an analysis of the work of different committees appointed since Independence to advise the Government of India on the country's health problems and their solutions. The recommendations of these committees have shaped the organisational structure of the health care services. Authors, however, feel that no one system has yet been able to encompass the large population of the country and hence there is a need for a comprehensive health policy compatible with the Indian conditions which lays emphasis on health care rather than the medical aspects.

Probing into the history and cultural origins of medicine and analysing the varying conceptions of health and diseases, A.L.Srivastava and S.D. Saxena tried to seek explanations from both the bio-physical as well as socio-cultural forces. The authors, therefore argue in favour of according a significant role to social scientists for better health care services and effective diseases control programmes.

K.L. Pokarna has noted the dominant role played by the traditional healers in the treatment of diseases through magico-religious, herbal and massage therapies. The existing beliefs and practices tend to make the prevention and control of disease difficult and hence need to be redefined so that they become culturally acceptable.

In their study of traditional healers, K.P. Shukla and C.P. Misra have observed that this profession is either a familial tradition or a person gains informal training in the profession. The wide use of magico-religious therapy with or without a combination of herbal treatment is commented upon. The preference of traditional healers over the institutional agencies has been attributed by them to the easy, prompt, cheaper and personal services.

In her paper on the patient and his illness, Madhu Nagla examines the social background of the patients and analyses the sick-role to gain an understanding of their behaviour and reactions towards treatment in the hospital.

Based on the Haryana experience, Pushpa Pasrija *et al*, attempts a sociological analysis of the health care delivery system. The study reveals that private practitioners are consulted more than community health volunteers and primary health centres, particularly in areas modestly covered by institutional services Beliefs in supernatural powers being the cause of certain diseases are widely prevalent, the study says.

Nirupama Prakash and A.L. Srivastava observed that delays in admission to the hospital and subsequently between admission and operation/treatment of patients with fractured neck of femur because of several prohibitive socio-cultural factors lead to the deterioration in the functional status of the patients.

Providing a psycho-social perspective to health, Praveen Kaur and M.L. Sharma report the profound influence of emotional factors like anger, anxiety, depression, helplessness and hopelessness on several diseases such as hypertension and asthma. The authors advocate the use of psychology in such cases.

Aneeta A. Minocha tries to examine a few key concepts pertaining the socio-economic equality in health and health care and concludes that the goal of equity in health is unattainable as economic status is not always related directly to health status.

Imrana Qadeer attempts to assess the standards of health with the advancement of medical sciences and the expansion of medical facilities to fulfil the objective of health for all. The author tries to trace the origin of poor health with the help of socio-cultural and environmental factors. Pointing to the distorted priorities in the health services, the author questions the justifications offered for the emphasis or curative and preventive fields at the cost of public health, thereby making health care rich and urban-biased.

Monica Sharma probes into the status and problems of maternal health care programmes and notes the negative effects of the socio-cultural practices and disparity in health care facilities. She calls for articulate policies and strategies to improve health which lay stress on changes in social prejudices and the provision of non-health facilities.

A socio-cultural analysis of maternity and child health has been attempted by Malkit Kaur. She notes that the beliefs and practices concerning the birth and care of the infant are governed by ignorance, conservatism and superstitions and calls for effective education to avert maternity and child mortality.

Sarla Mukhi in her assessment of the state of health status of the youth outlines the problems arising out of bio-drives and those arising due to the conflict between bio-needs and psycho-social forces in the wake of technological advancement. The strategies to cope with them are also discussed.

A systematic attempt to understand occupation related health problems was made by the National Commission on Self Employed Women and Women in Informal Sector by studying the various women-dominated occupations, the activities involved the working hours and effects of work on their nutritional status and physical and mental health. The study clearly brings out the type of physical stress the women workers are subjected to the damaging postural positions and their effects and the harmful effects of the noxious maternal used. While examining specific health problems involved in specific activity, the study offers suggestions to minimise health hazards.

In their analysis of the relationship between housing and disease, Sashi Srivastava and M.N. Srivastava observed the connections between types of houses and the diseases they foster. Such a relationship is not, however, perceived by the common man.

K.V. Ramana and B. Vijaya Lakshmi provide an insight into the gradual shift by the medical professionals from a purely clinical approach to a non-medical and psycho-social orientation in patient care. Social work which in the past showed a concern for interpersonal and social problems now provides the much needed social inputs in the field of medicine where success depends on the community approach to problems of health. The traditional beliefs and practices which are to blame for many health problems are structurally and culturally determined and hence can be changed only through community participation.

Recognising that the inability to provide timely medical treatment lies in a failure to communicate with the people Neerja Sharma probes into different aspects of the conversational approach in the doctor-patient relationship and examines its role in the treatment of diseases.

A.L. Srivastava and S.D. Saxena probe into the active participation and functional involvement of allied health personal of the hospital in the care and treatment of patients and note that though humanitarian considerations are discernible, a close interaction with the patient is lacking.

Ramesh Chandra tries to discern the relationship between population, family size and quality of life as measured in terms of income, food, health, housing, living space, education and recreation. A small family norm is stressed. Examining the issue of female survival,

Kuntal Agarwal considers the increase in sex determination tests, and abortion of female foetuses thereafter. The tendency is more pronounced among the highly educated in urban areas than in rural areas, and in the service class as compared to the business class. Women too are in favour of this procedure, the study underlines.

The relevance of population to health policies and programmes is examined by G.S. Somawat. He concludes that the current health projects are inadequate and advocates drastic changes.

An attempt has been made to assess the utilisation of health and family planning services by Malkit Kaur *et al.* Though the access and use are limited, the impetus given to these programmes has exerted a positive influence. The authors also highlight the role of socio-cultural factors in promoting and hindering the use of health innovations.

Neerja Sethi *et al.* attempt to assess the health needs of the older people in the context of the prevailing social and infrastructural framework and formulate an action plan within the available resources.

T.M. Dak and M.L. Sharma try to assess the deteriorating effects of the recent changes in the traditional social institutions of the elderly persons and examine the effects of various measures initiated for the persons and examine the effects of various measures initiated for the welfare of the aged.

Musafir Singh in his analysis highlights the profound influence of socio-cultural factors on food consumption and nutrition and argues further adoption of culturally acceptable approaches for effecting changes in food habits.

In her paper, Nila Chhatrapati attempts to examine the nexus between taboos, food and society and clarifies food interdicts on the basis of duration and volume of the interdict as also on the type of group to which it applies. The paper provides a cultural perspective on food behaviour in different societies and on different social occasions the knowledge of which according to the author may help in effective implementation of the nutritional improvement programmes.

The problem of malnutrition and undernutrition is examined in the context of social and economic framework of Indian society by Salil Sehgal and Asha Kawatra. The authors argue in favour of launching a multi-pronged attack on the problem involving changes in the production strategy, distribution system, nutritional education and a change in the beliefs and practices concerning foods.

Using the 32nd Round of NSS (1977-78), U.K. Pandey *et al.* draw a parallel between poverty and nutrition. The authors points to the deficiency in food and nutrition intake and the glaring inequalities in the food consumption in poor and rich areas. The intake of food tends to increase with the increase in food supply.

Sunita Gupta probes into the causative factors underlying the problem of malnutrition in India and examines the effects of malnutrition on brain functions and psycho-social behaviour as manifested in maladaptive, maladjusted and deviant behaviour

The problem of drug-abuse among university students is examined by Sailesh Darshan and M.L.Sharma. The authors concluded that while alcohol and tobacco are used by all sections of the society, psychotropic drugs are used more frequently by university students. While sex-differential were predominant, disturbing trend towards self-medication was noted. The breaking down of the traditional barriers of abstinence and other sociocultural restrictions have been found to be main reasons for the increase in drug-abuse.

References

1. Ackerknecht, E.H., "Primitive Medicine and Culture Pattern," *Bulletin of the History of Medicine*, XII, 545-574, 1942.

2. Banerji, D., *Poverty, Class and Health Culture in India*, Vol. I, Prachi Prakashan, NewDelhi,1981.

3. Banks, A. Laslie, *Social Aspects of Disease*, Edward Arnold and Co., London, 1953.

4. Basu, S. C., *Handbook of Preventive and Social Medicine*, Current Books International, 1977.

Becker, Marshall, H. " Psychosocial Aspects of Health-Related behaviour," In Freedman, Howard E. *et al.* (eds.), *Handbook of Medical Sociology*, Prentice-hall Inc., New Jersey, 1977.

6. Boek Walter, E. and Hilleboe, Herman E. "Role of a Social Scientist in Public Health." *Human Organisation* XIV, 25, 1956.

7. Brown, Esther Lucile, *Newer Dimensions of Patient Care*, Part - III, Russel Sage Foundations, New York, 1965.

8. Carstairs, Morris, G., "Medicine and Faith in Rural Rajasthan," in Paul Benjamin D. (ed.) *Health, Culture and Community*, Russel Sage Foundation, New York, 1955.

9. Coe, Rodney, M., *Sociology of Medicine*, McGraw-hill Book Co., New York, 1978.

10. Cornely, Paurl B. and Bigman, Stanley K. *Cultural Considerations in Changing Health Attitudes*, Harward University, (mimeographed) Washington, p.169, 1961.

11. Dharia, Mohan, "Population Problem," *The Hindustan Times*, New Delhi, July 20, 1989.

12. Dunbar, Helen Flanders, *Mind and Body; Psychosomatic Medicine*, Random House, New York, 1947.

13. Fillozat, J., *The Classical Doctrine of Indian Medicine*, Munshi Ram Manohar Lal, Allahabad, 1964.

14. Foster George M., "Public Health and Behavioural Science: the Problems of Team Work" *American Journal of Public Health*, LI (Sept.) 1290, 1961.

15. Gamson, William A. and Suchman, Howard, "Some Undercurrents in the Prestige of Physicians" *American Journal of Sociology*, LXVIII (Jan.,) 468, 1963.

16. Govt. of Haryana, *Economic Survey of Haryana*, 1988-89; *Economic and Statistical Organisation, Planning Department*, Chandigarh, 1989.

17. Govt. of India, *Health For All By 2000 A.D.: Report of the Working Group*, Ministry of Health and Family Welfare, New Delhi, 1981.

18. Govt. of India, *India's Population : Demographic Scenaried*, Department of FamilyWelfare, Ministry of Health and Family Welfare, 1988.

19. Govt. of Punjab, *Nutrition in Punjab*, Punjab Nutrition Development Project, Govt. of Punab and CARE, 1974.

20. Graham, Sazon and Reeder, Leo G., 'Social Epidemiology of Chronic Diseases ' In Freeman, Howard E., *et al.* (eds) *Handbook of Medical Sociology*, Prentice-Hall Inc. New Jersey, 1977.

21. Greenblatt, Milton *et al., From Custodial to Therapeutic Patient Care in Mental Hospitals: Explorations on Social Treatment*, Russel Sage Foundation, New York, 1955.

22. Grotjahn, Alfred, *Soziale Pathologie*, August Hirschwald, Verlag, Berlin, pp. 9-18, 1915.

23. Grotjahn, Alfred, *Soziale Pathologie*, quoted in George Rosen, "Approaches to a Concept of Social Medicine: A Historical Survey", Milbank Memorial Hall, New York, p.18, 1949.

24. Gu'erin, Jules, Medicine Social, Au Corps medicale de France, *Gazette Medicale de Paris* (March 11): 203, 1948.

25. Hasan, K.A., *The Cultural Frontiers of Health in Village* India, Manaktalas, Bombay, 1967.

26. Hall, Oswald, "Sociological Research in the field of Medicine" *American Sociological Review*, XV(Oct.) : 639, 1951.

27. Hindustan Times "*Billion-Mark Scare*", December 5, 1988, New Delhi, 1988.

28. Horton, Paul B., and Laslie, Gerald R., *Sociology of Social Problems*, Appleton, Century-Crofts, New York, 1970.

29. Hyman, Martind., "Medicine" In Lazarsfeld, Paul F. *et al.* (eds.) *The Uses of Sociology*, Weidenfeld and Nicolson, London, pp. 119-49, 1968.

30. ICSSR and ICMR, *Health for All : An Alternative Strategy*, Indian Institute of Education, Pune,1981.

31. Indian Council of Medical Research, *Dietary Allowances for Indians*, ICMR Special Report Series No. 60, New Delhi, 1971.

32. Kielman, A.A. and Oberoi, I.S., *Interaction of Nutrition and Infection : A Prospective Field Study on Children in Selected Villages of Punjab; Rural Health Research Centre*, Ludhiana, 1972.

33. Knowles, John H., "Introduction" In Howard E. Freedman, Sol, Levine and Leo. G. Reader (eds.) *Handbook of Medical Sociology*, Prentice Hall Inc. New Jersey, 1979.

34. Kroeger, G., *The Concept of Social Medicine* as presented by Physicians and other writer in Germany: 1919-1932, Julius Rosenwald Fund, Chicago, pp. 14, 15, 1937.

35. Leavell Hugh, R., 'Foreword' In : Benjamin D. Paul (ed.) *Health, Culture and Community*, Russel Sage Foundation, New York, 1955.

36. Marriott, Mckim, " Western Medicine in a Village in Northern India", In Benjamin D. Paul (ed.) *Health, Culture and Community*, Russel Sage Foundation, New York, 1955.

37. Mead, Margarett, cited in Macgregor, F.C., *Social Science in Nursing*, Russel Sage Foundation, New York, 1960.

38. Mechanic, David, *Medical Sociology*, The Free Press, New York, 1962.

39. Merton Robert, K.' Problem Finding in Sociology' In Robert K. Merton *et al.* (eds.) *Sociology Today*, Basic Books, New York, 1959.

40. Morris, J.N., *Four Cheers for Prevention*, Proceedings of Royal Society of Medicine, 66:225, 1973.

41. Mounting, Joseph W. 'Foreword' In Milton I., Roemer and Ethel A. Wilson, *Organised Health Service in a Country of the United States*, U.S. Public Health Service, Publication 197, Govt. Printing Office, Washington, 1951.

42. National Commission on Self-Employed Women and Women in Informal Sector, Shramshakti, Govt. of India, Deptt. of Women and Child Welfare, New Delhi, 1988.

43. Parsons, Talcott 1988, *The Social System*, The Free Press, Glencoe, Illinois, 1951.

44. Paul, Benjamin, D. (ed.), *Health, Culture and Community: Case Studies of Reactions to Health Programmes*, Russel Sage Foundation, New York, 1955.

45. Polgar, Steven, "Health and Human Behaviour: Areas of Interest Common to the Social and Medical Sciences," *Current Anthropology*, III, 159-205, 1962.

46. Pytlik, Edward C., Landa, Donald P., Johnson, David L., *Technology, Change and Society*, Davis Publications Inc.. Massachusetts, 1978.

47. Robinson, C.E.A., Social Sciences and Mental Health, *Canadian Journal of Public Health*, LIV, 157, 1940.

48. Roney, James G. Jr. "Social Sciences in the Teaching of Public Health" *Journal of Health and Human Behaviour*, I, 1940.

49. Rosen, George, The Evolution of Social Medicine, In Freedman Howard E. et al (eds.) *Handbook of Medical Sociology*, Prentice Hall Inc.. New Jersey, 1977.

50. Rosen, George, *A History of Public Health*, M.D. Publications, New York, 1958.

51. Rosenstock, Irwin M., "Public Acceptance of Influenza Vaccination," *America Review of Respiratory Disease*, p. 172, 1961.

52. Rosenstock, I.M., "Historical Origin of Health Belief Model," *Health Education Monographs II* (Winter): 328-35, 1974.

53. Rochoux, J.A., *These de Concours pour la chaire d'hygiene*, (presentee et Soutenue la Janvier,1938), De Rignoux et Cie., p. 28, 1838.

54. Sigerist, H.B., *The Great Doctors*, Doubleday Anchor, New York 1960.

55. Sigerist, H.B., *"On the History of Medicine"*, In Felix Marti-Ibanez (ed.) M.D. Publications, New York, 1960.

56. Straus, Robert, "The Nature and Status of Medical Sociology", *American Sociological Review*, April, 200-204, 1957.

57. Straus, Robert, and Clausen, John A., "Health,Society and Social Science", *Annals of the American Academy of Political and Social Science*. CCCXLVI, 6-7, 1963.

58. Suchman, Edward A., "Social Patterns of Illness and Medical Care, " *Journal of Health and Human Behaviour*, VI (Sprint), 2-16, 1965.

59. Suchman, Edward A., 'Public Health' In Lazarsfeld, Paul F *et al.* (eds.) *The Uses of Sociology.* Weidenfeld and Nicolson, London, pp. 567-611, 1968.

60. Thomas, Mc Keown, *The Modern Rise of Population*, Arnold Publishers Ltd., 1976.

61. UNICEF, *The State of the World Children*, UNICEF, 1987.

62. Virchow, Rudolf, *Scientific Methods and Therapeutic Standpoints*, 1849.

17

Low Utilisation of MCH Care Services–Suggestions for Improvement

With an objective to ultimately improve the M.C.H. care services in the country, the I.C.M.R. undertook a situational analysis study in 9 P.H.Cs, one in each State, with regard to the physical facilities existing, the services provided for by the staff and the community perception and utilisation of their services.

Orissa was included in this multicentric project and the present study was conducted in one of the blocks of the State serving a population of 1,20,509 in 154 villages.

Communication facilities in the block where the P.H.C. is situated was found to be extremely poor. Even when spread over both sides of the major district road, though unevenly, only 12 per cent of villages were served by Pucca and another 80 per cent by Kutcha roads. Rest had no road facilities at all. Bus and auto services were available in 18 per cent villages and telephone facilities extended to only 10 per cent villages and most of them were owned by private individuals.

Regarding the availability of health care services it was seen that nearly 12 per cent villages were within 5 km of P.H.C. Headquarters. But 90 per cent were within 5 km of their respective sub-centres indicating that minimum service facilities were available within walking distance.

The staff position of both P.H.C. and sub-centres was found to be reasonably good and most staff were in position.

In spite of this elaborate health infrastructure both the delivery and utilisation of services were extremely poor. To cite an example only 49 per cent of the expected pregnancies were registered by the P.H.C. staff. Record maintenance was equally poor. Of the 22 sub-centres under study only 3 sub-centres had trimester-wise registration of pregnancy cases.

Regarding antenatal and postnatal care services, all L.H.Vs and A.N.Ms, did abdominal palpation to find out the presentation and position of the foetus and conducted physical examination to detect anaemia and oedema of feet, but none examined the urine or checked blood pressure. None of the L.H.Vs, and A.N.Ms, enquired about fever during their postnatal visits.

Distribution of Iron and Folic acid tablets was unsatisfactory. Only 65 per cent of the registered pregnant women received 30-90 tablets of Iron and Folic acid, 62 per cent cases received 2 or more doses of T.T. and 63 per cent women were paid 2 postnatal visits.

Regarding delivery services it was observed that 80 per cent of deliveries were conducted by T.B.As or untrained *Dais* and all the recorded cases were domiciliary in nature.

All the L.H.Vs and A.N.Ms, did not monitor the weight of the child nor did they pay any attention to common infections of the baby.

Records were not available for births, deaths, maternal and neonatal deaths either at the sub-centre or at P.H.C. indicating extreme poor record maintenance system.

Regarding the background of the community served by the Health Centre, more than 98 per cent of the respondents were Hindus, the rest being Muslim. Majority of the families (64%) belonged to joint family and nearly 76 per cent respondents had a pre-school child in their family.

Regarding economic status it was seen that nearly 1/3rd of families had an annual income below Rs. 3,500 per annum.

Out of total 500 respondents, 50 per cent were males and 50 per cent were females (according to the design provided by I.C.M.R.). The mean age of male respondents was 35.17 years and that of females 29.4 years. The overall male and female literacy was 83.2 per cent and 58.4 per cent respectively.

It was satisfying to note that 87.0 per cent respondents were aware of the presence of birth attendants in the village.

Most of the deliveries were conducted at home by untrained *dais* because they were cheap and easily available and 93.8 per cent respondents stated that they had their last child birth at home. Hospital attendance for last delivery increased with increase of educational status.

Out come of last delivery was live birth in 98.4 per cent cases and still birth in 1.6 per cent and all still birth occurred in domiciliary deliveries.

It was interesting to note that 62.4 per cent females and 47.6 per cent males stated that the quantity of diet during pregnancy should be less. The reasons offered for taking less food was to keep the women fit, avoid lethargy and for smooth and easy delivery of the child. Only 7.2 per cent respondents advocated for more diet, the reason was to keep the women healthy and active and for better foetal growth.

Antenatal care was advocated and 69.4 per cent respondents stated that antenatal check up should be done. According to them it was necessary for safe and smooth delivery, to know about foetal growth and for seeking advice for complications.

Unfortunately 82.8 per cent respondents stated that they were not contacted by the government functionaries during last pregnancy. Only 17.2 per cent respondents were contacted. The reasons of contact were primarily to give Tetanus Toxoid injection and Iron and Folic acid tablets.

Majority of respondents preferred the homoeopathic private practitioners for their child's illness. The second preference was for M.B.B.S. doctors. The reasons of choice being better quality and efficient treatment.

Nearly 11 per cent mothers breast-fed their child on 1st or 2nd day and 1.6 per cent mothers did not breast-fed their child at all. These mothers had no idea about colostrum but still they breast-fed their child on 1st and 2nd day as a routine practice. In case of 24 per cent infants breast-feeding was prolonged for more than 2 years.

Only 4.6 per cent respondents stated that the baby's weight was recorded at birth and that too mostly by doctors or nurses. Regarding the size, 56.8 per cent respondents were of the opinion that the size of the baby should be big. Females comparatively preferred smaller babies than males. The preference for small baby was for easy and smooth delivery. The reasons for big baby was for rapid and luxuriant growth. The preference for bigger babies increased with educational level of respondents.

Almost half of the respondents pointed out that doctors should conduct delivery. Next they preferred the village *dais* and the trained *dai*. The preference for the doctors was due to their higher qualification and experience. Untrained *dais* were preferred for their easy availability and being less expensive.

Regarding place of delivery 52.6 per cent respondents chose home to be the preferred place for delivery. Next to home the other places were hospital, P.H.C., sub-centre. Female respondents preferred home while males chose P.H.C. and sub-centre for conducting delivery.

RECOMMENDATIONS

1. Record maintenance system needs to be improved both at Sub-Centre and P.H.C. levels. Recording of vital events such as birth, death (infant, maternal, neonatal), antenatal, post-natal, immunisation registers to be maintained.

2. The M.C.H. services are to be revamped. On the job training to be provided to the staff for better functioning. Domiciliary visits to be increased by the M.C.H. staffs. The importance of blood pressure measurements, urine examination and physical examination, growth and development monitoring should be emphasised.

3. The untrained *dais*, T.B.A.s are to be given training regarding asepsis and safe delivery practice.

4. Colostrum feeding to be promoted in the community by health education activities.
5. Importance for balanced diet during pregnancy is to be advocated.
6. Supervision and continuing education of staff members to be emphasised.
7. Management in the weakest link in the system, needs to be improved.
8. Inter-sectoral and multi-sectoral coordinations are to be promoted as non-health component in health care system are also equally important.
9. Drugs and equipments, supply line is to be maintained.
10. A regular system of feedback is extremely important to improve the services and such a mechanism needs to be ensured.

Finally accountability of the staff members have to be ensured.

18

On Utilisation of Rural Health Services in Madhya Pradesh

INTRODUCTION

Health is an important component of quality of life of the people; therefore health and family welfare services have been made as essential part of the economic and social developmental programmes in India right from the beginning of Independent era. The formation of network of these services was slow in the beginning (because of constraints of resources) but picked up momentum in successive five-year plans when services expanded rapidly. Today, we have one health guide and one trained *Dai* for every village (of about 1000 population), two para-medical workers–one male and one female—for a sub-centre of 5000 population and three medical officers, a large number of para-medical staff and a Block Extension Educator at Primary Health Centres for a population of 100,000. This rural infrastructure has support of extensive referral services at Taluka, District, State and National level; each successive level has greater sophistication in medical services. For backward and inaccessible areas like tribal populations and hilly terrains, the infrastructure is still more intensive and there is one sub-centre for 3000 population (instead of 5000). The efforts on to expand this infrastructure still further and have one Primary Health Centre for 30,000 population and one Community Health Centre with specialists' services for 100,000 people.

Though a vast network of health service infrastructure has been built, it is felt that its utilisation has not been adequate—rather it is under-utilised. People still either use their home remedies (reflecting less faith in the available services) or go to the private practitioners some of whom are not even adequately trained. It is particularly so in rural areas where large fraction of sub-centres and Primary Health Centres are ignored by the clients who crowd the Taluka, District, State or National health service units which should really be serving as referral units. This pattern of utilisation has affected quality of services at all levels—the low patronage of services in rural areas (sub-centres and Primary Health Centres) has disheartened the staff there who have lost interest in work in such areas and over-crowding in hospitals has affected degree of attention which is necessary for quality services.

It is therefore necessary to understand the reasons for under-utilisation of the health necessary to understand the reasons for under-utilisation of the health services in rural areas so that efforts can be made to improve its utilisation, thereby affecting overall quality of health services. This article has three-fold objectives : first to show the extent of utilisation of health services in rural areas, then to point out the reasons for under-utilisation and in the end to suggest how such utilisation can be improved.

OBJECTIVES

The broad objective of this article is to suggest how utilisation of health services in rural areas in India can be improved. This will be done in two stages, first by listing some indicators to show the degree of utilisation of the health services and then analysing the reasons why health services are not being utilised. More specifically the objectives of this article are :

(i) to determine extent of utilisation of health and family welfare services in rural areas.

(ii) to identify the factors affecting utilisation of health services, and

(iii) to determine how the utilisation can be increased.

The data from rural areas of eight districts of Madhya Pradesh, India, will be used for this purpose.

DATA AND METHODS

A study was conducted on different aspects of health services in the rural areas of eight districts of Madhya Pradesh in 1983. These eight districts were Bhind, Morena, Gwalior, Datia, Shivpuri, Sagar and Tikamgarh. They formed 13.5 per cent area and 14.2 per cent population of M.P. The specific objectives were (i) to determine the organisational and implementation aspects of the programme which needed strengthening, and (ii) to estimate certain programme indicators which could provide situational analysis of the programme.

A multistage stratified sampling design was adopted, villages being the first stage units and households in the villages as the second stage units. In each district, a sample of 24 villages was drawn with probability proportional to population size and from each selected village, a systematic sample of 48 households was selected. Thus a sample of 1150 households was drawn from each district, making a total of 8050 households for the study. Two schedules, one for the household and the other for each currently married women in the household, were canvassed to each sampled household. While the former collected information related to the household, the latter was mainly devoted to the information about the couple. In the former category, information was collected, besides other aspects of health services, on utilisation of health services by the households, their satisfaction with the services by the problems faced in utilising them. In the second schedule, similar information was collected from a couple regarding MCH and family planning services. In addition, discussion was held with the village community groups to know what they felt about health services. Separate detailed reports have been prepared.*

* Copies of the report can be obtained from the authors.

It may be pointed out that though data were collected from eight of the forty-five districts of M.P., the findings are by and large, applicable for the whole State. Also, though these data belonged to the State of Madhya Pradesh, the findings may hold true for other States with similar socio-economic and cultural background.

PROFILE OF THE POPULATION

Ninety-eight per cent of the sampled population was Hindu. About 28 per cent belonged to scheduled castes and seven per cent to the scheduled tribes. Seventy per cent males were engaged in agricultural labour. Among males of ages five years and over, 45 per cent were literate and among females, this percentage was only 15.

Most of the houses were kutcha (69%) and only less than one-tenth were pucca. Electricity was used by ten per cent of the households and tap water for drinking purposes only by than two per cent. The average age at current marriage of women was found to be 13.5 years and the first birth occurred at an average age of 18.6 years. It may thus be seen that population whose responses are being utilised are of poor socio-economic level.

FINDINGS

Degree of Utilisation of Health and Family Welfare Services

The utilisation of various health and family welfare services in rural Madhya Pradesh in 1983 has been shown in Table 17.1. It is obvious that utilisation ante-natal, natal care given by trained persons (though training status of dais who had conducted most of the deliveries is not known),status of dais who had conducted most of the deliveries is not known), post-natal care and child care services has been very poor — none of these services are utilised by more than 12 per cent people. The current practice of Family Planning in (1983) was also very low.

Table : 17.1

PER CENT RESPONDENTS UTILISING VARIOUS HEALTH AND FAMILY WELFARE SERVICES

	Type of Service	*Per cent respondents reporting use*
	1	2
1.	*Ante-natal Care*	
	Per cent couples used ante-natal care for previous child	
	a) Ante-natal check up	11.6
	Government infrastructure	10.3
	Private doctor	1.3
	b) Iron and Folic Acid Tablets	6.6
	c) Tetanus Toxoide	6.7

Contd.

1	2
2. *Natal Care*	
a) Per cent mothers with type of attention at last delivery	
Dai	70.4
Relative/Friend/Neighbour	24.5
LHV/ANM	3.1
Doctor	1.9
b) Per cent mothers with place of last delivery	
At house	96.6
At institution	3.4
3. *Post-natal Care*	
Per cent mother reported utilisation of post-natal care (in four months post delivery)	
a) Visit of health worker	2.1
b) Self-visit to health centre	3.7
4. *Child Care*	
Protection status of children below five years of age	
BCG	12.3
Polio	4.2
Triple Antigen	6.1
Vit.'A' administered	0.7
Nature unknown	3.5
5. *Family Planning*	
Per cent couples currently practising family planning methods	
Female sterilisation	8.1
Male Sterilisation	4.0
I.U.D	0.2
Nirodh	1.7
Oral contraceptive	0.1
6. *Utilisation pattern in case of sickness*	
Per cent persons reporting pattern of utilising health services during their sickness of last month	
No treatment	29.8
Government health services (including health guide)	20.1
Non-government health services—trained	41.8
Non-government health services—untrained	8.3

Contd.

1			2
7.	*Medical attention at death*		
	Per cent persons reporting type of medical attention at death		
		None	48.8
		Government health service	29.5
		Non-government health services—trained	10.8
		Non-government health services—untrained	10.9
8.	*General utilisation pattern of health and family welfare services*		
	a)	Per cent households usually utilised government health services	37.0
	b)	Per cent househods visited government health facility in last year	
		Hospital	23.8
		Primary Health Centre	12.1
		Sub-centre	2.9
		Allopathic dispensary	8.9
		Ayurvedic dispensary	3.2
	c)	Per cent households reported visit of any health worker in the last one year	61.0
		Male Health Worker	54.3
		Female Health Worker	4.0
		Others	2.7
	d)	Per cent households reported visit of Health Guide in the last one year	41.9

The pattern of health service utilisation in the case of sickness is shown in index 6 of Table 17.1. Thirty per cent sick persons do not take any treatment, another eight per cent go to untrained people. The remaining (about 60 per cent) sick people go to trained people for treatment—about 42 per cent to non-governmental infrastructure and 20 per cent to the government. In other words, only about 20 per cent sick people seek services from the governmental facilities. In the case of deaths (Index 7), almost 50 per cent people do not get any medical attention at death and about 11 per cent get attention from untrained people. Thus only about 40 per cent people get medical attention from trained people at the time of death—30 per cent from the governmental set up and 10 per cent private. Only about 37 per cent people had usually used the government health services whenever they felt need for it; the remaining were going to private practitioners.

Information was collected on utilisation of health services in the last one year; the indicators 8 (b), (c) and (d) show the results. The maximum percentage of people use hospital services, that too, only one-fourth of people. The lowest utilisation is that of sub-centres, only about three per cent people had reported its utilisation in the last one year.

Regarding domiciliary visits, about three-fifths of people had reported visit of the health staff, most of them of the male health worker. The visits by the Female Health Workers (ANM) was very disappointing—only 4 per cent people had reported their visit in the last one year though they have primary responsibility in the delivery of MCH services. This is reflected in poor level of MCH services. There is need therefore to ensure that female workers make more frequent visits; it is also necessary to build such an image of female workers that more and more women accept their services.

It is gratifying to note that 75 to 97 per cent of users of health and family welfare services had reported satisfaction with Government services (Table 17.2). It was only IUD users where satisfaction with the use of the method and after-care services was the order of 75 per cent compared to 84-97 per cent for others methods. In order to determine intensity of satisfaction, the users were also asked whether they had recommended the services to others. It was found that very few people recommended government health services to others. This is noteworthy finding.

Table : 17.2

PER CENT RESPONDENTS REPORTING SATISFACTION WITH GOVERNMENT SERVICES

	Indicator	*Per cent respondents*
1.	Per cent users reporting satisfaction with government health facility in last one year	
	Hospital	78.8
	PHC	84.7
	Sub-health Centre	83.9
	Allopathic dispensary	84.5
	Ayurvedic dispensary	85.4
2.	Per cent households reported satisfaction with the visit of health staff	91.0
3.	Per cent households reported satisfaction with services of Health Guide	93.0
4.	Per cent households reported satisfaction with the family planning methods they were using	
	Female sterilisation	84.0
	Male sterilisation	85.2
	IUD	75.0
	Nirodh	92.8
5.	Per cent couples reported after care services (of family planning methods) good	
	Female sterilisation	96.8
	Male sterilisation	92.1
	IUD	75.0

Factors Affecting use of Government Health and Family Welfare Services

Information on the factors affecting utilisation of government health and family welfare service has been collected in different forms. One set related to the responses of those who were not using the government services (Table 17.3). The other set was from those persons who had utilised the services; this group was asked whether they had any reasons for dissatisfaction (Table 17.4) — some of this information was directly asked and some was inferred from the quality of service as reported by the users. The information was also collected from the Medical Officers of the Primary Health Centres on the problems they were facing in giving satisfactory health services to people (Table 17.5). All these bits of information are suggestive of various factors which are responsible for poor utilisation of government health services.

Table 17.3 gives reasons why people did not accept the government health services. Two major points which came out of this table are : (i) people still did not see benefits of using health and family welfare services, and (ii) they faced problems when they wished to use the services. Responses like "health units at a distance" or "no facility nearby" are suggestive that people have not been strongly motivated to accept the family welfare services.

Table : 17.3

PER CENT DISTRIBUTION OF RESPONDENTS NOT UTILISING HEALTH AND MCH SERVICES BY REASONS FOR NON-USE

1.	Reasons for non-utilisation of Government medical services	
	No illness	50.5
	Home treatment	10.8
	Prefer private doctor because of better service	29.1
	Health units far off	7.6
	Others	2.0
2.	Reasons for non-utilisation of ante-natal care	
	No knowledge	32.9
	No facility nearby	33.6
	Felt no need	33.4

Table : 17.4

PER CENT RESPONDENTS REPORTING REASONS FOR DISSATISFACTION WITH THE GOVERNMENT HEALTH INFRASTRUCTURE

	Indicator	*Per cent respondents*
1.	Per cent respondents reporting problem in use of government services	
	No Problem	25.3
	Services not good/medicines not effective	29.1
	Too much time consuming	20.8
	Available services far off	19.9
	Charge money	4.9
2.	Per cent respondents reporting dissatisfaction with the visit of health worker	
	Medicines not supplied	5.7
	Medicine not effective	2.4
	Workers charge money	1.9
3.	Per cent users dissatisfied with the use of Nirodh because of irregular supply	6.3
4.	Reported problems related with health services Insufficient facility for major illnesses	51.2
	Insufficient visits of PHC staff	34.2
	Lack of medicines	17.6

Table 17.4 reports some of the answers which respondents about the type of dissatisfaction with the government services. The major factors responsible for dissatisfaction were: (i) poor services, (ii) long waiting time, (iii) lack of medicines or poor quality of medicines, and (iv) poor accessibility of the services; Almost thirty per cent had said that services were not good or medicine were not effective. Even accessibility of services had also been reported as problem by one-fifth of respondents. Two other factors which have been reported were (i) insufficient domiciliary services, and (ii) insufficient facilities for major illness. Some respondents even reported that government health staff charged money.

Some reflection on the quality of services came from the reports of respondents on the pattern of service. For instance, when women who had received ante-natal care were asked the number of visits made by health workers made by during their pregnancy, their responses were as follows :

No. of visits made by health workers during pregnancy	*Percentage of respondents*
One	43.7
Two	33.1
Three	15.2
Four or more	8.0

In other words, even women who received ante-natal care did not get desired quality service more than 75 per cent women were visited only once or twice during the whole ante-natal period—most of them received ante-natal care irregularly.

The assessment of medical officers on the problems they faced in organising PHC services is shown in Table 17.5. They reported lack of infrastructure like manpower, audio-visual aids and equipment as well as shortage of supplies of vaccines, medicines and contraceptives.

Table : 17.5

PER CENT MEDICAL OFFICERS REPORTING VARIOUS PROBLEMS IN ORGANISING PHC CLINICS

Problems	*Per cent MOs*
Staff inadequacy	64.5
Audio-visual aids	59.6
Accommodation	57.6
Medicines	51.1
Shortage of funds for miscellaneous activities	50.8
Including syringes	50.5
Vaccine supply	43.5
Records/Stationery unavailable	40.4
Transportation	27.0
IUD and Nirodh supply	5.8

Reasons for preference	*Government facility*	*Private facility*
Free treatment	51.4	1.1
Good Treatment	30.4	59.3
Medicines effective	4.8	12.6
Near to house	9.6	19.6
Less time for service	2.5	3.2
Better facilities	0.8	4.1
Others	0.5	0.1

Preference for Government Health Services Vs. Private Services

An attempt was made in this study to know the considerations of a client which lead him to go to the government or private health service facilities. Those who were using government or private services were asked the reasons for their choice. The table shown below gives the stated reasons for preferring government or private service.

One may note that major reason for preference of government facility is free treatment. In contrast, private facility is preferred because of good treatment, effective medicines and nearness to the house. It is desirable that all these qualities should be brought in the government services.

Factors which can Improve Utilisation of Government Health and Family Welfare Services

Different categories of health functionaries were asked how the government health services could be strengthened. Their suggestions have been listed in Table 17.6. Most of the suggestions relate to (i) more frequent contact with people, (ii) better infrastructural facilities, (iii) wide base by involving teachers and (iv) better preparation of workers by periodic orientation and improving their working conditions.

Table : 17.6

PER CENT OF HEALTH FUNCTIONARIES MAKING SPECIFIC SUGGESTION TO STRENGTHEN HEALTH AND FAMILY WELFARE PROGRAMME SERVICES

Suggestions	*Percentage Health Functionaries*
1	2
1. Health workers should make more frequent visits to build better rapport with people and let people know about theirvisits in advance	59.0
2. Have frequent meetings with villagers	50.5
3. Supply of more medicines	45.0
4. Strengthen infrastructural facilities	36.0

Contd.

1		2
5.	School teachers should be oriented and involved in the programme	34.1
6.	Re-orientation training to workers	34.0
7.	Intensive and extensive educational activities	33.5
8.	All the three medical officers should be answerable for work of PHC	30.8
9.	Improve working conditions and promotional chances of health workers	28.6
10.	Strengthen follow-up services to increase satisfaction	26.0
11.	Strong chain of supervision so that workers provide good service	18.2

SUMMARY, FINDINGS AND PROGRAMME IMPLICATIONS

The utilisation of health and family welfare services in rural areas is quite poor. Several factors are responsible for this. There is need to make efforts to ensure optimal utilisation of the infrastructure. This article has attempted to give indicators on the degree of utilisation of various health and family welfare services and factors responsible for them. The important findings emerging from this study are as follows :

1. The utilisation of post-natal, ante-natal, child care and family planning is very low in the population. The deliveries have been conducted mostly by untrained personnel. Only 37 per cent people utilise government health facility whenever they need. This under-utilisation of the services may be either due to non-familiarity of people with the services or the services have not yet come to the expectations of the people.

2. In regard to morbidity, only three-fifths of people seek medical assistance most of which comes from the non-governmental practitioners. In the case of mortality, most of the medical attention comes from the governmental organisations.

3. In domiciliary visits, more contacts have been reported by male health workers than females. The low contact by the female health workers is also reflected in low utilisation of MCH services which are female-oriented. Thus there is need to ensure that female health workers make visits frequently. The better quality of her services will also be helpful in increasing contacts of people with the female health workers.

4. Most of the users of health and family welfare services reported satisfaction with the services. But it was strange that the users did not become salesmen for the programme—they did not recommend use of the Government services to

others. This may suggest that the users are probably satisfied but they are not happy so as to be spokesmen for the government services. There is need to bring people to this stage of satisfaction when they can speak favourable of the programme services to others.

5. Various reasons reported for non-utilisation of government services suggested need for more health education. There is need to (i) educate people on benefits of using health and family welfare services, (ii) educate them about the disadvantages of not using the services, and (iii) inform them about the place of availability of services. Therefore there is need for heavy educational activities.

6. People have also reported some problems in the use of health and family welfare services. The important of these are poor quality of government services, non-easy accessibility of the government services, shortage of medicines and too much waiting time. Some of them even reported that the government workers charged money for the services they provided. There is need to remove these problems.

7. The medical officers of the Primary Health Centres had reported problems in the organisation of good medical/health services. The important types of problems were (i) shortage of staff, (ii) shortage of infrastructural support, and (iii) supply lines of medicines, vaccines and contraceptive. There is definite need to strengthen services on these counts.

References

Reports on Baseline Survey on Demographic Situation and Utilisation of Health and Family Welfare Services in Eight Project District of Madhya Pradesh :

Vol. 1	:	Levels of fertility, mortality, family welfare and utilisation of health and family welfare services.
Vol. 2	:	Role and functioning of Medical Officers of Primary Health Centres.
Vol. 3	:	Role and functioning of Health Supervisors.
Vol. 4	:	Role and functioning of Health Workers.
Vol. 5	:	Role and functioning of Health Guides.
Vol. 6	:	Role and functioning of Trained Dais.
Vol. 7	:	Existing organisations and various developmental activities in the villages.
Vol. 8	:	Health needs, health services and involvement of the community in health activities.
Vol. 9	:	Resources and activities of Primary Health Centres.
Vol.10	:	Inventory of medical and other public facilities at village level.

Talwar, P.P. and Bhandari, S.C., "Health and Family Welfare Services in Rural Areas of M.P.—An Assessment of Quality". Paper presented at the ORG Workshop on *Quality of Health and Family Services provided by PHC Sub-Centres in Rural India* (24th April, 1987).

19

Factors Responsible for Low Utilisation of Health and Family Welfare Services in India

INTRODUCTION

Independent India, while adopting the national constitution, pledged itself to the creation of a new social order based on equality, freedom, justice and dignity of the individual and to that end, decided to eliminate poverty, ignorance, and ill-health. Provision of the health services, therefore, became one of the basic and vital foundation of the free nation. Majority of Indian Population still lives in rural areas, the future of healthy India, therefore, could be built only on all-round development of Indian villages. It was to this effect that the integrated and comprehensive approach to our health and family welfare programme was made by establishing primary health centre and sub-centre infrastructure all over the country since our Independence.

GENESIS OF HEALTH AND FAMILY WELFARE PROGRAMMES

Ministries of Health were established in the Centre and States in 1947. Though both Bhore (1943) and Mudaliar (1962) Committees had strongly recommended a comprehensive approach to total health and family welfare care, most of the National Programmes got started as individual and unipurpose programmes at different points in time. A number of relevant changes have been made at the national level in various programmes. Also a separate department of family welfare was constituted in the Union Ministry of Health in 1966 to coordinate Family Planning programme at the Centre and State levels.

A number of the national uni-purpose health programmes have achieved good success in more than one front at Central as well as at the State level. A big net-work of dispensaries, sub-centres, primary health centres and hospitals have been established. Large health and family welfare manpower has been trained and placed in both the rural and urban areas. Mentionable advances have been made in the related fields of nutrition, maternal and child health care and family welfare awareness. There have also been considerable and periodical change in the approach of the Family Planning Programme since 1952 based on the feedback and evaluation reports from the community. Achievements of family planning have been higher in terminal methods like vasectomy and tubectomy than in various non-terminal spacing methods.

UTILISATION OF SERVICES

In spite of all the above gains one finds that the availability of comprehensive health service and benefits of primary health care to an average rural has not been met satisfactorily. Full success has also not been achieved in certain important basic health criteria which were laid down initially. This is seen from a number of evaluative and monitoring studies taken up from time to time by Government as well as other related organisations.

A joint base-line "survey on fertility, mortality and related factors in Maharashtra" was undertaken in July 1985 by I.I.P.S., Bombay and Marathawada University at Aurangabad in two districts namely Osmanabad and Parbhani. One of the objectives of the survey being to determine awareness about the availability of health services and their utilisation by the respondent families.

The respondents were asked whether any member of the household had taken advantage of the services of any health centre during the past one year. The centres included were: the Primary Health Centre, Sub-Centre, Government Dispensary, District Hospital, also Dispensary and Hospital run by Non-Government organisations. In order to avoid under-reporting, this question was asked by naming each person in the household. When it was found that not a single member in the households had utilised the services of any health centre during the past one year, the reason for non-utilisation were asked. Table 18.1 and 18.2 give some details of the findings.

Table : 18.1

PERCENTAGE DISTRIBUTION OF RESPONDENTS BY REPORTED UTILISATION OF HEALTH SERVICES BY MEMBERS OF THE HOUSEHOLD (DURING PAST ONE YEAR)

	Osmanabad (total)	*Parbhani (total)*
At least one person	49.09	37.49
Nobody	50.13	62.51
Total	100.00	100.00
Number of individuals	1989	1998

More than one reason was given by the respondents, "No need/Nobody fell ill/ Minor ailments are treated at home" was the reason put forward for non-utilisation of health services by the majority of respondents in both the districts; 60.34 per cent in Osmanabad and 48.28 per cent in Parbhani. The reason mentioned by the next largest group was "we take treatment from private doctors" 27.45 per cent in Osmanabad and

32.59 per cent in Parbhani. Author has rightly commented, that this finding was quite unexpected as it is generally believed that rural people are poor and hence would not desire to incur expenditure on medical treatment privately. One reason which has a direct bearing on the health services was, "proper medical treatment is not given/behaviour of the health staff is not good."

Table : 18.2

PERCENTAGE DISTRIBUTION OF RESPONDENTS REPORTING NON-UTILISATION OF HEALTH SERVICES DURING THE PAST ONE YEAR BY ANY HOUSEHOLD MEMBER BY REASONS FOR NON-UTILISATION*

		Osmanabad	*Parbhani*
1.	No need/Nobody fell ill/Minor ailments are treated at home	60.34	48.28
2.	Proper medical treatment is not given/behaviour of health staff is not good	16.55	23.86
3.	Medicines/Injections have to be bought from market	55.5	1.92
4.	Lot of time is spent in waiting	0.48	1.44
5.	Many times the centre is closed/there are no fixed timings	0.30	0.40
6.	Centre is far away from home, no time to go to far away Centre	3.43	5.44
7.	Centre is far away from home, no money for travel expenses	1.41	2.48
8.	Take treatment from private doctor	27.45	32.59
9.	Nobody to accompany patient to health centre	0.50	0.56

* As more than one reason was given the percentage do not add up to one hundred.

This reason was mentioned by 16.55 per cent in Osmanabad and 23.86 per cent in Parbhani. Other reasons were each put forward, by and large, by less than 4 per cent of those who reported non-utilisation of health services.

LOW UTILISATION-FACTORS RESPONSIBLE

India has one of the very good infrastructures for rural health care delivery system in whole of the world. The network of primary health centres, sub-centres, cottage hospitals, rural dispensaries, mini-rural hospitals etc. can deliver an excellent and effective comprehensive health service provided some of the following bottle-necks are removed and services are allowed to function at their maximum capacity.

For the purpose of discussion following factors are responsible for low utilisation of health and family welfare services being considered under separate sub-heads :

1. Policies and Programme Planning.
2. Personnel Management at Various Levels.
3. Implementation of Services.
4. Role of Community.
5. Status and Role of Women.

Policies and Programme Planning

National Programmes

Health and Family Welfare programmes have to be seen in Table 18.3 as positive investment for socio-economic development of a long range nature. These decisions need not always be based on immediate cost benefit results which are not easily evident in health programmes. Thus appropriate resource allocation need to be made for health and family welfare.

Table : 18.3

POSITIVE INVESTMENT FOR SOCIO-ECONOMIC DEVELOPMENT

Sector of Development	*5th Plan*	*6th Plan (1980-85)*	*7th Plan (1985-90)*
Economic			
Agriculture and Allied Sectors	11.0	7.40	5.87
Rural Development	—	—	5.04
Irrigation and flood control	10.7	12.5	9.43
Special area programmes	—	—	1.75
Energy	26.2	27.2	30.46
Industsry and Minerals	18.7	15.4	12.48
Transport and Communication	17.6	15.9	16.36
Science and Technology	—	0.9	1.37
Social			
Education	3.3	2.6	3.55
Health	1.7	1.9	1.89
Family Planning	1.3	1.0	1.81
Other	9.5	9.70	10.0
Total (per cent)	100.00	100.00	100.00
Public Sector Outlay in Crores of Rs.	39,322	97,500	1,80,000

The figures shown in Table 18.1 indicate that while there has been a steady increase over a period of time in total resources allocated to all development activities, there has been much increase in the amount allocated to education, health and family planning.

This disparity needs to be looked into and funds required for health and family welfare activities need to be strengthened accordingly.

Minimum needs programme, again a joint responsibility of Central and State Government was introduced in the country in the year 1973. It has been showing the following back-log :

Table : 18.4

MINIMUM NEEDS PROGRAMME—BACK LOG IN 1977-78

Sl. No.	*Items under minimum needs programme*	*Position in the beginning of the sixth plan(1977-78)*	*Backlog as in the beginning of sixth plan (1977-78)*	*Targets for sixth plan (1978-83)*
1.	Primary Health Centres	5,400	NIL	178
2.	Sub-Centres	38,115	5,713	38,566
3.	Rural Hospitals	315	978	545

Similarly back-log and low achievements are being seen in health impact indices like crude death-rate, infant mortality rate, maternal mortality rate and in the incidence and prevalence rate of most diseases and general morbidity pattern in the community.

An important factor which needs to be looked into detail is the duplication of similar health facilities by various Governmental and non-governmental agencies at some places. This leads to lot of waste in human energy and scarce resources available.

Various services from Primary Health Centres and Sub-Centres, Integrated Child Development Scheme (I.C.D.S.), Applied Nutrition Programme, additional programmes run by other voluntary agencies etc. are all funded from different financial heads, but very often doing a similar job needs to be well co-ordinated at the implementation stage. This may lead to dilution of the services, as each service may feel that others are providing the service and community is put at a disadvantage in spite of the multiplicity of the programmes in the area.

Comprehensive Health Care—An Important Concept

Though both the earlier Tables 18.1 and 18.2 confirms the notion that the services provided through various channels at the village level are not being utilised by the community to the extent expected, yet one must also infer that concept of positive health still has to make an impact on the community. Even though most of our programmes are public health-oriented, respondents still equate health services with treatment of sickness and first-aid. Respondents do not talk about visiting P.H.C., or a sub-centre (Comprehensive Health Centres), for a well-baby clinic visit, immunisation, anti-natal care, post-natal care, etc. One has to work towards this kind of change in our rural community and to motivate them in this direction of preventive health care, which is more in tune with our public health programmes. In the above Table 18.2, respondents from Osmanabad (60.34%) and Parbhani (48.28%), respectively, give reasons for under-utilisation as, no need, nobody felt ill, and as minor ailments being treated at home. A large majority of population still equates health services with medical treatment and not with preventive and promotive services. Curative services and first-aid is only one of the eight major functions of P.H.C.s and Sub-Centre. Rest of the seven functions are all related to promotive, preventive, and rehabilitative health services. This fact needs to be propagated much more with stress on these services. A beginning has to be made in this direction for future positive health outcome at the national policy planning level specially because of the fact that family planning programme is one of our vital preventive and promotive health programmes.

Health—A Joint Responsibility

Health is listed in the Constitution under Article 346, covering all the health subjects. These subjects have been enumerated in the seventh schedule under three Lists—Union Lists; Concurrent List and the State List. It is thus the joint responsibility of the State governments to implement the programmes as per the directives and policies received from the Centre. Because of the dual control, very often the priorities change at the State level. This is because only a part of financial allocations are received from Centre, as remaining is to be incurred by the State government from State funds. In October 1979, Community Health Volunteer Scheme was launched and States were asked to share 50 per cent of the expenses. Punjab, Rajasthan, Kerala and Tamil Nadu were among the States which refused to take on the responsibility, due to different reasons. Punjab did not want to spend its own money. Kerala, with a well-developed health delivery system and unemployed doctors saw no exceptional merit in the scheme. Jammu and Kashmir had its own alternative scheme involving teachers and community health workers. The result was that an all over National Programme did not find justification for its implementation in all the Indian states.

Programme Planning Vs Implementation

Most of the policies and programmes are formulated after considering various possibilities and are based on the studies and research undertaken in the field. The programme implementation details reach the grass-root level after passing through the State departments, district level offices and block level offices. Most of the time specific emphasis is stressed along with the lines, but by the time programme guidelines reach the implementation state at the periphery only part of the specific emphasis remains and the totality of the programme is lost. For example, in Multi-purpose worker scheme, a worker is supposed to look after all health care and family planning programmes, but very often they are seen performing only one or two of their total functions repeatedly. At a particular area the Malaria Control Programme fell short of the targets proposed, the instructions came to lay more stress on it, most of the M.P.W., even much later were seen only collecting blood slides for Malaria eradication, with the result other programmes got neglected.

This outcome is also due to non-implementation of integrated approach at the district levels. In most of the states still the district level offices are unipurpose, supervising their own individual programmes. Thus primary health centre acts only as a funnel of integration with programmes running as unipurpose at both the upper and lower ends.

Training Needs Assessment Vs Implementation

Training Needs Assessment are being carried out regularly by the Central Training Institutes to organise appropriate training programmes for Key trainers and other functionaries. Frequent changes in policies can affect the quality of the proposed programme and sometimes a lot of efforts go wasted. Very often a new programme or well-proven scheme is not given anytime to justify its success in the field. Training module for Block Extension Educators training in communication was prepared for a period of six months after a lot of deliberation and hard-work. After it was prepared a three-month module was suggested at the Central level which was also finalised and pre-tested. This too was changed and finally reduced to one month duration. By the time the one month modular-training-set was ready, previous enthusiasm of the trainers was at the lowest ebb, besides a lot of efforts, time and energy, being lost in the process and in preparing all the three modules.

Health Workers—Different Functionaries

The infrastructure of health services are different in States. In Maharashtra, there are no Block Extension Educators instead the work is carries out by the Block Co-ordinators. There is a B.E.E., per block in other states while as there can be more than one Block Co-ordinator depending upon the number of P.H.C. in a given block. Thus, for the complete success of training programme at national level either method of implementation at different States has to be different or the health infrastructure needs to be the same all over the country.

Personnel Management

Commitment to Job

In health care and family planning services, the personnel play an integral and important role as they are intermediaries between the planned programme and the beneficiaries, i.e., community. They are the contact point between services and the people. One of the most vital requirement for a Government as well as a non-government worker at any level of hierarchy is the total commitment to the job. This has been obvious from various successful experimental projects which have been taken up by various agencies. Whether the commitment is that of the team leader at top or of the workers at the peripheral level, the health and welfare programme have been successful. Many examples can be cited, Jamkhed in Maharashtra; Tilonia in Rajasthan; Pachod in Maharashtra etc. Unfortunately, this commitment seems to be lacking to a large extent both in governmental and in the non-governmental sectors. If one was to isolate one single factor which is most crucial but not always seen at all the levels, is the commitment of the individuals on the job, be it in government or voluntary sector, bearing a few exceptions. Put even one committed person at any level of the hierarchy and see the results and the positive outcome. This commitment generated positive results are as much true at advisory or senior-most level as at the peripheral or the grass-root level. Commitment to work seeps up and down, others not so committed also gear-up for the occasion and want to see that things move and work gets done. Few others may also work with fear of being watched. In any case real commitment or generated commitment both works towards a better and positive result. Thus with the same infrastructure and same budget provisions things can happen and matters can move at all levels. If some committed people and but on the job.

Selection and Aptitude

Most important factor for a peripheral worker and supervisor is to select individuals from the local village where they belong. This way no time would be lost in travelling and would help in rapport building with their known village community. In case of female worker selected locally, they would feel more secure being in their own village.

Selection of an appropriate person to a particular job is very crucial to the success of the health and welfare programmes. Even more than required educational qualifications and work experience, it is necessary that the person has an aptitude towards his or her job. Sometimes this aspect is neglected with the result that the workers are on roll but the output of work is minimum. This is an important criterion which even Government agencies should keep in mind while selecting an individual even for peripheral work. If the selected persons get job satisfaction it would also get reflected in their work behaviour with the community. Interest in work would mostly act as positive feed-back with advantage to both, service provider and the beneficiary.

Training, Continuing Education and Motivation

Appropriate selection helped with required training can create a good cadre of workers. Continuing education is a must for all medical, para-medical and grass-root workers. During these continuing education sessions stress has to be given to motivational training and basic concepts of behaviour sciences like interviewing techniques etc. even for multi-purpose workers and other community level workers. Training needs assessment needs to be emphasised and needs to be undertaken for all level workers from time to time.

A study on Training Needs Assessment of fertility, mortality and related factors by F.W.T. and R. Centre, Bombay revealed lack of knowledge and skills of F.P. amongst a number of trained *dais* and multi-purpose workers. In other areas of midwifery, ante-natal care and nutrition, except health worker female all other categories are lacking both in knowledge as well as in skills. They are very important categories of workers as they form a link between the P.H.C. and community. Training has been taken up on priority basis and a number of basis as well as in-service programmes are continuously being conducted by a number of P.H.C., rural Training Centres, Regional Health and F.W. Training Centres and various Central Training Institutes all over India. Often these centres get under utilised due to non-release of various workers for training programmes. Training has to be given more status and importance.

At some places *dais* are trained, but kits are not made available to them, so they use their old traditional ways even after their training. These are small things, but are very crucial from the point of impact on utilisation of services provided.

Trained Medical Officers for Medical Termination of Pregnancy procedures are not available in rural areas and thus many times people do not utilise the services when referred even to district centres, resulting in high drop-outs rates. Failures of cases handled by untrained staff can sometimes create fear amongst the community.

To remedy all these shortcomings, stress on proper initial training with frequent inbuilt continuing education is a must for confidence of the worker and acceptance of services by the community.

The Health Workers—Job Responsibilities

The health workers are expected to look after the health and welfare needs of the rural population in the area allotted to them. One indicator to assess whether this is actually being done is to find out whether the health workers make home visits for the purpose. In the Maharashtra survey, the respondents were asked whether the male and the female health workers had visited them during the past 3 months. Though the concept of time may not be very well defined in the minds of the rural population, the findings on this point give some idea of the extent to which the rural population had been reached by health workers as perceived by the people themselves. In Osmanabad about 43 per cent were visited by M.P.W. (Male) and 16 per cent by M.P.W. (Female) and in Parbhani about 66 per cent by male and 24 per cent by female health worker. This percentage was provided by respondents who reported that the male and female health workers had visited their homes during the past three months. The analysis was done separately for male and female respondents and presented separately as it was expected that the responses would differ. This expectation was not borne out by the findings and the percentages were not markedly different for the two groups. Another factor in relation to M.P.W. non-performance is that workers are not doing the jobs specified in the programme, but instead carry out the work as per the orders of the individual programme officers. Workers' job evaluation being based on target achievements is also one of the reasons for other jobs getting neglected, which reflects in the under utilisation of various services.

Very often the reasons for services being inadequate is due to the reason that a number of posts like multipurpose workers and supervisors being vacant at the peripheral place. For the optimal utilisation of the existing service these vacant posts have to be filled up expeditiously.

Supervision

Many times it is seen that female health workers and male workers, and other peripheral level staff do not carry out their job responsibility in a satisfactory manner often due to lack of proper supervision. It has to be changed to more of guided and supportive supervision and none of old policising type. Supervisory staff is to be exposed to basics of modern supervision. Supervisory techniques during training normally provided to a grass-root level worker is inadequate and in-appropriate. Supportive supervision at higher levels like district and block level is also essential for a smooth flow of activities up to the grass-root level. Often supervisory staff lacks the skill of direct supervisory techniques, thus training in supervision with a problem solving approach is a must for all such staff at all levels.

Incentives

Motivation for an optimum output can be maintained only with the help of various types of incentives for the workers and officers in far-flung rural areas. These may not always be monetary in nature. May by an opportunity for an out-of-state training in another State or a fellowship for training abroad. After servicing in a remote area or a village for a period of three to four years, worker may be given the choice for a transfer to a bigger township or a city. Very often once selected, a worker or even a Medical Officer, get stuck at one particular Primary Health Centre with no possibility of a transfer to a bigger town.

Of course, opportunity for upgradation in service is one of the best incentives for an individual. Unfortunately there are hardly any promotional avenues for peripheral health workers both male and female, specially once they reach the health supervisory status. Even the chance of that one promotion in total services span is limited to a very few. Health and Family Welfare departments have to evolve a long-term policy for promotions. There is a need for incentives for the families of the workers, like children's educational facilities, locally or in a district place, physical facilities of housing etc. Younger people having children of pre-school age may be preferred for rural jobs. Same holds true for medical graduates at the block level. Keeping in view the large number of vacant posts in rural set-up, an initial posting of first three years of the job could be made compulsory for most of the posts, once basic facilities are provided.

Because of lack of these facilities to workers in rural areas few people come forward for working and those who come have difficulty in finding houses which affects the work in long run. If workers are commuting from another village, a lot of time is lost in travelling. In such cases, drop-out rate and job change rate is very frequent and high.

An important factor which is not an incentive, but rather a service condition, needs to be improved tremendously. This is the settlement of travelling bills of the workers when they return from tours. Very often the workers are forced to spend out of their pockets and bill settlement takes a long time and results in a lot of dis-satisfaction with service.

Implementation of Services

Work Load of M.P.Ws.

Implementation of services determines its utilisation and achievements. A well-implemented programme is received and accepted by the total community. It also helps in creating effective participation from the community, specially if the local person has been chosen for the job.

One of the important factors which to a great extent would be responsible for low-utilisation of services is the work load that has been given to multipurpose workers and their supervisors both males and females. In a study undertaken by Gandotra and Patel on

M.P.W. scheme in Gujarat when workers were asked to opine regarding the feasibility of completing the present work load of the M.P.Ws, the Supervisors in a good majority (67%0 indicated that it was not feasible. The major reasons given were the greater population to be covered with respect to the multifarious activities which the workers are required to perform, and the increase in the workload with the increasing targets for various programmes. It is not possible for these workers to visit all the families allotted to them. This work load needs to be re-evaluated in relation to feasibility. Also needed is rescheduling of their work plan with the lesser number of houses. Keeping in view the multi-faceted activities of M.P.W., a relatively lesser coverage would enable them to make frequent house visits and generate community satisfaction and better rapport.

Provision of Medicines, Stationery and other Materials

To improve the medical, first-aid and emergency services enough basic drugs need to be provided not only with M.P.W. (Male and Female) but at sub-centre and P.H.C. levels. Absence of the workers and the non-availability of the prescribed medicines makes any service inadequate and unpredictable on day-to-day basis. For health educational activities specially for motivating the community for Family Planning and other preventive and promotive services, some simple aids like charts, booklets have to be provided to the workers.

Follow-up Services

Good follow-up services are a must for acceptance and continued utilisation of health services. Very often after family planning, ante-natal immunisation and other health camps, follow-up which is very essential is not given much importance. It is suggested that a camp approach to follow of cases may solve this problem. It would be a good try to have a follow-up camp organised for any service which had been initially taken up as a camp. This follow-up camp could be held on the day medical staff is expecting, any complications that may arise. For example, in case of an immunisation camp, call all the children on 2nd day for a follow-up. This would also help in clearing all the doubts the patients or the community may have had after the camp. This way the rumours can also be reduced to minimum and community would feel that health personnel are caring and feeling for them.

One of the major reasons that some of the tubectomy camps went into dis-repute was that private doctors would have major camp in a village with no follow-up services to back it up with the result that all the complications and follow-up was left to local Primary Health Centre medical officer, who is not always fully equipped with medicine etc. to do the needful.

Role of Community

Community Apathy

An active and energetic community plays a vital role not only by creating a demand in health services, but also by demanded an improvement in the existing health delivery set-up. A close monitoring by the formal and informal leaders of whys and hows of low-utilisation of health service can play a critical role in its improvement and utilisation. An essential factor for low-utilisation of health service is definitely an inert community. This total apathy of the people towards the services and the lack of involvement and complete non-participation can be major blocks for services reaching out to the people. Indian community needs to know and demand their rights along with their responsibilities in local health care set-up.

Community Beliefs

Attitudes and beliefs play an equally important part in low-utilisation of health and family welfare services. Some religious beliefs do not allow the use of contraceptives Illiteracy and lack of social awareness leads to fears, its growth and spread in the community, preventing people from utilising the health services. Others believe more in traditional type of medication. There are people who doubt any services provided free and provided by a Governmental agencies and look at it with suspicion. Workers have to create a positive motivation of the community towards the health care set-up.

Lack of Awareness

An important constraint on use of services, especially family welfare is the ignorance of people about family planning methods in India, as is evident from various evaluation projects which have been undertaken in the country. Lack of information is also an evident fact on various health aspects. As already stressed even though our health delivery has important components of preventive, promotive and rehabilitative service, people take advantage only of curative service. Health education on preventive aspects is a must.

Lack of Awareness about Services Available

Some of the studies have shown that nearly 50 per cent of the people in a particular village were not knowing about the various services available to them. They were only knowing about a part of the services. Lack of knowledge about availability reduces the utilisation. There is need to integrate health plans with those of socio-economic development, bringing in awareness about health care and its availability amongst the people.

Inter-Personal Communication Interspouse Communication

Several studies indicate that husband-wife communication on the number of children to have has a significant impact on acceptance as well as continuation of family planning. However, in India, particularly in rural areas, discussion of these issues is still considered to be a shameful act and, hence, the level of interspouse communication remains low.

In Khan *et al.*, study at the national (All-India) level in half of the cases the husband generally made the final decision on the number of children the couple should have. However, in more than one-third of the cases the decision was made jointly by husband and wife. In 9 per cent of the cases, an elder's decision was honoured. There would be a similar kind of lack of communication on health matters if a study of such a nature was taken up. Since no interspouse communication taken place, the advantage of a educated male view point would be lost, even in health matters as it is not communicated to the wife.

Status and Role of Women in India

One would like to quote often used quotations that "You educate a man only one person is educated, and you educate a woman, a family gets educated." Women from 50 per cent of India's adult population thus being direct representatives of health of the country. Besides having additional strain of motherhood, special care of women at this vulnerable reproductive age is vital for the health of these mothers and the future generation. With only 26 per cent female literacy, impact of health services being offered gets lost. Indian women are physically and nutritionally also weak. It is reported that when records of in-door and out-patients of medical institutions are inspected, it is found that for every three men who avail of health services, only one women does so, this is true for the bed allotment for male and female wards in a hospital also. Yet the percentage of sick women to sick men at any given point of time is always higher.

Women's poor health status is directly linked to her social status. High maternal mortality and morbidity, lower expectation of life, malnutrition, high mental dis-order and high suicide rates etc. are linked with women's status in society. Improvement of status of women in society has shown a remarkable and definite change in the health picture in State of Kerala. With this change in her status, the acceptable rate of family planning and improvement in health of the whole family has been evident in Kerala State. Since traditionally mothers is the one who takes care of the family and the children, it would be she who would utilise health services for them. Well-baby clinics, nutrition clinics, immunisation camps, ante-natal and post-natal care goes unutilised because either the women does not know its existence, or is too busy or too weak to take advantage of the service.

Thus, woman's status is an important factor which needs to be looked, into while both planning and as well as while implementing the national health programmes.

References

1. *Base-line Survey on Fertility, Mortality and Related Factors in Maharashtra*, International Institute for Population Sciences, Bombay, Department of Sociology, Marathwada University, Aurangabad, July, 1985
2. *Country Monograph series No. 10*, Population of India, 1987.
3. F.W.T. and R. Centre, Bombay, Report on *Training Needs Assessment in selected districts of Maharashtra*, U.S.Aid Project, 1982.
4. Gandotra, M.M., Patel, Gita C., "Multi-purpose Health Worker Scheme in Gujarat : An evaluation." *The Journal of Family Welfare*, Vol. XXXIV, No. 2, 1987.
5. Government of India (1946), *Report of the Health Survey and Development Committee*, Government of India Press, Simla.
6. Government of India (1962), *Report of the Health Survey and Planning Committee*, Ministry of Health, New Delhi.
7. Government of India, Planning Commission, *Sixth Five Year Plan*, 1980-85, New Delhi, Government of India Press, 1981, pp. 57-58.
8. Government of India, *Draft Five Year Plan*, 1978-83, New Delhi, Government of India Press, pp. 17-18.
9. Jha, Saroj S., *Women's Health*, Dhanwantri Oration XIV, Annual Conference I.A.P and S.M, Jaipur, February 1984.
10. Khan M.E. and Prasad C.V.S. "A comparison of 1970 and 1980 survey findings on Family Planning in India", *Studies in Family Planning*, Vol. 16, No. 6, Part I, December, 1985.

20

An Analysis of Causative Factors Responsible for Low Utilisation of Health and Family Welfare Services

THE BACKGROUND

Uttar Pradesh is the most populous State of the country having 12 divisions and 57 districts spread over in an area of 3.24 lakh square km. There are vary vast socio-cultural, ethnic, geographical and ecological variations. For raising of the quality of life and improving the living standards of its millions of people, there have been tremendous efforts for economic and social development through all the Five Year Plans. In health sector as well, massive financial resources have been allocated which has strengthened and augmented the service infrastructures. Presently a vast network of Primary Health Centres (2046), Sub-Centres (22020) , Post-partum Centres (203), Urban Family Welfare Centres (158), Tehsil and District level Male and Female Hospitals (200) and Medical College Hospitals (9) are available to cater to curative, preventive, promotive and rehabilitative medical, health and family welfare and services to teeming millions of men, women and children of the State. But in spite of all this, the health standards of the people are far from satisfactory. A perusal of the vital rates shown in Table 20.1 explicitly reveal the actual situation.

Table 20.1 very clearly shows the poor state of the health of the people in the State. The Birth Rate, Death Rate and Infant Mortality Rate should and must always be decreasing but their occasional increase in comparison with earlier period shows the inadequate efficacy and impact of the Health Programmes. Another indicator *i.e.*, Life Expectancy also illustrates this point. During the decades 1951-61 and 1961-71 at national level it increased from 41.2 to 47.7 years while in this State it increased from 38.9 to 43.0 years respectively. Review of these rates in comparison with national level indicates further towards the most sorry state of affairs. Similarly, more than two decades since family welfare was undertaken and launched as a national programme. But the Couple Protection Rate which should show a positive trend during the temporal sequences has decreased year by year after 1977 and has shown negligible increase in this decade which is approximately half of the national rate

(34.9) and lags much behind when compared to Kerala (41.1) and Maharashtra (53.1). Henceforth, it becomes of immense empirical as well as practical value to study causative factors which are responsible for inadequate utilisation of services and conspicuous impact negation of optimum resource allocation and maximum assiduous efforts.

Table : 20.1

VITAL RATES*

Years	*Birth*		*Death*		*Infant mortality*		*Couple protection*	
	Rate	*Increase (+) or decrease (–)*	*Rate*	*Increase (+) or decrease (–)*	*Rate*	*Increase (+) or decrease (–)*	*Rate*	*Increase (+) or decrease (–)*
1	2	3	4	5	6	7	8	9
1970	45.4		21.6		N.A		N.A	
1975	43.1	—	22.6		198		8.3	
1980	39.4	—	16.6	—	159	—	11.6	+
1982	38.6	—	15.1	—	147	—	11.3	—
1983	38.4	—	15.7	+	N.A		13.1	+
1984	38.8	+	15.8	+	154	+	15.5	+
1985	37.6	—	15.8		140	—	16.7	+

* U.P. at a Glance (Facts and Figures) published by Demographic and Evaluation Cell, S.F.W.B.U.P., Lucknow (1987).

THE STUDY

For enumeration and identification of problems and causative factors which are responsible for low utilisation of Health and Family Welfare Services, a study was conducted in 12 districts of the State. From each, two Primary Health Centres were selected on achievement/performance basis. All the functionaries of these centres were interviewed besides 50 villages living in two villages from each of the centre's operational area. Thus, a total number of 600 functionaries and 1200 villagers were interviewed. Discussions with senior officers of the districts and State Headquarters were also held besides scrutiny and examination of records, service statistics and reports. Observations from peripheral to onward levels were also made. The findings of this study are being presented subsequently. Suggestion based on the findings are also presented.

CAUSATIVE FACTORS/PROBLEMS RESPONSIBLE FOR SERVICES INADEQUACY

Officials

The functionaries enumerated the following problems and causes which in their opinion and experience were adversely affecting the adequate utilisation of services (Table 20.2).

Table : 20.2

PROBLEMS/CAUSATIVE FACTORS : MULTIRESPONSE TABLE

Sl. No. Particulars	*Frequency*	*Percentage*
1. Erratic and irregular supplies	336	56.0
2. Inadequacy of finance, resources and equipment	412	68.6
3. "Single Point" Accountability	516	86.0
4. "Targetism"	516	86.0
5. Inadequate supervision and guidance	376	62.6
6. Absence of Residential Accommodation	496	82.6
7. Paucity of Education, Information Communication (IEC) Literature Audio-visual Aids and resources etc.	432	72.0
8. Absence of a pragmatic and wholistic strategy	516	86.0
9. No opportunities for proper application of Health Education and Extension methodologies	516	86.0
10. Absence of community participation	336	56.0
11. Socio-cultural milieu and demographic characteristics of the villagers	522	87.0
12. Poor Service conditions leading to job dissatisfaction	522	87.0
13. Inadequacy of Training and Refresher Courses	337	87.0

Base : 600

Source : Direct Enquiry

Success or failure of health programme depends a lot on timely adequate and satisfactory supplies of medicines, equipments, vaccine and contraceptives. More than half of the functionaries (56.0 per cent) who found supplies erratic and irregular have correctly made the point. It is common experience that immunisation and contraception programme suffers a lot from delayed and inadequate supplies. A beneficiary to be given multi-doses for Tetanus, Polio, and many a times vaccine for subsequent doses is either not made available at all or supplied so late that immunisation schedule is not adhered and entire efforts are negativated. Such examples dishearten and serve as disincentive for prospective utilisers. Moreover a considerably high percentage (68.6 per cent) of functionaries have experienced financial and resources inadequacy. These constraints dampen the morale, zeal and will to work which when often repeated leads to frustration ultimately resulting into a "NO WORK" situations and propensities.

A large number of functionaries (516) have attributed two reasons "single point accountability" and "Targetism" which in their opinion are crucially important reasons for poor performance and/or success. As a national health policy, "Multi-purpose Working" Scheme has now been enforced at the sub-centres level. One male and one female health workers are now available for population of 50000 and 3000 in plain and hilly areas of the State, respectively. These workers are required to provide all the medical, health and family welfare services including Maternity and Child Health Services. Their job responsibilities are institutional as well as peripatetic. They are also required to impart health education and do motivation extension work for enabling people to accept small family norms. This is the programme strategy or the operational methodology which the workers should adopt and adhere. But in actual practice, the situation is just the reverse. Every worker supervisor and officer within a Primary Health Centres is given the targets (Family Welfare and Maternity and Child Health both). The sterilisation target achievement has the highest priority or rather the single priority. Functionaries work is assessed on this "single point". If he or she has motivated this fixed number of men or women and they have accepted sterilisation, then his or her assessment rating is very satisfactory and there are no questions asked about his/her other job responsibilities or duties fixed under the Multipurpose working wherein Malaria, TB and Cholera is also to be eradicated, environmental sanitation ensured, Anaemia, Blindness Eye diseases prevented and other promotive/rehabilitative health services rendered. Even if a worker has done wonderfully excellent job related to all these programmes and failed to motivate sterilisation cases in adequate number his/her performance rating is at the rock bottom and he/she may be fired. This anamolously contradictory working methodology has actually played havoc and has been adversely detrimental to all the programmes/services as the grass-root where peripheral worker has been made a "Automation" who has to produce by hook or crook sterilisation cases. All the time, efforts and labour is devotedly wasted in case finding and neither there is time nor willingness to establish rapport the community, strengthen interpersonal relationships and discharge other duties. Thus workers credibility stands lost and confidence in him/her eroded leading to little or negligent service utilisation.

Very closely related to this "single point accountability" the other reasons attributed by the respondents (516 or 86%) is 'targetism' which in their opinion is another very significant dampening or demotivating reason/factor. This needs further elaboration. The long-term and overall objective of our Family Welfare Programme is stipulated reduction in Birth Rate and betterment of quality of life by requisite health services to the mother, child and other family members. But fixation of the contraception methods targets in general and sterilisation in particularly highest importance and priority defeats this long-term and overall objective. Couples who have reproduced a fullest complement of children and have crossed fertile age period of their lives, when sterilised show a quantitative achievement with zero impact on Birth Rate. Since last three years, in this State, officials of other development departments (Revenue, Rural Panchayat Raj, Cooperative etc.) have been given sterilisation targets and since they are either in a position to dole out a benefit (loan, aid) or cancel a utility they get elder couples sterilised motivated by anything but the acceptance of small family norm. Very strict enforcement of this cult of "Targetism" has not only dwindled the efficacy of sterilisation but has further created opening for falsification of achievements of other methods like intrauterine devices, condoms and oral pills users. The functionaries have shown ample awareness about this jeopardizing situation and have correctly identified this as a major cause/reason.

A significant number of respondents (496) attribute absence of residential accommodation to be another important cause/similarly paucity of Education, Information and Communication (IEC) Material qualitatively and quantitatively has been another stimbling factor attributed by 72 per cent of the respondents. The functionaries are also well aware of the lack of adequate supervision and guidance and 86 per cent of them pointed out towards absence of an adequate strategy of working. The preceding analysis is closely related with this reason as the practical strategy adopted is greatly at variance with long term and overall objectives. High rate of illiteracy in general and in women in particular, socio-cultural taboos, moves, customs, traditions (like male child preferences) and conspicuous absence of peoples participation are some other crucial causes of inadequate success.

A very large number of functionaries (522 or 87%) have mentioned improper service condition leading to job dissatisfaction and thus lowering the work morale. Astonishingly majority categories of functionaries have no promotion avenues. Job security is very flimsy due to 'Targetism'. Moreover 33.7 or 56 per cent respondents have revealed that adequate arrangements for training and refresher courses are also lacking, which do not enable them to keep pace with rapidly developing technologies and operational methodologies. Cumulative effect of these causes/reasons jointly and separately leads to low utilisation of existing services as the persons charged with the responsibility of its delivery find themselves working under adverse circumstances and coping with insurmountable problems.

Villagers

The villagers interviewed for identification of causative factors were 1200 and out of their responses, Table 20.3 is prepared related to the service infrastructure aspects.

Table : 20.3

PROBLEMS/CAUSATIVE FACTORS

(Multi-response Table)

Sl. No.	*Problems*	*Frequency*	*Percentage*
1.	Inadequate Service Infrastructure	410	34.2
2.	Supply shortages/irregularities	682	56.8
3.	Paucity of Staff	328	27.3
4.	Recalcitrant attitude and behaviour of functionaries	592	49.3
5.	Exhortation for money	607	50.6
6.	Inadequate follow up	702	58.5
7.	Great distances	480	40.0
8.	Inadequate home visits	612	51.0
9.	Inadequate supervision	507	42.3
10.	Others	615	51.3

Base : 1200

Source : Direct Enquiry

The foremost finding of the above table is that villagers are howsoever illiterate, ignorant and superstitious they are fully conversant with the problems which they think are acting as great impediments for adequate delivery of Medical, Health and Family Welfare Services. Regarding shortage of supplies, they were very vociferous in complaining that they never get any medicines at the service centres and whatever medicines they are supplied ineffective. A very significant percentage (56.8) of them complained about the undersirable and recalcitrant attitude and behaviour of the functionaries. The main reason for this situation is that workers positioned at the centres, consider themselves hospital/clinic staff only and this attitude results into unbecoming behaviour to the persons who visit these service centres or are contacted at their homes. The other contributory factor to this phenomenon is that the majority of these workers hail from urban areas and they consider it very disgusting and dissatisfactory to live and work in rural areas which are sometimes very distant from cities and towns and all the good living facilities are not available there. These villagers also complained about the follow up services which as per their version were very inadequate. These respondents by a percentage of 42.3 were also aware that these service centres and its functionaries were not properly supervised and guided. In this connection it was observed that all the 3 Medical Officers posted at the Primary Health Centres are required to be available at the centre for 3 days of the week and for 3 days to visit the field. But in actual practice, this procedure was not followed and taking example from them other staff members also paid lesser field visits. Moreover, the district level senior officers like the Chief Medical Officers, Deputy Chief Medical Officers did visit the centres occasionally but they hardly went to the villagers, except very rarely visiting a sub-centre. This evidently showed the inadequacy of supervision and guidance and the respondents were very correct and right when they reported this fact.

More than half *i.e.*, 51.3 per cent respondents enumerated some other problems like absence of transport means, inadequacy of roads and routes, socio-cultural milieu and superstitious of the villagers and misutilisation of financial and other resources by the officials. Regarding organisation of Orientation Training Camps for village leaders, they complained great malpractices were adopted in this work.

SUGGESTIONS

The aforementioned causes enumerated by officials and beneficiaries clearly indicate that their Total impact jointly and singularly involves a cyclical phenomenon. Hence the services are not utilised or are under-utilised leading to poorer health standards. To remove these causative factors following set of action may be suggested based on the finding of the study :

(i) Service conditions of the functionaries should be improved. Personnel management procedures need study and appraisal as to make it effective in creating job-satisfaction. Service matters should be promptly attended for which sanction and decision taking powers need further decentralisation. Workers mobility also needs improvement.

(ii) As regards finances, medicines, equipments, vaccine and other resources adequate provision should be timely made. The delays and shortages should not occur.

(iii) Requisite modification in the programme strategy should be made. In spite of 'single point' absolute weightage to sterilisation programme, all the other programme components should be given due weightage and functionaries evaluation should be based on his/her total performance. Ensuring qualitative aspects of the programme/services is as important as fixation of quantitative targets. The prevailing tradition of deriving immense satisfaction on the achievement of quantitative targets on the cost of its quality should be discontinued.

(iv) Functionaries lack knowledge and skills to adequate delivery of services. Arrangements for adequate pre-and in service training and refresher courses should be made. It should be ensured that the functionaries capabilities are sharpened and improved keeping pace with fast developing service-delivery and extension methodologies from day to day. This training should also consist of theoretical/practical concepts and values which should ensure due regard to and amicable dealing with the acceptors who so far have been not given even the minimum consideration for human-dignity. Development, thus, of an abidingly proper conceptual framework is of greatest importance.

(v) Information, Education and Communication (IEC) and Mass Education and Media (MEM) are the weakest links of the programme. Though immense funds have been and are still frittered away on this yet it has not created the desired impact. Adequate modification in the strategy and implementation methodologies should be made on scientific lines.

(vi) Conspicuous absence of adequate supervision and guidance is another great stumbling block. Job assignments are neither communicated in black and white not otherwise made understood by the functionaries. The supervision also lack much in knowledge and skills. The supervision and guidance work further suffers a lot due to confusion, overlapping and in frequency. This aspect needs looking into and adequately improved and strengthened.

(vii) Programme monitoring and evaluative have a lot to improve. There is no systematic scientific and pragmatic built-in mechanism for concurrent and/or terminal evaluation. It is undertaken as an off and on exercise. Further absolute absence of any mechanism to ensure implementation of evaluation findings is another big impediment. So whatever evaluation is done it becomes in vain and a futile exercise. The situation should be modified and improved accordingly.

21

An Approach to Public Health

THE COMMUNITY DIAGNOSIS.

The diagnosis of an individual patient is a fundamental idea in medicine, but applied to the community, it is a public health concept that will be new to many readers. The meaning of 'community diagnosis' is, however, well worth grasping, for its provides fresh insight into the disease pattern of a population and makes it possible to take more efficient action to improve the health of the group. The easiest way to describe the community diagnosis is to compare it with the individual diagnosis.

In caring for a sick individual the first step is to look for signs and symptoms, the next is to infer causation from them—to make the diagnosis. After this comes treatment and then follow-up to see whether this treatment has been effective. There are similar stages in caring for a sick community.

The first stage is to gather epidemiological data, the next is to make inferences from it—to make the 'community diagnosis'. The third is to prescribe community treatment, or as it is usually called, 'community health action' as part of a 'community health action programme.' Finally, the effect to this health action is followed up and evaluated.

With the individual, the term diagnosis is usually used to cover both the eliciting of signs and symptoms and the making of inferences from them. The same is true of community diagnosis which includes both the collection of data and deductions to be drawn from them.

The community diagnosis may be defined as the pattern of disease in a community described in terms of the important factors which influence this pattern. When this definition is examined it is seen to incorporate, the essential feature of the community diagnosis. This is the inferences to be drawn from the data because, unless such inferences have been drawn, the factors responsible cannot be described nor can their relative importance be assessed.

An Aid To Understanding the Community Diagnosis of Kwashiorkor

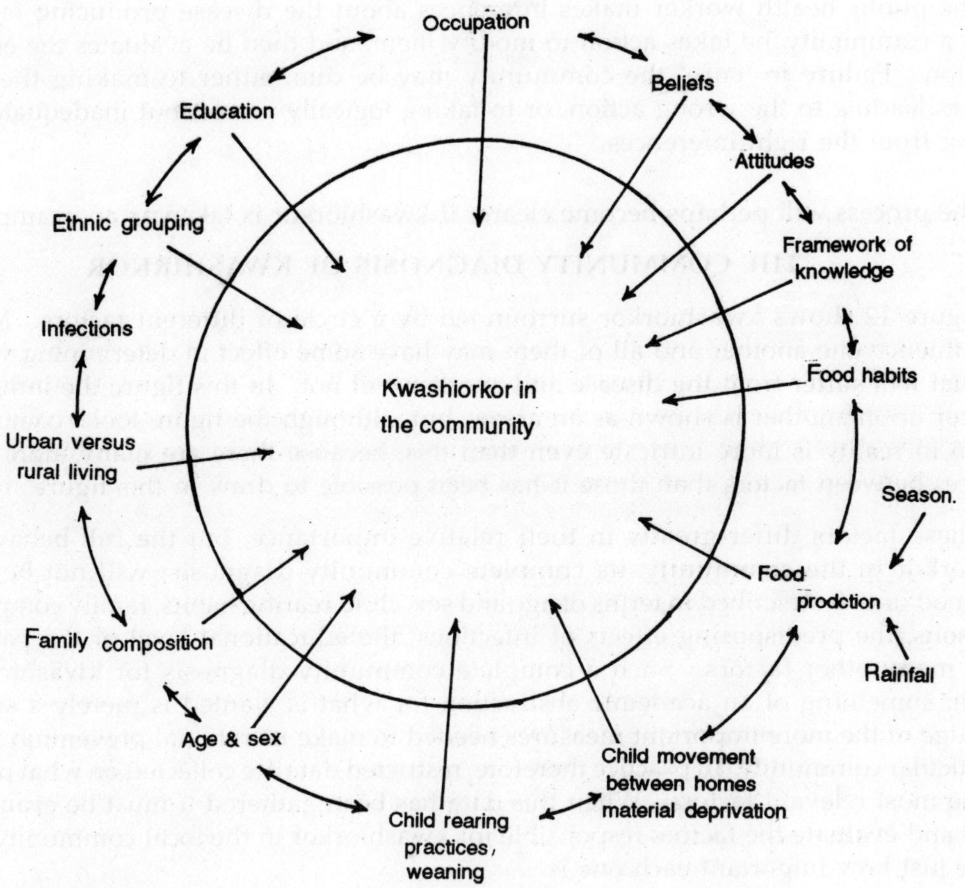

Fig. : 21.1

This is an attempt to describe in diagrammatic form the relation of kwashiorkor in a community to some of the factors which are responsible for it, and to give some idea of their intricate relation to one another. All the factors in this diagram have an effect on the prevalence of kwashiorkor in a community, and most of them also influence one another.

In gathering his data and making inferences from them, the public health worker is merely applying the scientific method termed 'induction'. This is to gather data, to make inferences from them as to why things happen and then to construct experiments with which to test the truth of these inferences. Hypothesis is the term more often used instead of inference, but in this context they mean the same thing. The critical part of the process is the 'inference,' which is really an intuitive guess, but what distinguishes science from mere guesswork is the ability to design experiments to test the truth of the guess.

The public health worker makes inferences about the disease producing factors at work in a community, he takes action to modify them, and then he evaluates the effects of this action. Failure to 'cure' the community may be due, either to making the wrong inferences leading to the wrong action, or to taking logically correct but inadequate action following from the right inferences.

The process will perhaps become clearer if kwashiorkor is taken as an example.

THE COMMUNITY DIAGNOSIS OF KWASHIRKOR

Figure 12 shows kwashiorkor surrounded by a circle of different factors. Many of these influence one another and all of them may have some effect in determining why one individual will suffer from the disease and another will not. In this figure the influence of one factor upon another is shown as an arrow, but, although the figure looks complex, the situation in reality is more intricate even than this, because there are many more mutual influences between factors than those it has been possible to draw in this figure.

These factors differ greatly in their relative importance, but the full behaviour of kwashiorkor in the community, its complete community diagnosis, will not be wholly understood until is described in terms of age and sex, child rearing habits, family composition, the seasons, the predisposing effects of infections, the educational level of the parents as well as many other factors. Such a complete community diagnosis for kwashiorkor is, however, something of an academic abstraction for what is wanted is merely a sufficient knowledge of the more important measures needed to make its rational prevention possible in a particular community. In practice therefore, restricted data are collected on what promises to be the most relevant factors. When this data has been gathered it must be examined to confirm and evaluate the factors responsible for kwashiorkor in the local community, and to estimate just how important each one is.

To illustrate the kind of inferences that can be drawn an example from Zambia can be quoted. Two doctors there observed, when analysing data from their children's ward, that, whereas malnutrition in all its forms was more common in the heat of October, in the cold of June cases of kwashiorkor comprised a much larger fraction of all the malnourished children. From this they inferred that cold might be an important factor in precipitating the oedema which is such a striking feature of this form of malnutrition. The 'health action' that this led to concerned therapy more than prevention and, with other observations has done much to emphasise the importance of keeping these children warm, of leaving them close to the heat of their mother's bodies and of nursing them in a warm room.

Table : 21.1

AN EVALUATION OF THE EFFECT OF HEALTH ACTION ON A GROUP OF MALNOURISHED CHILDREN

The health action taken was that involved in starting an under-fives clinic (16:1), Data from Sierra Leone (39).

	The Average Weight of the Children					
	6 months		*12 months*		*18 months*	
Initial Data	lb.	oz	lb.	oz	lb.	oz
Before starting the clinic	14	2	16	8	18	4
Evaluation Data						
One year after starting the clinic	14	6	18	6	19	2
Two years after starting the clinic	14	8	18	8	20	8
Three years after starting the clinic	14	10	18	2	20	10

In a disease influenced by as many factors as kwashiorkor, a sudden dramatic drop in incidence must not be expected to follow even the most vigorous community health action. Slow steady improvement is all that can be hoped for. This is evaluated in Table 21.1 where the average weights of children in an under-fives clinic in Sierra Leone are shown, both before and after the starting of this clinic. The health action taken was of various kinds of which health education was the most important. It will be seen to have caused a progressive rise in the average weight of the children towards the optimum and illustrated in Table 21.1. Before the clinic was instituted children between 9 and 18 months were conspicuously underweight with many cases of frank kwashiorkor, but, as their average weight increased, this became less common.

Both these examples have been criticised as much less than ideal, the first one in particular because the writers did not rule out all the other factors that might have precipitated kwashiorkor, such for instance as a winter increase in infections, or a seasonal alteration in the foods available. These provisos further illustrate the complexity of the community diagnosis of this disease, and the editor can find no better examples.

'Hard' and 'Soft' Points in the Culture. Having collected the data and made the inferences from them, a community diagnosis is still incomplete, for 'community health action' tries to alter peoples' practices in relation to their health. The community diagnosis must therefore contain information on just how susceptible to change these practices are. Some alternations involve 'soft' points in the culture that are easily changed while others are so deeply established, so 'hard' as to be quite unchangeable. Often, there are alternative approaches to the eradication of a particular disease, and, whereas one will involve a 'hard' point another may involve a 'soft' one. The first is likely to fail, the second may succeed. Thus most people are very 'hard' on the point that their particular staples is the best of foods and nobody would be advised to try to make them live on anything else. However, such people can often be persuaded to *add* other acceptable foods to this staple—a 'soft' cultural point and, in trying to make the change like this, food habits can often be improved and the incidence of kwashiorkor reduced. Community diagnosis is therefore, completed by the inclusion in it of information on the capacity for change by a community at the critical points in its cultural pattern. In such community studies social scientists can make a very useful contribution.

The Community Diagnosis Need not be Complete. Kwashiorkor has been taken as an example, and it has been shown that, even with this one disease, a complete community diagnosis is impracticable. But kwashiorkor is only one of many diseases that afflict the human group. What then of the total community diagnosis—all the diseases in terms of all the relevant factors ? This is an impossibly compete entity. Nevertheless, as an idea and in a limited form applied to some of the major factors influencing the more important diseases, community diagnosis is at the same time useful, straightforward, and intimately related to the daily practise of hospitals and health centres. In the tropics the community diagnosis is of special value, for the common tropical condition of malnutrition and infection are particularly susceptible to control by the established methods of public health.

It may be argued that such an apparently complicated process of data collection and analysis is not required and that clinical impression alone suffice. This is not true, although clinical impressions do provide valuable leads in suggesting what data might usefully be collected. By themselves they are usually inadequate, and they are sometimes entirely wrong.

The Defined Area. In the second two chapters much was said about the extent of territory for which a health centre can be responsible—about 'the immediate area', 'the extended area' and 'special effort' area. A fourth area is also needed—the 'defined area'. This is an area of intensive study from which is gathered the data of community diagnosis and in which health action is most easily evaluated. In well staffed health centres responsible for comparatively small area it can be the whole territory served by the centre, but, in developing countries where resources are extended, it is usually better if it is less than the total area assigned to a centre. In general, it should be in this area alone that data should be gathered and health action evaluated, because unless it is limited and defined in this way, it may be difficult to gather data that are complete enough to be useful. The general work of a centre must of course go on throughout the territory assigned to it. To avoid confusion that records of patients from the defined area should be distinguished carefully from the rest.

A recent report emphasised the great value of carefully collected data and contained the following passage :

> 'Irrespective of whether one is dealing with disease in the urban or the rural areas of Africa, the outstanding obstacle to a rational approach to disease control is the complete lack of valid statistical data relating to the African population, and describing its distribution, birth rates, death rates and incidence of disease in terms of mortality and morbidity... Before any plan for the control of disease in Africa can be soundly formulated, it will be necessary to establish studies to several substantial data on the actual incidence of disease.., in both rural and urban areas.' (21)

Clearly, valid data from defined areas have a value which transcends their usefulness to an individual hospital or health centre, and thus deserve publication so that they can be fitted into the overall public health picture of the continent.

Community Health Action. This is the sum of the steps decided upon to remedy the critical features revealed by the community diagnosis. Action takes various forms; health education is the most important and is described. Immunisation is perhaps the next and is described. Other forms of health action are legislation, especially that relevant to such things as motor accidents and alcoholism, the issue of health-promoting foods, such as dried skim mile (14:14), the improvement of water supplies and campaigns against specific infectious agents. These are all different forms of community health action and in almost all instances simultaneous action of several different kinds is required. This action must be co-ordinated as a 'community health action programme' and, though it is only possible to give a few general ideas about it here.

Action should be directed towards the particularly susceptible groups in the community and to those aspects of the environment that have been found to be related to their health. Action is taken at three levels, at the level of the individual patient himself, at the level of the family and at the level of the community as a whole.

Individually directed action is taken at the various clinics, curative and preventive, in the midwifery unit, and in the domiciliary care of the sick. At this level hospitals and health centres function in the same way and should work together, especially in the follow-up of hospital patients, a task which is often best done by health centre staff.

Home and family directed action seeks to modify and improve home and family living and is carried out in the home itself by any workers who visit it, be they public health nurses, health visitors or midwives. But action directed at the home and family can also be taken at clinics or in community groups such as women's clubs.

Community directed action involves the community as a whole through its leaders, formal and informal and its various natural groups. Here, it is important to realise that community directed action is not merely action directed at the community at large by professional health workers of various kinds, but, that it seeks to promote health action by groups within the community led by the community's own natural leaders. In a developing country, schoolmasters, especially primary schoolmasters, are among the most important natural leaders in this respect.

Because the resources for health action vary so much from one society to another, the local society should be studied very carefully before any community health action programme is planned. Close liaison needs to be established with organisations of various kinds, such for instance as tribal chiefs and community development workers.

The was in which these different types of health action can work together is best illustrated by an example taken from a boys' club in Israel which involved a community that was not well advanced. Shigella dysentery and infantile gastroenteritis were endemic in the area and very difficult to counter with public health measures. A Health Education therefore approached the leader of the club, explained the problem to him and spoke to the boys, telling them of the disease, how it is spread and how it could be countered. Thereafter, the boys under their own leadership carried out a survey of sanitation and refuse disposal in their area, tabulated their own data and did much to educate their friends and families in fighting it. The whole project lasted several months, and is a good example of community directed health action led and organised by members of the community themselves with the help of a trained Health Educator. At the same time as it was being carried out, individually directed health action was intensified in the various clinics, and public health nurses and others stressed the same problems in the families they visited.

Evaluation. All health action has to be evaluated. This means that data must be gathered to measure the improvement in the health of the community by methods similar to those originally and used in making the community diagnosis. This evaluation has to be thought about before any action is taken so that methods of doing it can become an integral part of the health action programme itself. This is shown in Table 21.1 where the clinic weight charts were used for this evaluation.

The Role of the Health Centre. So much for the public health sequence of data collection, inference making, community health action and evaluation—who is responsible for it and in what units does it take place ?

Though it must also operate on a national and a district scale, it is at the health centre that the process is most relevant, for public health work of this kind is the main purpose of a district medical officer in his role as supervisor of a group of health centres. Medical assistants are not usually capable of making the relevant deductions themselves but they can at least gather the data for him and put into effect most of the health action he plans.

The Role of Hospital. Though the full public health sequence of community diagnosis, followed by a wide range of different forms of community health action is properly the responsibility of the health centre, limited health action, notably health education and immunisation, must be undertaken by hospitals. If this health action is to be planned wisely, community diagnosis is essential. Added to this, circumstances often compel a hospital to assume the health centre role, however imperfectly. Community diagnosis and some community health action thus have a real part to play in the thinking and practice of a hospital.

Some Practical Suggestions. So much for theory, but what are the first steps in actually making the community diagnosis ?

The first thing to realise is that some at least of the data needed for community diagnosis are usually present in the records that are already being kept by most hospitals and health centres. As an example of how useful such ordinary hospital data can be, though in this case it was not used for community diagnosis much of that required for the plotting of the care gradients was easily extracted from the ledgers of the hospital and dispensary concerned. Hospital data have however to be interpreted with caution and information is usually more accurate if it is collected prospectively for a specific purpose. With little extra effort clerks can readily be trained to extract additional information from the patients they see and record it in a suitable form for analysis.

Hospitals and health centres are therefore encouraged to make good use of their opportunity for data collection, and, having done so, to use it creatively in planning community health action, particularly health education.

Method : making a community diagnosis.

Choose a defined area limited by convenient natural boundaries from which data can be collected. This area should include the hospital or health centre itself and not be too big—say 2-4,000 people.

Mark out this defined area on a map with a 'felt pen', fasten it to a piece of 'softboard' that easily takes pains and hang this up on the wall.

See if any basic data on the population of the villages in the defined area is available from the records of the provincial administration or the tribal headquarters.

Make arrangements to add to this information by recording births and deaths within the defined area, and, if possible, encourage the population to come up and register these events themselves.

Distinguish the records of patients from within the defined area by the use of cards of a special colour, some distinguishing mark or a special prefix to their record numbers.

Choose one or two diseases of particular interest or importance, think about them and decide what data would be of greatest value in studying their behaviour in the community or might most usefully point the way to effective community health action.

Explain the idea to the record clerks, and get them to collect the required information by questioning the patients and recording their data for analysis, preferably after the manner suggested in 26:12. Where relevant, record the location of the cases being studied by sticking coloured pins into the map.

Plot the data obtained in graphical or tabular form and put it on the wall.

When sufficient data has been collected, analyse it carefully, form some judgement as to its accuracy, see if it needs amplifying or extending and see what conclusions it leads to.

Then plan the necessary health action accordingly.

Data that have been carefully gathered and analysed have a value that extends beyond that to the health centre of hospital where they were originally collected (21:5). A place must be found where they can be made available to others, and one of the functions of a local medical journal should be to record data of this kind. It is advisable, however, not to waste time writing an article until the advice of the editor has been sought as to the general suitability of the material for publication.

Such a study of community health and the effect a health centre or hospital is having on it adds greatly to the interest of medical work. But in studies of this kind, look upon what the textbooks say should happen with a certain caution, because diseases behave differently in different area, and an open mind is required if interesting local variations are not to be passed over.

22

The Organisation of Health Services

INTRODUCTION

In the developing countries disease will only be reduced to the fullest degree possible, when the twelve axioms of the first chapter are put into action. They must be applied to every aspect of medical care from the large issues of policy down to the smaller details of daily practice. Countries vary in their educational and economic resources, in the present organisation of their health services as well as in other ways which affect health planning, but even so, it is only too obvious that the available resources of many of them are badly deployed, and that this is in part because some of the basic axioms have been given too little attention.

This chapter suggests how these axioms relate to the large scale organisation and development of health services and makes some basic generalisations governing the provision of medical care in developing countries. But before considering organisation, it is necessary to look at what scientific medicine has to offer in the way of preventive and curative services, the relationship between them and what the villager thinks about them.

Prevention and Cure. The most important preventive measures in the rural areas are health education directed towards improving environmental sanitation and modifying personal immunisation, and the routine examinations of the ante-natal and under fives clinics. These form the main work of the health centre as it is described in the next chapter. But there are other preventive measures also, such as campaigns against specific infections, trypanosomiasis and malaria for example, as well as legislation concerning such things as alcoholism, building standards and accidents, particularly burns.

Curative services also take many forms : Some patients come to hospitals or health centres to be cured of illness in a mild enough form for them to be treated as outpatients. Common among such conditions are minor trauma and sepsis, upper respiratory infections and malaria. Other patients present themselves when so ill as to need admission to a hospital ward under the supervision of a doctor and at times need also the services, both emergency and elective, or a surgeon as well as the facilities of an operating theatre, a laboratory and an X-ray plant. In the rural areas these are the limits of curative medicine.

Between prevention and cure, they are in practice closely interwoven in almost every part of the medical endeavour, and nowhere perhaps in this better shown than in the account of the under-fives clinic. It is for this reason that there is no special section devoted to organising preventive medicine apart from curative medicine. Rather, it has seemed better to emphasise the health centre as a unit whose major function is prevention, and health education has been considered as an important part of the practice of both health centres and hospitals, which should be places for educating people and not only for curing them. All through these pages, as through medicine itself, prevention and cure are intimately linked.

Prevention and cure are also often linked in the way the tropical villager looks at scientific medicine. When a community is new to it—and this is becoming increasingly rare—some dramatic cures may be necessary to win the confidence of the people and to persuade them to come for medical attention of any kind. In other communities people will attend a hospital for cure of their disease and then go to a traditional healer for the removal of its cause. Many villagers are sensibly pragmatic in what they accept, and soon come to know which illnesses a particular hospital or surgeon can cure, and what diseases it is useless to attend with. The same pragmatic attitude may extend to preventive medicine also, and there are even some indigenous systems of medicine with a decidedly preventive outlook. But with the passage of time, scientific medicine as a whole is coming to be held in ever higher esteem by the present communities of developing countries, and there is an ever increasing popular demand for medical services and above all for the provision of doctors and hospitals.

These in brief are the preventive and curative services that medicine has to offer, and the staff and facilities that patients and politicians clamour for. The fundamental question is therefore this. *How, in the rural areas in particular, can preventive and curative services be planned so as to provide the maximum return in human welfare from limited resources of money and skill ?*

Distance, population, finance and staff are the four main determinants of medical care, and, although other issues are often important, these four usually predominate. Before considering just how critical they are, it is necessary to consider very briefly the kind of units that have been devised to provide this care, the relationship between them, the dimensions and units in which medical care be measured and in both urban and rural conditions, but it is rural services, particularly as they involve problems of distance and transport, that are mainly the concern of the next few sections.

The units of medical care. Ideally, the first and simplest 'unit' of medical care should be a person with some medical skill, however little, in each and every village. He or she should act as the local representative of the health services at the periphery of the health service. Whatever their exact status, these local representatives must be visited regularly by mobile teams from the health centres, they must be given instruction and encouragement and progressively upgraded with every visit. They need a few drugs and dressings so that they have something to give away, but their main function should be to spread health knowledge in their village. They are discussed further, for want of a better term, they are called 'station masters', as being the persons in medical charge of the 'station' where a mobile team stops to hold a clinic.

Unfortunately, these local representatives usually exist in theory rather than in practice. They are not part of the otherwise excellent Kenyan scheme of health centres described in the next chapter, and at present most health services omit the village worker altogether. Instead, health services usually start at the periphery with the 'aid post' which is followed up by the 'dispensary' and the 'one doctor hospital'. These units represent the initial attempt to provide medical care in the rural areas and, though theoretically outmoded by 'health centres' and more substantial hospitals, they are still typical of many developing countries.

An 'aid post' is really no more than a rendezvous visited weekly by a medical representative who comes armed with a box of drugs, and is helped by a nurse who gives the injections. Between them they may see some hundred patients at each visit, but the treatment they offer is minimal, and any health education they can give is usually inadequate.

The dispensary is a small building staffed by a medical assistant a nurse and also perhaps by a midwife. As many as three hundred out-patients may be seen daily, and a dozen or so inpatients treated during short illnesses or pending their transfer to hospital. Many dispensaries run aid posts in their vicinity, but apart from this, their work is restricted to the minor curative activities that can go on within their walls. Dispensaries have neither the staff nor the facilities to do anything more.

By contrast the ideal unit of medical care near the periphery of a health service is described separately elsewhere. There it is defined as a unit which provides a family with all the health services it requires, other than those which can only be provided by a hospital. Each health centre is responsible for a specified area, and, ideally, the whole country, urban and rural, should be divided up between health centres. Great emphasis is laid on the importance of health centres extending their influence throughout the territory they are responsible for, and on their role in health education.

Dispensaries and health centres are often confused, but, though a poorly developed health centre may be little more than a good dispensary, these two units are really quite different. They are distinguished by the range of services they can provide, by their activity in the surrounding area and by the emphasis placed on health education. Dispensaries are not converted into health centres, as has been attempted in at least one country, merely by changing their names in order to keep up with the latest fashion. A true conversion from a dispensary to a health centre demands both the expansion, and the thorough retraining of existing staff, with increased emphasis on preventive activities, especially those outside the centre.

There is a wide measure of agreement on the theory and functions of a health centres, but there is some difference of opinion on the size of the unit for which the term should be used. It is applied to a unit without a doctor led by a specially trained medical assistant and staffed by half a dozen other auxiliaries. In some countries a health centre refers to a larger unit run by a doctor who administers a number of smaller satellite clinics with the same functions.

The relationship between units of medical care - the 'Referral System'.

The concept of the health centre is closely bound up with that of the 'referral system'. This system is based on the idea that patients are to be treated as close to their homes as possible in the smallest, cheapest, most simply equipped, and most humbly staffed unit that will still look after them adequately. Only when a particular unit cannot care for a patient adequately is he to be referred to a unit higher up in the chain : the chain being the health centre, the district hospital, the regional hospital and the national hospital.

Treatment at the periphery of a service is much cheaper than that at the centre; this is the great advantage of the referral system. The following table from Kenya shows how greatly the cost of treating an illness increases, the closer it is referred to the centre of a service. Even when allowances made for the longer stays in the regional and national hospitals, due largely to their treating different kinds of case, the difference in average cost is considerable (13)

Institution	*Average stay*	*Average cost per illness*		*Average cost per day*	
		Shs	*$*	*Shs*	*$*
Health Centre		4/-	0.56		
District Hospital	7 days	84/-	11.80	12/-	1.68
Regional Hospital	10 days	170/-	24.00	17/-	2.40
National Hospital	22 days	370/-	52.00	17/-	2.40

Does the referral system work? Only in part; it often fails peripherally because few hospitals have health centres close enough to them, to screen their general outpatients so that the hospital deals only with referred cases. Transport difficulties also greatly impede the efficiency of the system and inevitably regional and national hospitals have mainly to act as district ones. For example, about 80 per cent, of the patients admitted to the New Mulago Hospital. Uganda's national hospital, come from the neighbouring districts of Mengo which contains only 20 per cent, of Uganda's people. Even so, the referral system is very important, particularly at its lowest level in which health centres refer cases to the district hospitals.

Dimensions and levels of care. There are many dimensions to medical care. This is well shown by the wide range of services provided by the health centres, but, as convenient dimensions for measurement and as illustrating the points at issue, only two will be considered here—total outpatient attendances and the availability of hospital beds.

Before either of these can be discussed with profit they have to be seen against some level of reference; some level of outpatient care is required and likewise some level for the provision of hospital beds.

As a realistic, if somewhat arbitrary level of outpatient care, it has been suggested that two adult and three child attendances per person per year constitute a convenient basis for planning. To some readers this may seem unrealistically high, and it is certainly seldom achieved, but, when it is realised that this should include attendances at clinics for antenatal mothers and the under-fives, as well as repeated attendances for dressings and injections, it will not seem excessive, particularly when infectious disease and malnutrition are usually to prevalent. The under-fives clinic requires more attendances than this, but, until more is known about the levels of outpatient care that should be attained by tropical communities, this figure will have to serve. If, as is usual, about half the population are under fifteen this level of attendance implies an average of roughly 22.5 attendances per person per year.

As a way of measuring the availability of hospital beds the total number per 1000 people is chosen here. This is a well accepted dimension, gross national averages, ranging from 10.6 in the United Kingdom to 0.12 in Nepal—almost a hundredfold difference. Here again little is known about the number of beds which should be available to tropical communities.

It is to be noted that both outpatient attendances and hospital beds are merely means to an end—the reduction of disease. They are chosen here as convenient dimensions or parameters of medical care for discussion in the sections which follow, but increasing the availability of health facilities should never be confused with improving the health of the people.

OUTPATIENT CARE

The inequality of access to outpatient care. In a developing country distance is a critical determinant of medical care, and it is widely realised that only those close to a medical unit can derive the full benefit from its services. While this may seem obvious, it is not generally appreciated just how inequitable this way of distributing medical care really is. For example, it was found in Kenya that 40 per cent, of the outpatients attending a health centre lived within five miles of it, 30 per cent lived between 5 and 10 miles from it, and a further 30 per cent, lived more than 10 miles away). What these figures imply about the distribution of medical services can best be appreciated by expressing them in terms of the areas from which patients were drawn. When this is done it will be seen that approximately four times as many people came from each square mile within the 0-5 mile zone as came from one in the 5-10 mile zone. The same grossly inequitable distribution of outpatient services has been observed in Uganda in the study based on Mityana hospital. Here data were obtained from a hospital, a dispensary and an aid post, and it was found that the same principles governed outpatient attendance at all three of these units.

Because distance and the difficulty of transport have such a profound effect on the availability of medical care, the purpose of the following sections is to present arguments for the importance of providing mobile services so as to take medical care closer to the homes of the people. Arguments are presented based on 'outpatient care gradients', on population density and on economy.

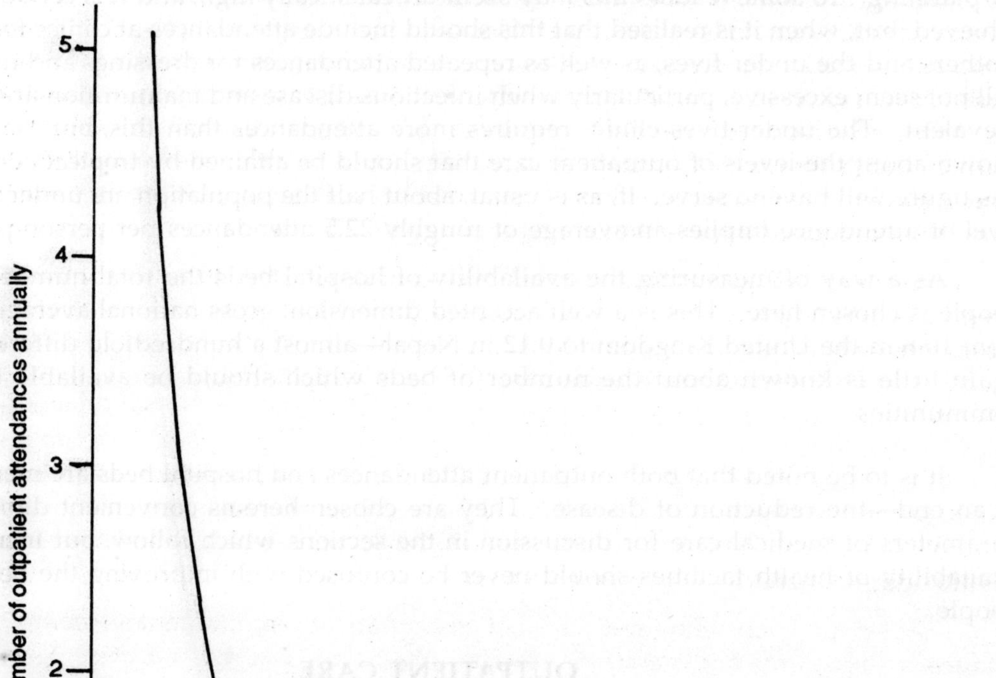

Fig. 22.1: Outpatients attendances per person per year related to the distance he lives from the hospital.

TAKING SERVICES TO THE PEOPLE

The argument from outpatient care gradients. Figure 22.1 shows how the average member of outpatient attendances per person per year falls precipitously the greater the distance that separates the patient's home from the hospital. The relationship is in fact exponential which means that attendance drops by a constant percentage with each additional mile that separates the patient's home from the hospital. If a graph is drawn showing distance and outpatient attendances on a logarithmic scale, the relationship between attendance and distance becomes a linear one, and the slope of the line measures the 'outpatient care gradient' for this hospital (Figure 22.2).

Outpatient care gradients have also been measured for a dispensary and an aid post. These have been plotted with that from the hospital in Figure 22.3. Comparative data obtained from a dispensary in India are also shown on the same graph. The slopes of the outpatient care gradients for the dispensary and the hospital differ slightly and are at different positions on the graph, because the number of outpatients seen by these two units differ widely (about 100,000 attendances annually for the hospital and 52,000 for the dispensary). The average number of outpatient attendances per person per year will be seen to halve itself about every 2 miles (3.2 km) for the hospital and the dispensary, and every mile (1.6 km.) for the aid post. The slope of the gradient for the dispensary in India is the steepest of all—attendance there halves every half mile.

The factors determining the slopes of an outpatient care gradient are complex, but the distance that patients are prepared to walk appears to be a major factor. Few Ugandan patients were prepared to walk more than five miles. The cost and availability of different kinds of transport is another important factor and is well shown in the same figure. Perhaps the most important factors of all are the severity of the patient's disease, and the quality of the care available—the better the medicine the further will people be prepare to go for it.

The information contained in the graphs can also be expressed as a map. Figure 22.4 is a map of the Mityana area on which lines have been drawn joining points where outpatients care is equal—points of equal care or, as they might be called, points of 'isocare'. These 'isocare lines' make it possible to see at a glance the distribution of outpatient care within a given area, and on this map lines have been drawn representing 2.5, 0.25 and 0.025 outpatient attendances per person per year.

Certain simplifications have been necessary in drawing this map. Communications, such as roads, are assumed to be uniform throughout the area, the same gradients have been assumed for all similar units, the allowance is made for differing population density. For instance, it might be that the large majority of the population closely clustered round the various medical units and that a steep fall of in outpatient attendance is of little matter because few people live far away from a medical unit. This is not in fact the case, for in the area shown the population density is fairly even at about 250 persons to the square mile.

Despite the comparatively large number of medical units in the region shown on the map, in only about a tenth of its area does the level of care attain or exceed the suggested standard of 2.5 attendances per person per year. In a smaller but still significant area the

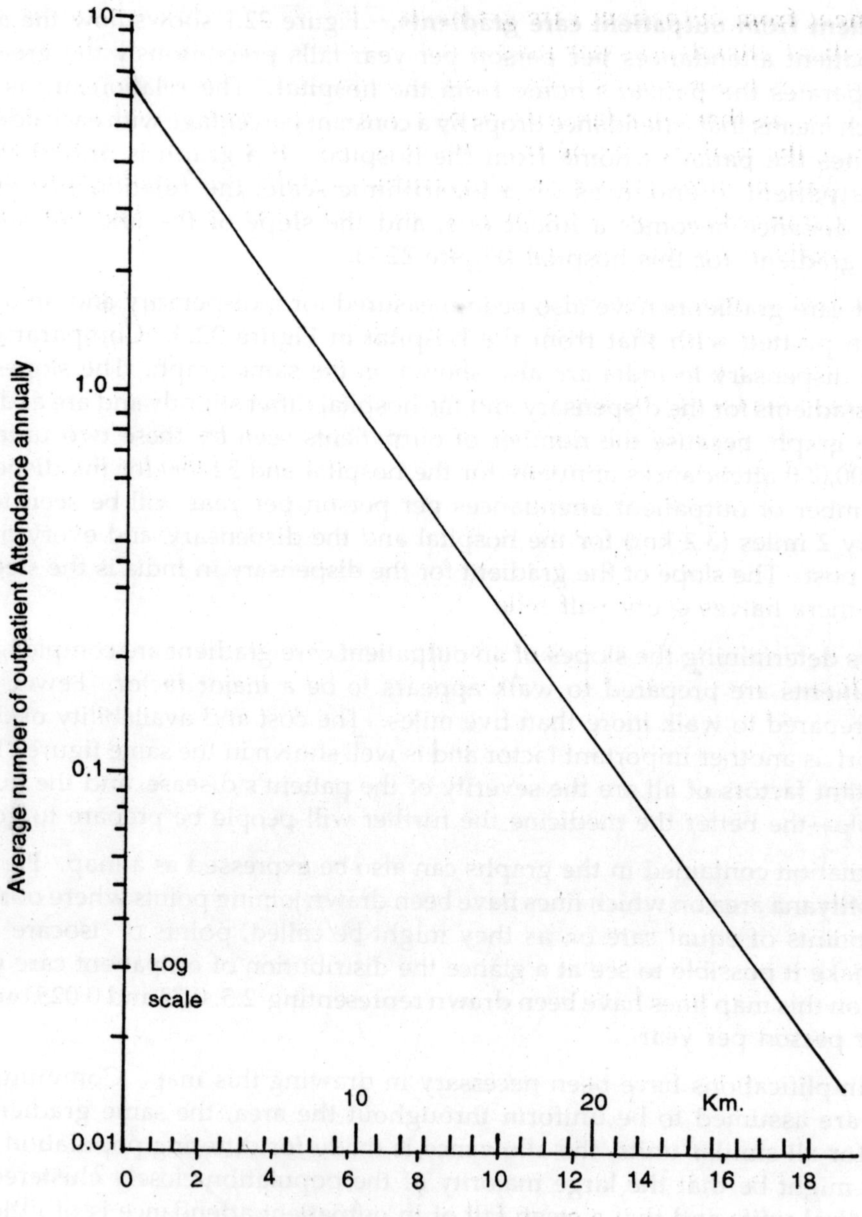

Fig. 22.2: Outpatients attendances per person per year (log. scale) related to the distance he lives from the hospital.

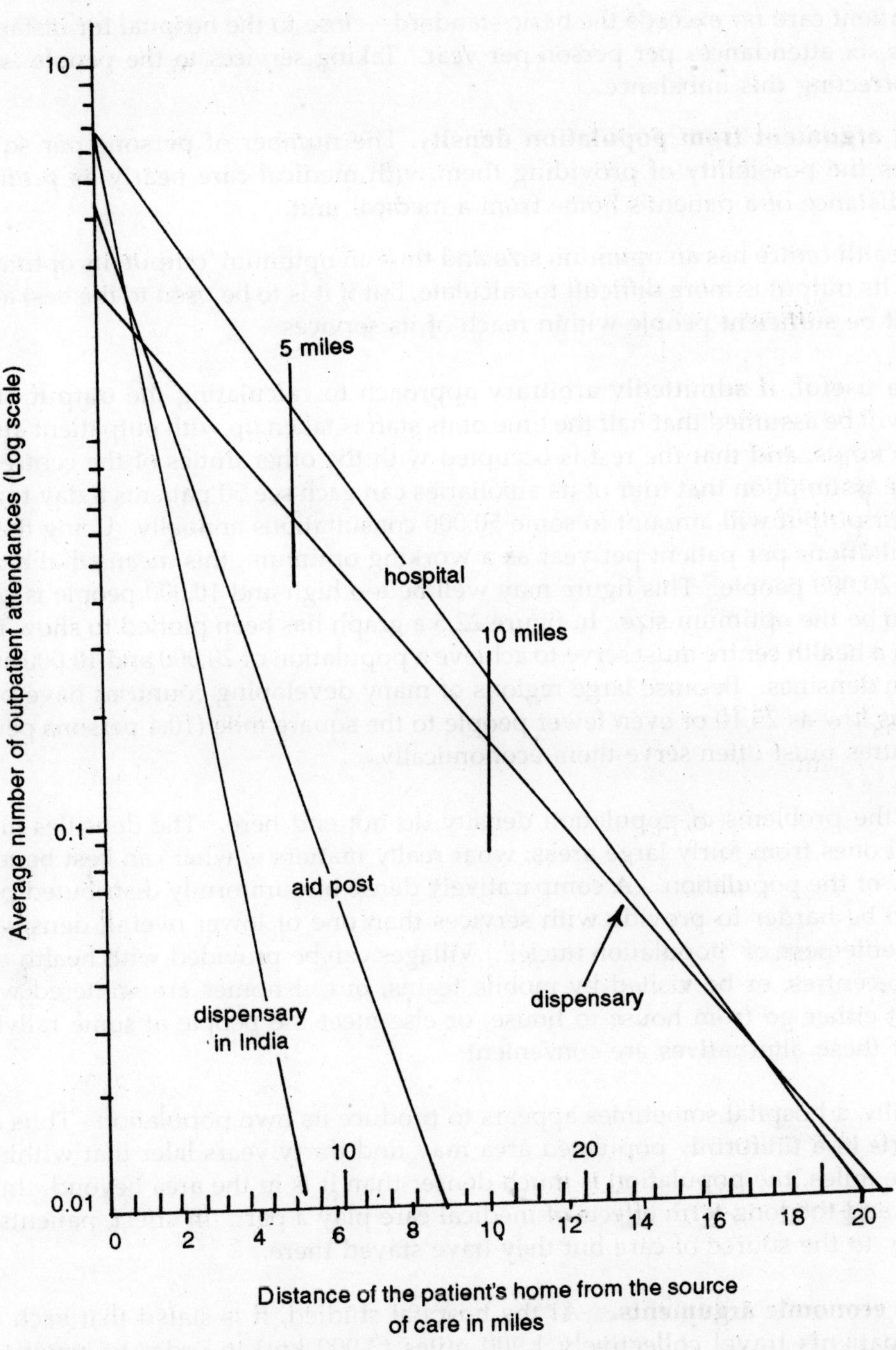

Fig. 22.3: The average number of times annually outpatients attend for medical care related to the distance they live from the source of this care.

level of patient care far exceeds the basic standard—close to the hospital for instance it rises as high as six attendances per person per year. Taking services to the people is the main way of correcting this imbalance.

The argument from population density. The number of persons per square mile determines the possibility of providing them with medical care nearly as profoundly as does the distance of a patient's home from a medical unit.

A health centre has an optimum size and thus an optimum 'output' its optimum size is probably. Its output is more difficult to calculate, but if it is to be used to the best advantage, there must be sufficient people within reach of its services.

As a useful, if admittedly arbitrary approach to calculating the output of a health centre, it will be assumed that half the time of its staff is taken up with outpatient attendances of various kinds, and that the rest is occupied with the other duties of the centre. Making the further assumption that four of its auxiliaries can each see 50 patients a day for 250 days a year, their output will amount to some 50,000 consultations annually. Using the figure of 22.5 consultations per patient per year as a working optimum, this means that a centre can look after 20,000 people. This figure may well be too high and 10,000 people is considered by some to be the optimum size. In figure 22.5 a graph has been plotted to show the radius of the area a health centre must serve to achieve a population of 20,000 and 10,000 at different population densities. Because large regions of many developing countries have population densities as low as 25,10 or even fewer people to the square mile (10.4 persons per sq. km.), health centres must often serve them economically.

But the problems of population density do not end here. The densities just quoted are overall ones from fairly large areas; what really matters is what can best be termed the 'nuclearity of the population'. A comparatively dense but uniformly distributed population is likely to be harder to provide with services than one of lower overall density living in compact settlement of 'population nuclei'. Villages can be provided with health centres, or health sub-centres, or be visited by mobile teams, but, if homes are scattered widely, the team must either go from house to house, or else meet the people at some rallying point. Neither of these alternatives are convenient.

Finally, a hospital sometimes appears to produce its own population. Thus a hospital which starts in a uniformly populated area may find thirty years later that within a radius of, say five miles, the population is much denser than it is in the area beyond. In this both migration and the long-term effects of medical care play a part. In effect, patients have not only come to the source of care but they have stayed there.

The economic arguments. At the hospital studied, it is stated that each day three hundred patients travel collectively 1,900 miles (3,000 km) in order to benefit from the services of two medical assistants and a doctor half time. The average distance each patient travelled was over 6 miles (10 km). Sheer economy demands that this travelling be minimised by making a few stall cover most of the distance so that patients need travel less.

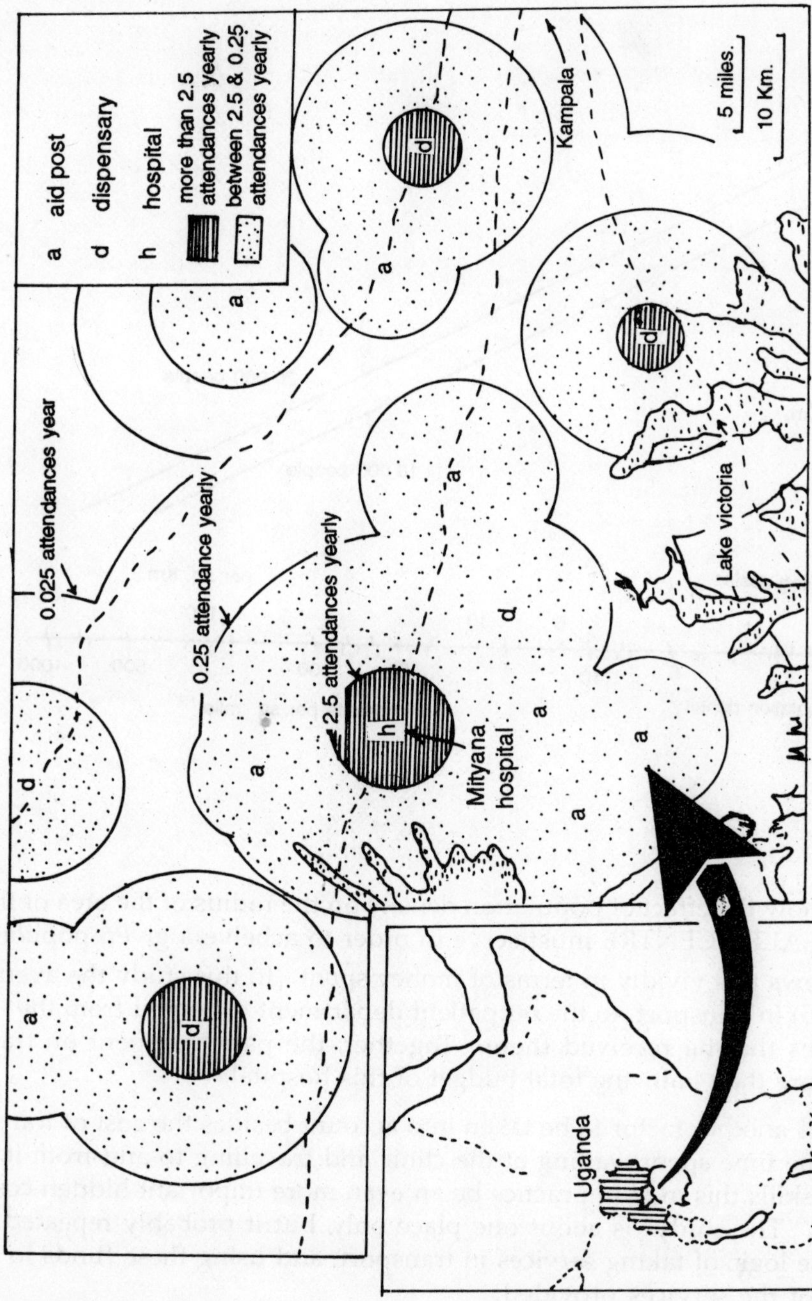
AN PUTPATIENT 'ISOCARE MAP' FOR THE MITYANA AREA OF UGANDA
a aid post
d dispensary
h hospital
more than 2.5 attendances yearly
between 2.5 & 0.25 attendances yearly
0.025 attendances year
0.25 attendances yearly
0.25 attendance yearly
2.5 attendances yearly
Mityana hospital
Kampala
Lake victoria
5 miles.
10 Km.
Uganda

Fig.: 22.4

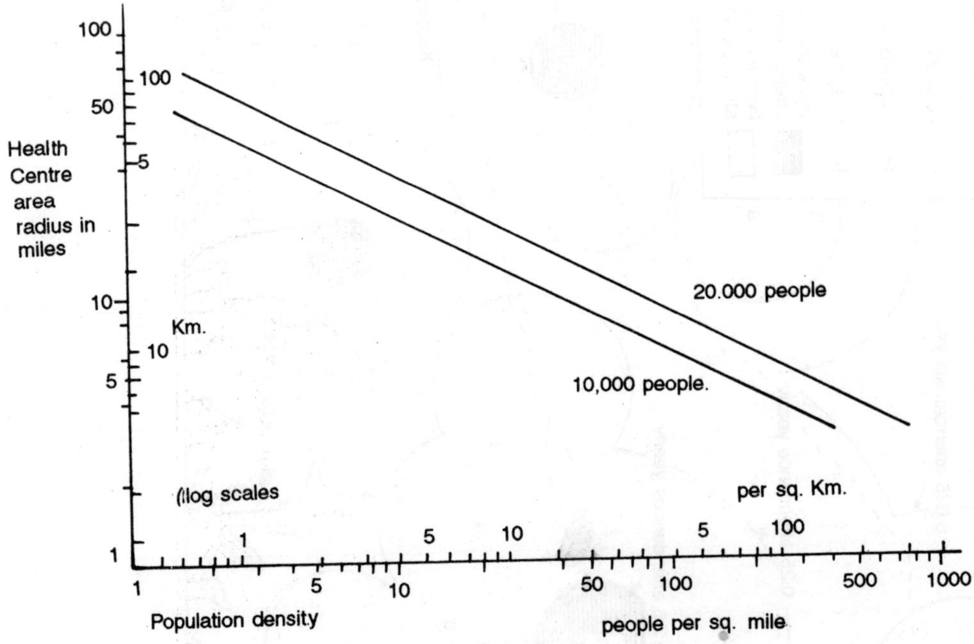

Fig. 22.5 : To show the effect of population density on the radius of the area of the territory a HEALTH CENTRE must serve in order to acheive a given population

It also shows this vividly in terms of money spent. In this study the average patient spent 2/50 ($0.35) in transport to the outpatient department to benefit from the -/81 ($0.11) worth of services that he received there. Together, the patients spent on transport the equivalent of more than half the total budget of this hospital.

But there is another factor to be taken into account besides the cost of transport. This is the value of the time spent waiting at the clinic and travelling to and from it. For adult Ugandans with skills this may in practice be an even more important hidden cost than that of the transport. The study is about one place only, but it probably repeated elsewhere, and points to the logic of taking services in transport, and using these funds to pay for the additional cost of the services provided.

The desirability of making a charge is further supported by the diagram depicting total health expenditure. Several developing countries spend as little as 7/- ($1) annually per head on all forms of medical care. This does not provide much, and it may be that some of the people might be able to pay the 1/- ($0.14) that the average health centre attendance costs. Considering that the annual per capita income (GNP per head) in many developing countries is of the order of £ 25 ($70) or more, this would appear to be possible.

Charges are beset with many administrative, political and educational difficulties. If charges are difficult there are other alternatives; the additional expense can be met through a special local association, from employers (who will save their employees 'working time), from the general revenue or from some simple health insurance scheme (1:9). But, in the last resort the choice is this: either some way is found to pay the cost of bringing services to the people or the people will pay their own way to hospital.

Mobile outpatient services. In general, mobile services can be of two kinds. Such teams require several vehicles and are expensive; they are not very manoeuvrable and there is an enormous amount of packing and unpacking to be done every time they break camp. In some areas they are the only possible form of medical care, but, as their applications are limited, they are not considered further here.

The second type of mobile services are those provided by a health centre, or sometimes by a hospital within its own region, particularly in its extended area, and especially in regions of low population density. It is services of this kind that the steep outpatient gradients in Figure 22.3 show to be so necessary. It is fortunate therefore that, with the exception of the few holding beds and the labour ward, all the services of a health centre can be made mobile.

Theory. Mobile services what is said here is complementary to what is said later. Mobile services should be based on health centres, for it is health centre services that they exist to provide: but, if there is no system of health centres in the area, then hospitals may have to provide them instead, and fulfil as much as they can of the health centre role in doing so.

Right at the start it must be made clear that mobile services have to be provided by auxiliaries, who must between them offer a range of skills and know how to organize themselves. Another important point is the multipurpose nature of the services that a team from a health centre or a hospital have to provide at any one visit. They will usually be able to visit each village only once a week, and, to be effective they must bring with them a wide range of facilities each time they come, including general outpatient services, antenatal and under-fives clinics as well as drugs to a particular patients. The demand for these services is likely to be heavy which such services as those for tuberculosis and the under-fives take preference. Visits must be regular and should make the most of the natural gatherings at markets or local government headquarters. It is best if the mobile clinics visit definite 'stations' in regular rotation, each of these stations having a local health representative of 'station master' of the kind.

While the general arguments for mobile clinic objections are sometimes raised which it will be useful to deal with specifically. First it is argued that mobile services can at the most visit each centre once a week, and that this is insufficient, particularly for urgent cases.

This is in fact a confusion over what the alternatives really are. The choice is likely to be between (a) a large daily clinic at the health centre, run by general staff; (b) the division of this into two smaller fixed clinics, one at the health centre and one somewhere else, at a health sub-centre for instance; (c) one fixed clinic at the health centre with a mobile team serving different points in the area on each of the five working days of the week. Without mobile services, most villagers will have to travel considerable distances to reach treatment, and experience shows that only a few will do so. With mobile clinics the medical care is likely to be available near at hand at least once a week. And, if it is not possible to wait, a patient can travel, either to the mobile clinic which is operating somewhere in the area, or to the health centre itself. For most people, this is no worse than before and—on one day a week at least—far better

Second, it is argued that mobile clinics would make it impracticable to refer cases to a doctor and would thus lower the standard of medical care provided. But, if the mobile team is run by a health centre, patients are not going to see a doctor anyway, and they can if necessary be referred to a hospital for a doctor's opinion direct from a mobile clinic. If the mobile team is run from a hospital, and is in effect serving as its outpatient department, patients can still be referred to the hospital for a doctor's opinion. It may even be possible for the team to take one or two patients back to the hospital with them, depending on the size of the vehicle they are using.

There is another objection which, although not widely considered may arise in the minds of those concerned with the economics of mobile clinics. In countries short of capital with much unemployed man-power, are not mobile clinics too 'capital intensive', using too much capital and relatively too little labour? The short answer is that the real economic alternatives are not whether to run the health services with transport or without, but whether many forms of private transport should be used to bring patients to the clinics, or whether the health services should use its own transport to take the services to the people.

Practical detail. There are many practical points to make mobile clinics easier. One is the vehicle itself, and although an ordinary ambulance or Land Rover can be used, a specially fitted vehicle may well be want the extra expense. Thus one group propose to use a one ton 'pick up' truck with side opening cabinets each side of its main load compartment (CHE). These trucks are made primarily as mobile workshops for such people as telephone linesmen and plumbers : they cost little more than the standard type of 'pick up', and may prove to be the ideal vehicle for the provision of mobile services. The cabinets with which they are fitted are already water-proof and can be made dust proof and lined with plastic foam to prevent their contents rattling. When the vehicle stops these are immediately available without lengthy unpacking. The cab seats three, or even four, and can be completely fitted and equipped with four wheel drive for £1,650 ($4,600). Such a vehicle could, it seems, do much to make mobile services practicable, and if their price seems excessive this should be compared with what some patients will spend on private transport, if services are not made mobile. A special mobile clinic conversion of the Land Rover is also available (PIL).

A major point of organisation is the distance mobile team has to travel. The less of their time the staff spend travelling the more of it will be available for treating patients.

Thus, if a vehicle can travel at 20 miles an hour (32 km/hr), it can reach a village ten mile (16 km) away in half an hour—mobility within this radius if thus highly practicable from the point of view of time. Transport needs to be economical if it is to be used on the necessary scale without becoming inordinately expensive.

Numerous minor details could also make mobile services easier. It may be found convenient to get the patients to keep their own records in polythene envelopes, though additional records may have to be kept for patients within the 'defined area'. Other useful points are to bring drugs prepacked in envelopes, and mixtures in plastic bottles which will be broken in transit. If a microscope, a centrifuge or lighting are needed, the vehicle's own battery can be used. Only simple accommodation is required for the station; it can be borrowed for the occasion and need be little more than a roof of thatch or corrugated sheeting and a few cubicles of 'mud-wattle-and-whitewash'. Some tables and chairs will be wanted, a source of water and also latrines. If the local community cannot provide anything else they can usually provide these bare essentials.

Such mobile services are the key to outpatient care in the rural areas. Their organisation provides a challenge that has been met in very few developing countries so far. While the detail and form of the service may have to vary considerably, there is little doubt that, in large areas or most developing countries, mobile clinics have an important part to play in bringing medical care to people who would otherwise have none.

INPATIENT CARE

The need to concentrate impatient care. Figure 22.6 shows the inpatient care gradient for the same hospital in Uganda from which the outpatient care gradients were derived. It shows the decline in the hospital beds the greater the distance that patients live from hospital. The graph was plotted by calculating the average number of days spent in hospital each year by persons living in a number of concentric zones around it. As a hospital bed is able to provide 365 bed-days each year, this figure can readily be converted to the number of beds used per 1,000 of the population. The graph has the same exponential form as the outpatient gradients, but, compared with the outpatient care gradient for the same hospital its slope is much less steep—the use of inpatient facilities halves every three miles (5 km.) while the average number of outpatient attendances halves every two miles (3 km.). Inpatient care is thus spread somewhat more equitably than outpatient care. Furthermore, because so many inpatients are selected directly from those who originally attend as outpatients, it is probable that inpatient facilities would become even more uniform if outpatient care could be distributed more evenly.

The comparatively flat slope of the inpatient care gradient, with its expected further flattening if outpatient care could be made more equitable, is a major reason for providing a few comparatively large hospitals rather than many small ones. But there are other good reasons for concentrating inpatient facilities at the same time as spreading outpatient services more widely. One is the support offered by health centres; a major advantage of an efficient network of health centres is that they permit hospitals to be large, fewer and more efficient.

This they do by providing minor curative services to many outpatients, and some inpatients, by sorting patients generally, so that only those deserving hospital attention are referred there, and by helping to provide transport for such patients as are referred to hospital.

The concentration of inpatient services is also supported by the small part that transport plays in the total cost of a hospital admission—in the study, transport accounted for only 10 per cent of an average inpatient admission, as against 75 per cent of the cost of an average outpatient attendance. Looked at in another way, only about one inpatient journey was made for every twenty outpatient journeys.

When contrasted with a hectic 80-bedded one-doctor hospital, a reasonably sized district hospital of 250 beds staffed by at least three doctors is a much more satisfactory place for a doctor to work in. When there are several doctors in a hospital, they can relieve and consult one another and specialise some what among themselves. A hospital of this size also makes better radiological and pathological facilities possible, and it reduces overheads as well as the time and money spent on administration. So great are the benefits to be drawn from having doctors working in units of more than one, that the one-doctor, 80 or 100-bedded hospital must now be considered an anachronism. The smallest practical size for a hospital is one with two doctors, and the 250 bed three or four doctor hospital should be the norm.

It is not possible to leave the subject of hospitals without defining just what a hospital is and what it is not. At its humblest a hospital is held to be a medical unit with beds, staffed by someone capable of doing at least some emergency surgery and equipped with a theatre, a laboratory and if possible an X-ray plant. Thus the use of the terms' rural hospital', or even 'district hospital', for units staffed only by a medical assistant and devoid of a theatre is to be condemned, for a 'hospital' which cannot, for instance, provide a Caesarian section or a blood transfusion plainly is not one. Politically, it may be useful to call such units hospitals, functionally they are not so.

Such then are, or should be, the district hospitals which need to be backed up by regional hospitals, each with a range of specialist services which are in their turn supported by a national teaching hospital in the capital city.

SOME MAJOR ADMINISTRATIVE MATTERS

The comparison of hospital and health centre costs. Certain working estimates have to be made in attempting to compare hospital and health centre costs, and although they are considered individually elsewhere, it is convenient to bring them together here.

As a working assumption a health centre is considered to cost £ 8,000 ($22,000) to build , £ 4,000 ($11,000) to run each year and to provide an adequate level of service for 10,000 people. Similarly, an equipped hospital bed is reckoned to cost £ 3,000; about the price at which they are currently being provided in several African countries. Once provided, such a bed is reckoned to cost £ 300($850) a year to service, and to be capable of being used for 68 inpatients a year.

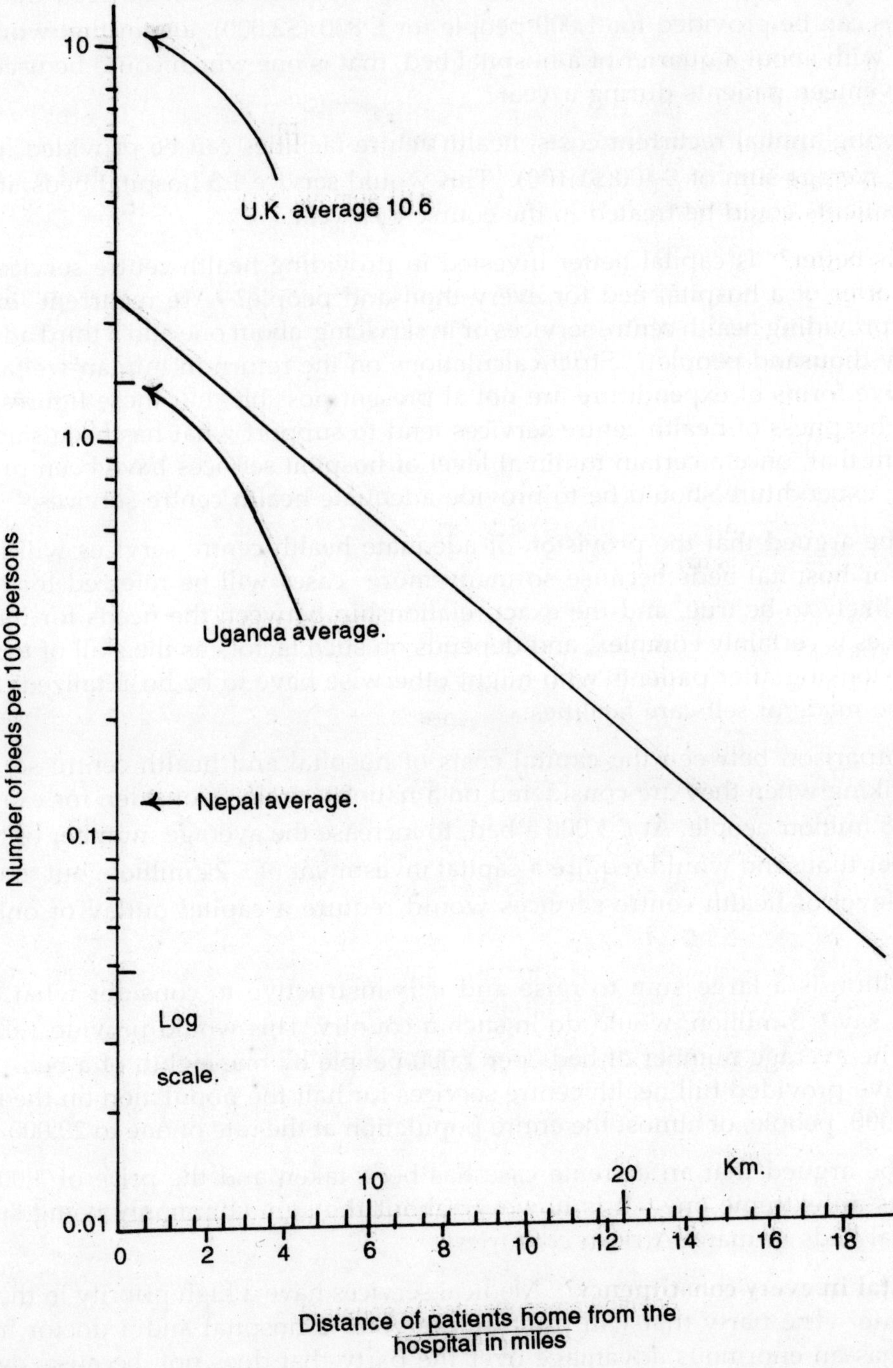

Fig. 22.6: The number of beds per 1000 persons and the distance they live from hospital.

Comparing the two units and considering capital costs, it will be seen that health centre facilities can be provided for 1,000 people for £ 800 ($2,000), a sum that would only provide them with about a quarter of a hospital bed, that is one which could be used for an average of seventeen patients during a year.

Considering annual recurrent costs, health centre facilities can be provided for 1,000 people for an average sum of £ 400($1,100). This would service 1.3 hospital beds, in which about 100 inpatients could be treated in the course of a year.

Which is better? Is capital better invested in providing health centre services or an additional quarter of a hospital bed for every thousand people? Are recurrent expenses better used in providing health centre services or in servicing about one and a third additional beds for every thousand people ? Strict calculations on the return in human welfare from these alternative forms of expenditure are not at present possible, but these figures for the comparative cheapness of health centre services tend to support what has been said under the sixth axiom that, once a certain minimal level of hospital services have been provided, then the next expenditure should be to provide adequate health centre services.

It may be argued that the provision of adequate health centre services will increase the demand for hospital beds because so many more cases will be referred for hospital care. This is likely to be true, and the exact relationship between the needs for these two kinds of services is certainly complex, and depends on such factors as the skill of the health centre staff in looking after patients who might otherwise have to be hospitalized, and the use that can be made of self-care facilities.

The comparison between the capital costs of hospital and health centre services is even more striking when they are considered on a national scale. Consider, for example, a country with 8 million people. At £ 3,000 a bed, to increase the average number of hospital beds by one per thousand would require a capital investment of £ 24 million, but to provide an adequate level of health centre services would require a capital outlay of only £ 6.4 million.

£ 24 million is a large sum to raise and it is instructive to consider what a more realistic sum, say £ 3 million, would do in such a country. This would provide 1,000 beds and increase the average number of beds per 1,000 people by one-eighth of a bed. Such a sum would have provided full health centre services for half the population on the basis of a centre to 10,000 people, or almost the entire population at the rate of one to 20,000 people.

It may be argued that an extreme case has been taken and the price of 3,000 for a hospital bed is an extreme one. It is however about the sum commonly being spent on district hospital beds in many African countries.

A hospital in every constituency? Medical services have a high priority in the minds of the electorate. The party that will promise the voter a hospital and a doctor in every constituency has an enormous advantage over the party that does not, because, even if it were possible, such a promise might not be the best health strategy. The dilemma is a real one. Most voters will know what dispensaries are but may not think much of them; they are unlikely to know what health centres are until they are well established—they have become very popular in Kenya. Voters well realise that money is short but will probably not appreciate the great difference between the costs of hospital and health centre services. In this situation there is a strong temptation to give the electorate what it wants instead of attempting to explain what is better. Too often this leads to many promises of little hospitals in numbers that make it impossible to staff and equip them properly, even if they were the most efficient unit.

Sometimes the electorate has a very firm idea that what it wants is doctors and will not be satisfied with medical assistants. Many voters do not understand the value of the work done by well trained medical assistants in health centre, the impossibility of producing doctors in sufficient numbers, the difficulties of paying them, and their reluctance to work in the rural areas.

In the long run the answers to the problems lie in a change of attitude and a new understanding from both voters and parliamentarians. Health education in schools should therefore include elementary ideas on the organisation of health services as well as on the diseases themselves.

The administration of hospital and health centre services. So far hospital and health centre services have been considered as if they were entirely separate. They are however complementary parts of the same health service, and must work together. Patients are referred from health centre to hospital and vice versa; all levels of their staff should on occasion visit the other part of the service; some at least of their workers are interchangeable; both owe final allegiance to the same directorate, and it is often convenient for a hospital store to supply health centres with drugs and equipment. If this close integration is so necessary, how is it to be achieved, and how are these two sides of the service to be administered?

When trying to provide the best solution, one almost universal danger has to be borne in mind; it is that hospital services almost invariably come to take undue precedence over health centre ones. There are several obvious reasons why this should be so. Prevention is never so dramatic as cure, and its results, though enormous, are not every easily measured. As has already been said, electorates and their politicians are well aware of hospitals but usually know little of health centres. Added to this most doctors prefer hospital work and few enjoy continued travelling that the supervision of health centres requires. Furthermore, in preparing plans for development, the emphasis is too often on large prestigious capital projects which lead to preoccupation with two or three large hospitals rather than with many humbler health centres. All these factors combine against the health centre and it is thus little wonder that among developing countries so few have established them effectively the great exception being Kenya.

Because of the likelihood of erosion of health centre services in favour of those of the hospitals, the first administrative principle should be to support the health centre wherever possible. Some have said that this is best done by separating them administratively, while others equally eminent and experienced hold exactly the opposite view !

The writers are hardly in a position to mediate, but wonder if the answer may be for hospitals and health centres to be administratively separate on the district level, but under the same direction at provincial level This is implied where a regional hospital and health centre are drawn close to one another but separate, one supervised by the district medical officer and the other by the medical superintendent. It has been pointed out that the possibility of rivalry and disputes in the district can be minimised if it is made quite clear who is the senior of the two officers in the service, the district medical officer or the medical superintendent. This would vary from time to time, depending upon the seniority of the officers who happened to be occupying these posts. The provincial medical officer would on the other hand be in charge of both parts of the service.

The place of the private authority hospital and the private practitioner. The health scheme that has been described is an organisation to which a variety of medical units may adapt themselves. It is but a historical accident that missions, or 'voluntary agencies' as some prefer to call them, have usually provided only hospitals, while governments have sometimes organised health centres as well. Provided some member of their staff has public health training, missions might well supervise a group of health centres and so complete their medical service to the area. To help them in this, it should be the aim of the state to supply funds to the limit of its capacity, and, if need be, auxiliary staff also, so as to make the best use of the medical skills that a mission has to offer.

So far the private practitioner has not been mentioned, and health services have been described here as being staffed entirely by salaried employees of the community through their agent, the State. It is one of the main themes of this symposium, than, in the developing countries, a doctor is at his most efficient in the service of the sick as a teacher, organiser and consultant to a team of auxiliaries, and that this is the best way in which his skills can be used when doctor-patient ratios approach those at the top of scale A.

It should be a doctor's role to see those outpatients referred to him by auxiliary staff, to bring his skills to the bedside of the sick, to undertake major operations and to supervise, administer, encourage and teach his many helpers. Working like this a doctor fulfils the third axiom '...obtain the maximum return in human welfare from the limited...skill available'. It is his skills that are short, and only by working with a team of auxiliaries does he make the most of them.

In his urban consulting room the private practitioner is without the help auxiliaries provide in the building of an efficient team, and he is usually also denied the beds, services and equipment needed for the most effective use of his skills. Too often he is but a provider of expensive palliatives to the few with the money to pay his fees. Though he will enjoy the amenities of the urban life, and is apt to grow rich, he will be of much greater value to the community, who provided the means of his education, if he serves them from a district health centre or in a district hospital.

If a doctor in a developing country leaves the government medical service, which is in effect the community's medical service, where he is of the greatest value, and starts to practice privately, it is only fair that he should refund to the community the complete sum that it spent in training him. This is reported to vary between £ 3,000 and £ 20,000 ($8,500 and $56,000) and may sometimes be even more. To introduce such a payment would not only be fair, but it would provide a major incentive for working within the government health service, thus leading to a more efficient allocation of a country's medical resources.

If a government finds it difficult to persuade doctors to work in the rural areas, it is well entitled to bond those to whom it has given a scholarship to a period of service in these areas. It can also give a salary differential for up-country work, and there is something to be said for tying an unpopular post to a very popular house.